T0263956

Spinal Cord Injury

Editor

JOHN L. LIN

PHYSICAL MEDICINE AND REHABILITATION CLINICS OF NORTH AMERICA

www.pmr.theclinics.com

Consulting Editor
SANTOS F. MARTINEZ

August 2020 • Volume 31 • Number 3

ELSEVIER

1600 John F. Kennedy Boulevard • Suite 1800 • Philadelphia, Pennsylvania, 19103-2899

http://www.theclinics.com

**PHYSICAL MEDICINE AND REHABILITATION CLINICS OF NORTH AMERICA Volume 31, Number 3
August 2020 ISSN 1047-9651, ISBN 978-0-323-75639-6**

Editor: Lauren Boyle
Developmental Editor: Nicole Congleton

© **2020 Elsevier Inc. All rights reserved.**

This periodical and the individual contributions contained in it are protected under copyright by Elsevier, and the following terms and conditions apply to their use:

Photocopying
Single photocopies of single articles may be made for personal use as allowed by national copyright laws. Permission of the Publisher and payment of a fee is required for all other photocopying, including multiple or systematic copying, copying for advertising or promotional purposes, resale, and all forms of document delivery. Special rates are available for educational institutions that wish to make photocopies for non-profit educational classroom use. For information on how to seek permission visit www.elsevier.com/permissions or call: (+44) 1865 843830 (UK)/(+1) 215 239 3804 (USA).

Derivative Works
Subscribers may reproduce tables of contents or prepare lists of articles including abstracts for internal circulation within their institutions. Permission of the Publisher is required for resale or distribution outside the institution. Permission of the Publisher is required for all other derivative works, including compilations and translations (please consult www.elsevier.com/permissions).

Electronic Storage or Usage
Permission of the Publisher is required to store or use electronically any material contained in this periodical, including any article or part of an article (please consult www.elsevier.com/permissions). Except as outlined above, no part of this publication may be reproduced, stored in a retrieval system or transmitted in any form or by any means, electronic, mechanical, photocopying, recording or otherwise, without prior written permission of the Publisher.

Notice
No responsibility is assumed by the Publisher for any injury and/or damage to persons or property as a matter of products liability, negligence or otherwise, or from any use or operation of any methods, products, instructions or ideas contained in the material herein. Because of rapid advances in the medical sciences, in particular, independent verification of diagnoses and drug dosages should be made.

Although all advertising material is expected to conform to ethical (medical) standards, inclusion in this publication does not constitute a guarantee or endorsement of the quality or value of such product or of the claims made of it by its manufacturer.

Reprints. For copies of 100 or more of articles in this publication, please contact the Commercial Reprints Department, Elsevier Inc., 360 Park Avenue South, New York, NY 10010-1710. Tel.: 212-633-3874; Fax: 212-633-3820; E-mail: reprints@elsevier.com.

Physical Medicine and Rehabilitation Clinics of North America (ISSN 1047-9651) is published quarterly by Elsevier Inc., 360 Park Avenue South, New York, NY 10010-1710. Months of issue are February, May, August, and November. Business and Editorial Offices: 1600 John F. Kennedy Blvd., Suite 1800, Philadelphia, PA 19103-2899. Customer Service Office: 3251 Riverport Lane, Maryland Heights, MO 63043. Periodicals postage paid at New York, NY and additional mailing offices. Subscription price per year is $313.00 (US individuals), $633.00 (US institutions), $100.00 (US students), $366.00 (Canadian individuals), $833.00 (Canadian institutions), $100.00 (Canadian students), $429.00 (foreign individuals), $833.00 (foreign institutions), and $210.00 (foreign students). Foreign air speed delivery is included in all *Clinics* subscription prices. All prices are subject to change without notice. **POSTMASTER:** Send address changes to *Physical Medicine and Rehabilitation Clinics of North America*, Customer Service Office: Elsevier Health Sciences Division, Subscription Customer Service, 3251 Riverport Lane, Maryland Heights, MO 63043. **Customer Service: 1-800-654-2452 (US). From outside of the United States, call 314-447-8871. Fax: 314-447-8029. E-mail: JournalsCustomer Service-usa@elsevier.com (for print support); JournalsOnlineSupport-usa@elsevier.com (for online support).**

Physical Medicine and Rehabilitation Clinics of North America is indexed in *Excerpta Medica, MEDLINE/ PubMed (Index Medicus), Cinahl, and Cumulative Index to Nursing and Allied Health Literature.*

Contributors

CONSULTING EDITOR

SANTOS F. MARTINEZ, MD, MS
Diplomate of the American Academy of Physical Medicine and Rehabilitation, Certificate of Added Qualification Sports Medicine, Assistant Professor, Department of Orthopaedics, Campbell Clinic Orthopaedics, University of Tennessee, Memphis, Tennessee, USA

EDITOR

JOHN L. LIN, MD
Director, Spinal Cord Medicine, Shepherd Center, Adjunct Assistant Professor of Rehabilitation Medicine, Emory University School of Medicine, Clinical Assistant Professor, Department of Medicine, Medical College of Georgia, Athens, Georgia, USA

AUTHORS

BENJAMIN A. ABRAMOFF, MD, MS
Department of Physical Medicine and Rehabilitation, University of Pennsylvania, Perelman School of Medicine, Philadelphia, Pennsylvania, USA

MATTHEW AMODEO, MD
Department of Physical Medicine and Rehabilitation, University of Pennsylvania, Perelman School of Medicine, Philadelphia, Pennsylvania, USA

JOHN R. BACH, MD
Professor, Department of Physical Medicine and Rehabilitation, Professor of Neurology, Rutgers New Jersey Medical School, Newark, New Jersey, USA

LINDSAY BURKE, BA, MD
Resident Physician, Department of Medicine, Morristown Medical Center, Morristown, New Jersey, USA

WESLEY CHAY, MD
Physical Medicine and Rehabilitation, Shepherd Center, Emory University School of Medicine, Atlanta, Georgia, USA

MICHAEL CHIOU, MD
Resident Physician, Department of Physical Medicine and Rehabilitation, Icahn School of Medicine at Mount Sinai, New York, New York, USA

LOREN T. DAVIDSON, MD
Clinical Professor, Department of Physical Medicine and Rehabilitation, University of California, Davis Health System, Shriners Hospitals for Children – Northern California, Sacramento, California, USA

DONALD F. DISTEL, MD
Department of Physical Medicine and Rehabilitation, University of Pennsylvania, Perelman School of Medicine, Philadelphia, Pennsylvania, USA

TREVOR DYSON-HUDSON, MD
Director, Center for Spinal Cord Injury Research, Kessler Foundation, West Orange, New Jersey, USA; Associate Professor, Department of Physical Medicine and Rehabilitation, Rutgers New Jersey Medical School, Newark, New Jersey, USA

EDELLE C. FIELD-FOTE, PT, PhD, FAPTA, FASIA
Director, Spinal Cord Injury Research, Crawford Research Institute, Shepherd Center, Professor, Department of Rehabilitation Medicine, Emory University School of Medicine, Professor of the Practice, School of Biological Sciences, Georgia Institute of Technology, Atlanta, Georgia, USA

DAVID R. GATER JR. MD, PhD
Professor and Chair, Spinal Cord Injury Fellowship Director, Department of Physical Medicine and Rehabilitation, Medical Director of Rehabilitation, Jackson Memorial Hospital, Co-Director, NIDILRR South Florida Spinal Cord Injury Model System, University of Miami Leonard M. Miller School of Medicine, Miami, Florida, USA

LANCE L. GOETZ, MD
Staff Physician, Spinal Cord Injury and Disorders, Department of Veterans Affairs, Hunter Holmes McGuire VA Medical Center, Associate Professor, Department of Physical Medicine and Rehabilitation, Virginia Commonwealth University, Richmond, Virginia, USA

CLAES HULTLING, MD, PhD
CEO, Spinalis SCI Unit, Solna, Sweden; Professor, Department of Neurobiology, Care Sciences and Society (NVS), Karolinska Institutet, Stockholm, Sweden

SHAWN JOSHI, BS
Drexel School of Medicine, Philadelphia, Pennsylvania, USA

STEVEN KIRSHBLUM, MD
Kessler Institute for Rehabilitation, Kessler Foundation, West Orange, New Jersey, USA; Rutgers New Jersey Medical School, Newark, New Jersey, USA

ERIC LAUER, MPH, PhD
Project Director, Institute on Disability/University Centers for Excellence in Disabilities Education, Research, and Service, College of Health and Human Services, University of New Hampshire, Durham, New Hampshire, USA

MARK S. NASH, PhD, FACSM
Professor, Departments of Neurological Surgery and Physical Medicine & Rehabilitation; Associate Scientific Director for Research, The Miami Project to Cure Paralysis; Vice-Chair for Research, Department of Physical Medicine & Rehabilitation; Co-Director, DHHS-NIDILRR South Florida SCI Model System, University of Miami Leonard M. Miller School of Medicine, Miami, Florida, USA

JOHN O'NEILL, PhD
Director, Center for Employment and Disability Research, Kessler Foundation, East Hanover, New Jersey, USA

LISA OTTOMANELLI, PhD
Clinical Psychologist, Research Service, James A. Haley Veterans' Hospital and Clinics, Associate Professor, Rehabilitation and Mental Health Counseling Program, Department

of Child and Family Studies, College of Behavioral and Community Sciences, University of South Florida, Tampa, Florida, USA

ALLAN PELJOVICH, MD, MPH, FAOA
Hand & Upper Extremity Program, The Hand & Upper Extremity Center of Georgia, Shepherd Center, Medical Director, Hand & Upper Extremity Program, Children's Healthcare of Atlanta, Clinical Instructor, Orthopaedic Surgery Residency Program, Atlanta Medical Center, Atlanta, Georgia, USA

MARY SCHMIDT READ, PT, DPT, MS, FASIA
Magee Rehabilitation Hospital, Jefferson Health, Philadelphia, Pennsylvania, USA

RÜDIGER RUPP, PhD
Spinal Cord Injury Center, Heidelberg University Hospital, Heidelberg, Germany

MICHAEL SAULINO, MD, PhD
Associate Professor, Sidney Kimmel Medical College, Director of Neuromodulation, MossRehab, Elkins Park, Pennsylvania, USA

ERIK SHAW, DO
Medical Director, Shepherd Spine and Pain Institute, Atlanta, Georgia, USA

BRITTANY SNIDER, DO
Rutgers New Jersey Medical School, Newark, New Jersey, USA; Kessler Institute for Rehabilitation, West Orange, New Jersey, USA

JOSHUA A. VOVA, MD
Director of Rehabilitation, Department of Physical Medicine and Rehabilitation, Children's Healthcare of Atlanta, Atlanta, Georgia, USA

Contents

> Neurogenic bowel has received surprisingly little attention. Among individuals with spinal cord injury, bowel function is considered a major physical and psychological problem that stems from the severe negative impact on social life and mobility. With transanal irrigation, individuals with neurogenic bowel have received an additional tool that may simplify life and improve independence. A recent survey showed that as many as 37% of the spinal cord injury patients interviewed had not heard about transanal irrigation. It should be a high priority at spinal cord injury centers to support patients with the right tools for proper bowel management and care.

> The International Standards for Neurologic Classification of Spinal Cord Injury (ISNCSCI) are the most widely used classification system in spinal cord injury medicine. The purpose of the ISNCSCI is to ensure accurate and consistent communication among patients, clinicians, and researchers. Since its first publication in 1982, the ISNCSCI has continued to evolve with the latest updates and revisions published in 2015 and 2019. The updates were incorporated into the 2019 ISNCSCI worksheet and booklet, and the International Standards Training e-Learning Program. This article details the ISNCSCI update from 2015 and revision in 2019.

> The aim of this article is to provide an overview of prognosis and outcomes after spinal cord injury (SCI), including variables that have an impact on neurologic assessment, extent and time frame of natural recovery, specific factors having an impact on prognosis of ambulation, the role of imaging and modalities for assessing the injured spinal cord, and strategies on presenting information to patients and families. The ability to predict outcome

after spinal cord injury is important not only for individuals who sustained traumatic SCI and their families but also for rehabilitation professionals and researchers.

Cognitive dysfunction (CD) is pervasive in individuals who have chronic spinal cord injuries (SCI). Although classically associated with concomitant traumatic brain injuries, many other causes have been proposed, including premorbid neuropsychological conditions, mood disorders, substance abuse, polypharmacy, chronic pain and fatigue, sleep apnea, autonomic dysregulation, post-intensive care unit syndrome, cortical reorganizations, and neuroinflammation. The consequences of CD are likely widespread, affecting rehabilitation and function. CD in those with SCI should be recognized, and potentially treated, in order to provide the best patient care.

Traumatic spinal cord injury (SCI) often results in several life-altering impairments, including paralysis, sensory loss, and neurogenic bowel/bladder dysfunction. Some of these SCI-related conditions can be accommodated with compensatory strategies. Perhaps no SCI-associated condition is more troublesome and recalcitrant to the treating physiatrist than chronic neuropathic pain. In addition to the expected challenges in treating any chronic pain condition, treatment of SCI-related pain has the added difficulty of disruption of normal neural pathways that subserve pain transmission and attenuation. This article reviews selected treatment strategies for SCI-associated neuropathic pain.

Respiratory complications often result from acute spinal cord injury. Ventilatory assistance/support is often required 12 hours to 6 days after admission and is typically delivered via translaryngeal tubes. When not weanable from ventilatory support, tracheostomy tubes are placed. Supplemental O2 is often provided irrespective of whether or not the patient is hypoxic. This renders the oximeter ineffective as a gauge of alveolar ventilation, airway secretion management, and residual lung disease, and can exacerbate hypercapnia. Thus, hypoventilation and airway secretions must be effectively treated to prevent lung disease and to maintain normal O2 saturation and CO2 levels without supplemental O2.

Intubated ventilator-dependent patients with high-level spinal cord injury can be managed without tracheostomy tubes provided that they have sufficient cognition to cooperate and that any required surgical procedures are completed and they are medically stable. Intubation for a month or more than extubation to continuous noninvasive ventilatory support (NVS) can be safer long term than resort to tracheotomy. Noninvasive ventilation (NIV) is not conventionally being used for ventilatory support. Noninvasive interfaces include mouthpieces, nasal and oronasal interfaces, and intermittent abdominal pressure ventilators. NIV/NVS should never been used without consideration of mechanical insufflation-exsufflation for airway secretion clearance.

The risks and health hazards of the cardiometabolic syndrome (CMS) are commonly reported in persons with spinal cord injuries (SCIs) and disorders. Overweight/obesity, insulin resistance, hypertension, and dyslipidemia are highly prevalent after SCI. Both the CMS diagnosis and physical deconditioning worsen the prognosis for all-cause cardiovascular disease. Evidence suggests a role for physical activity to address these risks, although intense exercise may be required. A lifestyle plan incorporating both exercise and nutrition represents a preferred approach for health management. Improved surveillance for CMS risks and exercise and nutritional management are essential for the preservation of optimal health and independence.

Mobility is essential for quality of life and social participation. Some individuals with spinal cord injury have sufficient residual lower extremity motor control to walk. Improving walking function incorporates practice and training, and assistive devices or stimulation to augment function and balance. Overground robotic exoskeletons may have the potential to transform upright mobility in the future. Most individuals with spinal cord injury use a wheelchair for at least some of their mobility needs. Wheelchair skills training can open up new possibilities for participation. Regardless of the means of mobility, developing habits that protect joint health are essential for optimal lifelong mobility.

With improvements in medical care, pediatric patients with spinal cord injuries with tetraplegia are living into adulthood. The goal of rehabilitation following loss of upper extremity function caused by tetraplegia is to maximize function and independence. Physiatrists must be aware of appropriate timing of referral for upper extremity surgery because it can have significant ramifications on the outcome. This article discusses the 2 most commonly used surgical strategies to restore upper extremity function: upper extremity tendon transfer and nerve grafting/transfer. Patient selection, physical examination, electrodiagnostic evaluation, and optimization of postoperative rehabilitation are important.

Allan Peljovich

Comprehensive programs for children who sustain traumatic spinal cord injury should incorporate optimizing hand and upper extremity function along with the other traditional pillars of rehabilitation. Children's smaller anatomy, open growth plates, and future skeletal growth, combined with the age-related psychosocial impact of these injuries, require protocols suited to these age-related issues. There is a role for surgical reconstruction, as is the case for adults with traumatic tetraplegia, and surgical outcomes are equally beneficial and long lasting. Strict adherence to surgical indications, and surgical strategies and protocols that incorporate their age-related challenges, are the keys to successful management.

Lisa Ottomanelli, Lance L. Goetz, John O'Neill, Eric Lauer, and Trevor Dyson-Hudson

The Americans with Disabilities Act, passed in 1990, represented landmark legislation and led to significant improvements in accessibility, such as prohibiting discrimination based on disability in public life, including employment. Now 30 years later, however, employment rates for persons with disabilities, including spinal cord injury, remain low. This article discusses why employment is so important for persons with spinal cord injury and challenges that remain. Presented are previously unpublished employment data from a nationally representative US sample. Finally, the state of the art of vocational rehabilitation, including models proven to facilitate this critical rehabilitation outcome, is discussed.

PHYSICAL MEDICINE AND REHABILITATION CLINICS OF NORTH AMERICA

FORTHCOMING ISSUES

November 2020
Integrative Medicine and Rehabilitation
Blessen C. Eapen and David Cifu, *Editors*

February 2021
Dance Medicine
Kathleen L. Davenport, *Editor*

RECENT ISSUES

May 2020
Pharmacologic Support in Pain Management
Steven Stanos and James R. Babington, *Editors*

February 2020
Cerebral Palsy
Aloysia Leisanne Schwabe, *Editor*

SERIES OF RELATED INTEREST

Orthopedic Clinics
Neurologic Clinics
Clinics in Sports Medicine

VISIT THE CLINICS ONLINE!
Access your subscription at:
www.theclinics.com

PHYSICAL MEDICINE AND REHABILITATION
CLINICS OF NORTH AMERICA

Foreword

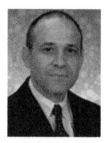

Santos F. Martinez, MD, MS
Consulting Editor

The field of Rehabilitation is proud and indebted to Dr Lin for his contribution to the Spinal Cord field as a clinician, researcher, and activist. As Dr Lin alludes to, we are in an exciting era with technology merging with clinical applicability. We must remain vigilant, however, to keep our basic core values and concepts that have developed over decades. I offer a personal thanks to Dr Lin for taking on the challenge of this issue. As customary, he has superseded expectations.

Santos F. Martinez, MD, MS
American Academy of Physical Medicine
and Rehabilitation
Campbell Clinic Orthopaedics
Department of Orthopaedics
University of Tennessee
Memphis, TN 38104, USA

E-mail address:
smartinez@campbellclinic.com

Phys Med Rehabil Clin N Am 31 (2020) xiii
https://doi.org/10.1016/j.pmr.2020.05.001
1047-9651/20/© 2020 Published by Elsevier Inc.

Preface

Facing the Reality: Confronting the Challenges of Spinal Cord Injury Sequelae in 2020

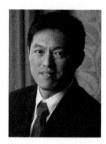

John L. Lin, MD
Editor

Since the turn of the millennium, excitement has been abuzz in the field of spinal cord medicine. Much like in the preceding decades that heralded in methylprednisolone, GM1 ganglioside, and 4-aminopyridine, the subspecialty is now again ebullient with the untold promises of neurologic recovery from stem cells to gait improvement associated with spinal cord stimulators. While the limelight for spinal cord medicine focuses on infinity and beyond, at least a quarter of a million Americans, and many more around the world, face the reality of living with a spinal cord injury (SCI) and the myriad of comorbid conditions challenging them daily now.

In this issue of *Physical Medicine and Rehabilitation Clinics*, we tackle these mundane, and sometimes overlooked, daily conditions when we gather life-long dedicated scientists, researchers, academicians, clinicians, and advocates to share their passion and knowledge. To lead us in, Dr Hultling, with the backdrop of his personal story with SCI, gives us a European perspective on neurogenic bowel management and an in-depth, first-hand discussion on transanal irrigation.

In the article by Dr Kirshblum and colleagues, updates from 2015 and 2019 on International Standards for Neurological Classification of Spinal Cord Injury are discussed in detail along with worksheets of sample impairments highlighting changes leading to new classifications. With the more nuanced classification, prognostication of neurologic recovery and functional improvement has also concordantly become more precise over the years. To that effort, Drs Chay and Kirshblum take us through evidence-based literature on prognosis over the decades, demystifying some conventional "wisdoms" that have been passed on through academic generations, perhaps in good faith, although not entirely based on science.

Phys Med Rehabil Clin N Am 31 (2020) xv–xvii
https://doi.org/10.1016/j.pmr.2020.04.009
1047-9651/20/© 2020 Published by Elsevier Inc.

Traumatic brain injury, drawing national attention with increased recognition among those who serve to protect this nation in combat and those who battle on the gridiron, has long been associated with those sustaining traumatic SCI. However, cognitive dysfunction from a myriad of other causes has been less appreciated in those with SCI despite decades of work by dedicated researchers. Dr Distel and colleagues shine the spotlight on these secondary comorbidities and how they may complicate diagnostic challenges in the setting of SCI. As pain and its associated treatment may lead to cognitive dysfunction, Drs Shaw and Saulino give us an update on the latest treatment approaches to pain associated with SCI.

Pulmonary impairment and respiratory dysfunction have long been recognized as leading morbidities associated with cervical and high thoracic SCIs. While mortality has improved since the iron-lung days, this improvement appears to be stagnant compared with the advancement in other parts of spinal cord medicine and especially compared with European countries. Dr Bach and colleagues, in their 2 articles, review fundamental pathophysiology, discuss current state of treatment interventions, and explore obstacles to overcome to advance pulmonary management to the next level, while examining the role of noninvasive ventilation. In the meantime, Drs Nash and Gater discuss how pulmonary comorbidities along with a whole host of comorbid conditions compound and exacerbate SCI-associated cardiometabolic syndrome and the current state of treatment despite the mitigated role exercises may have in this population. As important as exercises will always be, Dr Field-Fote reviews therapeutic interventions to improve mobility during the post-SCI phase.

Life-changing is often used to describe the transformative improvement in daily function that upper-extremity reconstructive surgeries give. In this issue, the challenges of making this transformation a reality for the pediatric population are discussed in 2 parts, first with the nonsurgical perioperative management by Drs Vova and Davidson, followed by detailing surgical management intricacies by Dr Peljovich.

Even more transformative on a societal scale is the effect of the Americans with Disabilities Act (ADA). Remarkable in today's atmosphere of heightened partisan rancor, ADA was passed 30 years ago with 90% of the US Senate and 95% of the US House of Representatives voting in the affirmative in this overwhelmingly bipartisan effort in leveling the playing field for those with disabilities to integrate into society. Although critics mocked it for legislating morality, this one single Act catapulted the United States into the global vanguard of disability rights and maintained its title as the most accessible nation on this planet to date. Like me, some of the authors of the last article in this issue are the direct beneficiaries of the legacy of ADA. In this article, Dr Ottomanelli and colleagues take us through the decades of transformation in employment of persons with SCI under the governance of ADA.

While I echo the sentiments of my fellow SCI survivors in cheering on those who dare to boldly dream to take spinal cord medicine into the new millennium, we are truly grateful to those who devote their profession to making each day in surviving with an SCI a better day than before. Medical management of comorbid conditions after SCI continues to improve yet is still far from being perfected. With the continued dedication of clinicians, academicians, scientists, and researchers, such as each of the authors in this issue of the *Clinics of Physical Medicine and Rehabilitation*, the future of spinal cord medicine is in good hands and is brighter than ever.

John L. Lin, MD
Medical Staff Office
Shepherd Center
2020 Peachtree Road, NW
Atlanta, GA 30309, USA

E-mail address:
john.lin@shepherd.org

Neurogenic Bowel Management Using Transanal Irrigation by Persons with Spinal Cord Injury

Claes Hultling, MD, PhD[a,b],*

KEYWORDS

- Neurogenic bowel management • Transanal irrigation • Spinal cord injury

KEY POINTS

- The neurogenic bowel has received surprisingly little attention, especially compared with urine incontinence.
- Among individuals with spinal cord injury, bowel function is considered a major physical and psychological problem.
- With transanal irrigation, individuals with neurogenic bowel have received an additional tool that may simplify life once they have got used to it.
- It should be a high priority at spinal cord injury centers to support patients with the right tools for proper bowel management and care.

INTRODUCTION

During early summer of 2018, I was invited to give a talk at Shepherd by Dr Anna Elmers. I was then approached by my colleague and friend Dr John Lin, who is the director in spinal cord injury medicine at the Shepherd Center in Atlanta, Georgia. I felt honored and acknowledged and I did not spend very much time in accepting the offer to be part of this edition. John and I met the first time during The International Spinal Cord Society meeting in Maastricht in the Netherlands, when we were introduced to each other by my even longer old friend Dr Don Leslie.

First, after accepting this task—I thought I was going to sit down and sort out the latest references and try to build up a spectacular 5000-word review article regarding the latest on neurogenic bowel dysfunction and how to embark onto the problem of

[a] Spinalis SCI Unit, Solna, Sweden; [b] Department of Neurobiology, Care Sciences and Society (NVS), Karolinska Institutet, Stockholm SE-169 89, Sweden
* Department of Neurobiology, Care Sciences and Society (NVS), Karolinska Institutet, Stockholm SE-169 89, Sweden.
E-mail address: claes@spinalis.se

Phys Med Rehabil Clin N Am 31 (2020) 305–318
https://doi.org/10.1016/j.pmr.2020.04.003
1047-9651/20/© 2020 Elsevier Inc. All rights reserved.

becoming obstipated when being a tetraplegic. After taking out more than 30 volumes of textbooks from the mid-1940s up until today and spending a weekend going through all the articles dealing with obstipation and neurogenic bowel dysfunction, I found myself being so fascinated by what Sir Ludwig Guttmann wrote back in 1946. With this in mind, I decided to make this a different article and take its origin from my own experience after living with a cervical spinal cord injury for more than 35 years and also after treating more than 3000 spinal cord injured patients in that timespan.

Let me start with some history. The last day of May 1984 I dove in shallow water. I dove in once and when I dove in the second time, I hit a concrete pillar and I fractured my C6 cervical vertebrae. I was together with friends, who rescued me from about 3 m of water and brought me up on the jetty. The rescue helicopter from my own hospital Karolinska came and brought me in to the Karolinska University Hospital in Stockholm, where I at that time worked as an anesthesiologist and was involved in intensive care. I was 31 years of age and I was going to get married to my wife Barbro in 2 weeks' time. She worked as a pediatrician and we had lived in sin for more than 5 years; we were going to crown our life with this wedding out in the Swedish archipelago.

That did not happen. Instead, I was in a Stryker bed for 5 days, I was then operated with a bone sponge between my fifth and my seventh vertebrae. I had to wear a thoracocervical collar for 12 weeks, but I embarked into a very active life, despite my disability. The first thing I did, against the will of the University Hospital, was to speak to my "chopper" friends who were running the helicopter service at the hospital. I wanted to go out from the hospital to the outskirts of the Swedish archipelago, where the Hultling family have had a summerhouse for decades. The officer who was in charge of the helicopter service was of course at first questioning whether this was appropriate or not but, taking into consideration the circumstances and the need of intense rehabilitation during the summer of 1984, we were on.

I started to work on September 1, 1984, in the intensive care unit. I could not be in the operating theater and I could not be in the emergency or acute care center. I wanted to be part of the crew and I felt it was important to me with the scrub clothes, white gowns, stethoscope, and pager—all the attributes that constitutes a real doctor on the ward. I focused on speaking to families and patients; I was writing referrals and prescriptions and I was being responsible for the early morning round at 07:30. That was a true challenge with a new tetraplegia to get up at 5 o'clock every morning and be at the hospital and try to do my task. After doing that for half a year, I realized that I was not going to continue with this type of work; I was instead going to work with spinal cord injuries.

WHAT HAPPENED NEXT?

During the first International Spinal Cord Society meeting—in 1985 in Edinburgh—I met with Sir George Bedbrook, who at that time was heading the unit in Perth in Western Australia. He had been asked by the Minister of Health in 1952 to transfer to Western Australia and establish this unit. He had done remarkable work in establishing a large, very comprehensive spinal cord injury unit in Shenton Park in Perth. It had long been doing very well, and they were taking care of more than 120 spinal cord injured patients at any given time. The catchment area was all the way up to Darwin in north and the entire western part of Australia. For his excellent job, he was knighted and became an Officer of the British Empire. When I met him together with my wife Barbro in Scotland, he became interested in finding out whether I could train with him. The first thing he did was to spend 1 hour with my wife to figure out whether she thought that we could handle this sort of situation. After that, he spoke urgently with me and was very insistent, stating that I should come and train with him. In the summer of 1986, I traveled together with my best friend and colleague professor Richard Levi and we stayed in Perth at his unit for more than 1 year. We were offered housing in the matrons flat over at the hospital; we worked long hours and had to stick with the British aristocracy, as well as a hierarchy with a quite formal way of delegating various task on the ward. Nevertheless, we learned the craftsmanship the hard way and came back to Stockholm in the summer of 1987.

SPINALIS

We were obsessed by the idea of starting a true spinal cord injury unit in Sweden and specifically in Stockholm. We approached the local municipality of health authority, but they were quite reluctant. They were not interested in facilitating this work for us. We approached the private industry and managed to get in contact with one of the most important Swedish entrepreneurs, Kinnevik, part of the Stenbecks' financial sphere. The constitution for Spinalis was signed by Jan Stenbeck, Jan Stenbecks' mother Märtha Stenbeck, and me. Kinnevik chipped in a large sum of money and I chipped in a very minor sum of money, and the foundation was created and up and running in 1989. After that, the foundation has gone through various developing phases and a new era has evolved; as of January 2020, the Rehab Station Stockholm/Spinalis is operating in brand new buildings with 56 inpatients about 3 km away from the main Karolinska Hospital. Situated in a park by the ocean, the Spinalis outpatient unit cares for 1437 spinal cord injured patients living in our catchment area (which constitutes 25% of the Swedish population). Hence, we serve one-quarter of all spinal cord injured patients living in our country.

During these years, I have also been able to work for 6 months with the Miami project in Florida as well as as a visiting professor at Stanford University from 2009 to 2010 in Palo Alto in California, where the clinical work was conducted in the Veterans Affairs unit connected to Stanford University.

LOW ATTENTION TO NEUROGENIC BOWEL

Anyway, this article is supposed to be dealing with the neurogenic bowel and the various types of treatment or approaches that the patient can use to make this huge problem less severe and then specifically regarding the use of transanal irrigation (TAI). But before going there, it has always fascinated me why the neurogenic bladder has been receiving so much more attention over the decades as to why the neurogenic bowel has been extremely neglected. Among individuals with spinal cord injury, bowel function is considered a major physical and psychological problem, likely owing to the severe negative impact bowel problems have on social life and mobility in general.[1] I remember traveling especially in the United States during the mid and late 1980s and how frustrated I was when I tried to establish contact with well-known professional paraplegics and tetraplegics. I could not reach them for a meeting—all because they were "doing their bowel program." It turned out to be that their entire life was steered and conducted by when they were forced to spend 3, 4, or even 5 hours on the toilet seat waiting for that stool to finally pass the anal sphincter. It does not only hold true for the United States; it holds true for most developed countries in the world. Although these countries were treating spinal cord injured patients after the Second World War and had them embarking into comprehensive rehabilitation, bowel management remains a great challenge for many patients and may severely limit their quality of life.

PATHOPHYSIOLOGY OF THE NEUROGENIC BOWEL

As a result from the spinal cord injury, nerves that allow a person to control bowel movements are often damaged. If the spinal cord injury is above the T12 level (thoracic 12 vertebrae), the ability to feel when the rectum is full may be lost.[2] The anal sphincter muscle remains tight, however, and bowel movements occur on a reflex basis. This means that when the rectum is full, the defecation reflex occurs, emptying the bowel. This type of bowel problem occurs with upper motor neuron injury. With a spinal cord injury below the T12 level, the defecation reflex may be impacted, and the anal sphincter muscle may be relaxed and nonfunctional. This is known as a lower motor neuron injury.

Commonly after a spinal cord injury, the patient experiences what is called "spinal shock."[3] During that time, the anal sphincter is atonic, and there is no reflexive activity in the sphincter or any part of the bowel. After 3 to 4 weeks, the reflexive activity comes back and for the upper motor neuron lesion patients that implies that they become semi-incontinent (they do not leak or need an anal plug that some lower motor neuron injury patients do). Bowel management is initiated in the acute phase after injury and then throughout life. Patients are informed concerning the importance of diet, fluids, physical activity, and medications to strive to achieve a scheduled bowel care. This training is complemented with other training on facilitating techniques, stimulation techniques, monitoring bowel movements, and other educational activities.

NEUROGENIC BOWEL IN REAL LIFE

How does it feel when you need to go to the bathroom and evacuate your stool or how do you perceive full ampulla, or how does your body react when you really feel an urge for bowel movement?

In the beginning after your spinal cord injury, most people do not sense the fact that they need to pass stool or poop and during these days involuntary accidents are quite common. You are right in the middle of something else and then you become aware of the certain smell, and then you realize that you goofed. It is very embarrassing; it has a huge effect on your psyche and your self-esteem. You feel miserable and you get to the point where you realize that life is unfair. You have to deal with it, and you have to get into a special, rational effective mood to proceed. Cleaning yourself, cleaning your wheelchair, cleaning your cushion, and eventually cleaning your underwear, your jeans, your T-shirt, and your sweater. If the catastrophe is there, there is no reverse gear. You have to deal with the extraordinary situation, and you have to do it without having it affect your emotions to that degree that you will give up. It is not easy, but over time you will learn. After months, and after additional time, your body will get tuned in and you will learn how to detect the small afferent impulses that indicate that something is happening. Not always, but most of the times. You will learn how to distinguish between a full bladder and a full ampulla. Usually, the full bladder signal indicates that you have a very limited time before the involuntary contractions of the detrusor muscle will end up in you passing urine. The idea is then of course to try to find a toilet or a hidden place where you can perform intermittent catheterization and to do that before you pee in your pants.

Back to our neurogenic bowel and the interesting afferent impulses that give rise to this odd feeling of colon and ampulla fullness. It is difficult to describe that very subtle feeling and it is more like a soft shudder that might result in something like a pre-autonomic dysreflexia reaction. You will get a tendency to goosebumps, you will get a tendency to sweat on your forehead, and you feel in your body that something is going on. In the most ideal cases, you can even distinguish between a fart and a full colon ampulla.

The normal procedures among tetraplegics and paraplegics are that they try to get into a formal pattern of emptying their bowel every second day, every third day, or even every fourth day. If you decide to do that the body will start to "learn" that your bowel emptying pattern is semiregular, and for a lot of people that works out fairly well. That means that you get up in the morning on the days that you have your bowel program days, get on your commode chair or the toilet, and introduce some kind of suppository to trigger the rectocolic reflex. The entire idea of stimulating the anus region and the para-anal region is to trigger the rectocolic reflex. The rectocolic reflex is of course the key element in having a proper defecation when you transport the content of your intestines from proximal to distal and eventually have a relaxation of the anal sphincter, which is usually done when the sigmoideum is distended. The routine is then to trigger while using a very mild, "benign" suppository such as a glycerin suppository. What is happening is that, if that does not work, a lot of paraplegics and tetraplegics move on to bisacodyl, which is known as Dulcolax and Magic Bullet. That agent has a much stronger effect on the tissue, and it penetrates the wall of the colon and effects the Meisner and Auerbach's plexa directly. It states very clearly that this drug should not be used for more than a maximum of 10 to 14 days. Even though those are the regulatory instructions, I have met individuals who have been using it for 15 years and they have developed colon descendant and caecum and an ampulla that is like a downpipe. If you have an overambitious nurse on the ward, she might also move on to bisacodyl, not only as an oral drug, but also as suppositories. The same nurse persuades the patient to take sodium picosulphate as droplets, and then we have used most of the chemicals we can use to evacuate the ampulla. If you look at the problem from another angle, one way is to increase the bulk (the volume) of the stool, which can be done by using polyethylene glycol (known as Miralax). All these attempts or techniques have the same goal: to facilitate the rectocolic reflex and move the contents of the intestines proximal to distal and eventually also out through your anus.

BOWEL MANAGEMENT INTERVENTIONS PYRAMID

If you try to sort out bowel management interventions, you can think of a pyramid (**Fig. 1**) indicating the degree of invasiveness of the treatment option.

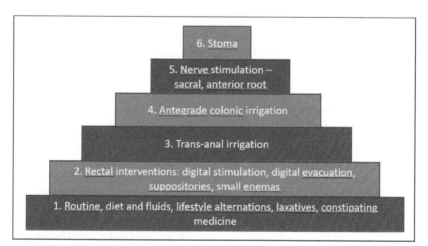

Fig. 1. Bowel management interventions pyramid.

At the bottom, you have the routines for diet, fluids, the lifestyle alterations, the laxatives, and the constipating medicine. That is level 1, at the very bottom. Level 2, the next step up, is rectal intervention, which includes digital stimulation, digital evacuation, suppositories, and small enemas. On level 3, there is TAI. We will definitely get back to TAI elsewhere in this article. On level 4 of this pyramid is the antegrade colonic irrigation through an enema technique that is, antegrade colonic enema. We return to that as well. On level 5 is the sacral anterior root stimulator. As a last option, on level 6 is the stoma, where you can have a colostomy or an ileostomy depending on the injury. Levels 4 to 6 include more invasive treatment options, such as nerve stimulation implants and surgical colonic irrigation.

THE CLAES HULTLING TECHNIQUE

During an early stage of my spinal cord injury, I learned that if you direct a jet of water toward the perianal region, and if the jet is not too strong but gentle and hot enough (not burning), you trigger the rectocolic reflex. It might trigger immediately; it might need a couple of minutes to trigger, and it might also be that you have to introduce small anal probe/catheter through the sphincter to get the acquired or desired effect. A prerequisite for this is that you have access to this small shower water device when you are traveling. That means that, in my case, I always bring a hose about 4 to 5 m long and that tubing helps me in almost any bathroom in the world. I carry with me a large number of connectors so that I can connect my hose to the faucet or the tap. It has worked extraordinary well for 35 years in most cases. However, as a complement to this method, every now and then (maybe once or twice a week), whenever I am "insecure" about whether I actually have emptied my lower part of the colon properly, I use TAI.

WHEN IS IT APPROPRIATE TO START USING TRANSANAL IRRIGATION?

The general idea is to avoid embarking onto a bowel emptying procedure that is more high-tech than the patient needs. If the individual has good, well-functioning reflex emptying of the ampulla and if the time on the toilet does not take more than 30 minutes every other day, it is fine and everyone should be happy and not try to change things that are working well. However, because the bowel procedure usually takes much longer time and frequently is unsatisfying, I think it would be a good idea to try TAI for a period of 3 months—and see if it suits the individual better. If that procedure can improve life quality—which it often does—then go for it.

Interestingly, in a recent survey by the Danish Spinal Cord Injuries Association, it was shown that as many as 37% of the patients with a spinal cord injury interviewed had not heard about the TAI method.[4]

THE TRANSANAL IRRIGATION METHOD

The idea of cleansing the gastrointestinal tract through colon hydrotherapy likely stems from ancient history. As early as 1500 BC, there are ancient Egyptian documents called the "Ebers Papyrus" (Georg Ebers was a German Egyptologist) that describe colon cleansing as beneficial. The Egyptians assumingly used a combination of techniques, such as purgatives, enemas, diuretics, heat, and steam. In the early 1900s, colon hydrotherapy and irrigation was again tried as a remedy, for example, by Dr John H. Kellogg. In 1936, Kellogg filed a petition for his invention of improvements to an "irrigating apparatus particularly adaptable for colonic irrigating, but susceptible of use for other irrigation treatments."[5] By the 1920s, enemas were standard practice in many hospitals.[6] The modern TAI technique was subsequently introduced at the end of the 1980s, initially to treat children with spina bifida.[7]

There are several TAI devices on the market including Qufora Irrisedo Mini/Cone/Klick/ Balloon/Bed systems (MacGregor Healthcare Ltd, Macmerry, UK), Peristeen (Coloplast A/S, Humlebaek, Denmark), and Navina Classic (Wellspect Healthcare/Dentsply IH AB, Mölndal, Sweden). These devices use a manual pump. There is also Navina Smart (Wellspect Healthcare/Dentsply IH AB, Mölndal, Sweden) with an electronic pump and a capacity to store the patient's technical data on the TAI procedure, including an app to allow access to this information. The devices are displayed in **Figs. 2–5**.

For patients who can use such a device, it does help in preventing constipation and fecal incontinence, and can also give the individual control over the time and place of defecation. It can be used both for patients with upper motor neuron and lower motor neuron injuries. Importantly, the TAI enables a more predictable bowel function and

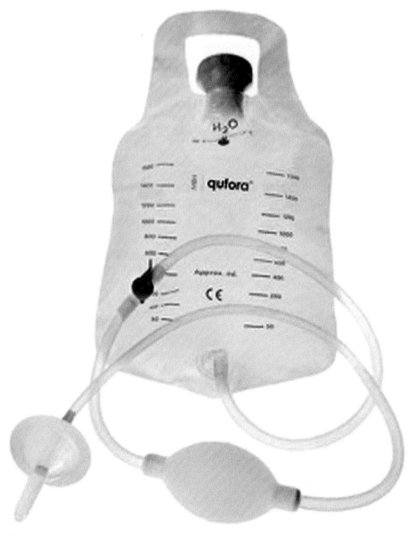

Fig. 2. The Qufora Irrisedo. (*Courtesy of* MBH-International A/S, Allerød, Denmark.)

may provide a level of independence for some patients compared with traditional methods. The consideration of using TAI should always be in a dialogue with the spinal cord injury medical team (including the nurse and the doctor), who check if it is suitable for the patient to test and who also ensure that the patient does not have any of the listed contraindications for TAI (**Table 1**). The spinal cord injury medical team also supports training in the technique.

In short, the TAI method facilitates evacuation of stool from the rectum and lower part of the colon by passing water into the bowel (irrigation) via the anus in a sufficient volume enough to reach beyond the rectum. Regular irrigation of the bowel empties the colon and rectum so effectively that new feces will not reach the rectum before the next scheduled management episode. This pattern not only prevents fecal incontinence, but it also prevents constipation through the insertion of water, which creates a mass movement from the transverse colon.

Once the training period is over and the bowel has adapted, the aim is to use TAI every second day so that the whole TAI process takes 20 to 40 minutes. For some individuals, a longer time is required.

The Navina Smart device is a more updated model compared with the other TAI devices; it has more automatic functions through its electronic pump and control unit, ensuring that each irrigation is the same—the same balloon size and the same water level in the bowel. It can be stopped earlier, but it cannot pass a fixed maximum volume of the balloon or a fixed maximum water volume. The electronic control unit enables the individual to track his or her own irrigation results and the opportunity to optimize the bowel emptying process.

HOW TO USE TRANSANAL IRRIGATION

The patient who is about to start using TAI should read the manual and should spend time with an urotherapist or a neurogenic bowel nurse to get the necessary hands-on

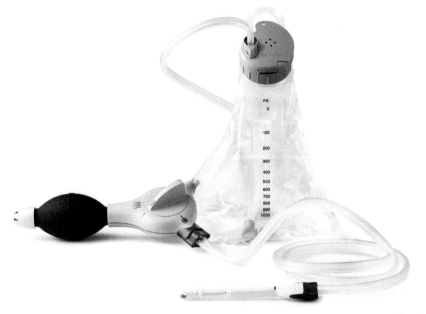

Fig. 3. The Peristeen device. (*Courtesy of* Colorplast AB, Sweden, Kungsbacka, Sweden.)

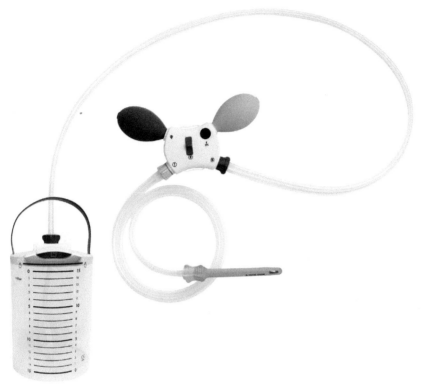

Fig. 4. The Navina Classic device. (*Courtesy from* Wellspect Healthcare/Dentsply IH AB, Mölndal, Sweden.)

information before starting on his or her own. There are also videos that may be useful in dialogue with the patient.[8,9]

Manual Transanal Irrigation

The simplest equipment for performing TAI is to use the Qufora system. It has a water bag, a tube with a manual pump, a lubricated tip, and a cone. You fill up your water bag with a maximum of 1500 mL and, after that, when seated on the toilet, you introduce the lubricated tip at the end of the tube that is about 5 cm long and ends with a cone into your rectum. Using this system requires good hand function and you need to have 1 hand on the outside of the cone while keeping the catheter into your rectum. The other hand could be used to pump water from the water bag through the tube into ampulla recti. Subsequent versions of TAI equipment available on the market are the Peristeen and Navina Classic. Both systems rely on a water container with tubing and a valve, so that you can increase the air pressure in the container for the water to flow from the container through the pipe into the anal catheter. The Qufora system uses gravity. The Peristeen and the Navina Classic systems use hyperbaric pressure and have an inflatable air balloon in the catheter mounted roughly 25 mm from the tip. The balloon keeps the anal catheter in place. After turning the handle on the device, you can go from a mode where you introduce air to the container to a mode where you introduce air into the balloon, and then water into the pipe and the anal catheter.

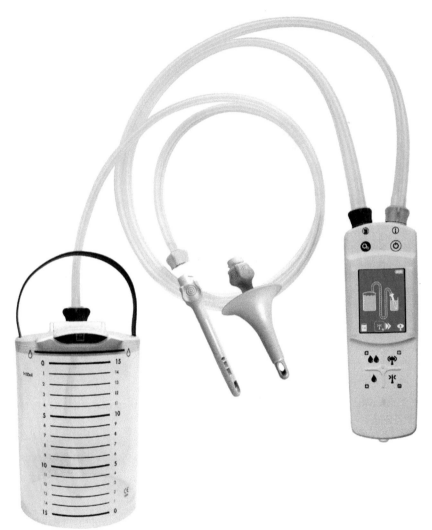

Fig. 5. The Navina Smart device. (*Courtesy from* Wellspect Healthcare/ Dentsply IH AB, Mölndal, Sweden.)

Electronic Transanal Irrigation

With electronic TAI (Navina Smart), the patient fills the container with roughly 1 L of water and adds some soap to make it a little bit softer. The normal procedure holds true, as when introducing every rectal catheter, that it is good to lubricate the area surrounding the anus. The patient should be very careful when pushing the catheter in place. The Navina catheters have a hydrophilic coating that makes additional lubricant unnecessary. When the catheter is in place, the patient starts to fill the balloon with air. With the manual version the patient has to estimate how much air is inflated, but after some training sessions the patient will learn roughly how much air that should be in the balloon. An advantage of the Navina Smart device is that it can be set for the correct amount of air before the catheter is introduced. The patient will after a while realize whether it is enough air to keep the catheter in place.

Table 1
Contraindications to TAI

Absolute Contraindications	Relative Contraindications
Anal or rectal stenosis	Severe diverticulosis Diffuse disease Dense sigmoid disease Previous diverticulitis or diverticular abscess
Active inflammatory bowel disease	Long-term steroid medication
Acute diverticulitis	Radiotherapy to the pelvis
Colorectal cancer	Prior rectal surgery
Within 3 mo of rectal surgery	Fecal impaction
Within 4 mo after endoscopic polypectomy	Painful anal conditions
Ischemic colitis	Current or planned pregnancy
	Bleeding diathesis or anticoagulant therapy (not including aspirin or clopidogrel)
	Severe autonomic dysreflexia

Data from Christensen P, Bazzocchi G, Coggrave M, et al. A randomized, controlled trial of transanal irrigation versus conservative bowel management in spinal cord-injured patients. Gastroenterology. 2006;131(3):738-47; and Passananti V, Emmanuel A, Nordin M, et al. Short term evaluation of a novel electronic transanal irrigation system in patients with neurogenic bowel dysfunction previously exposed to transanal irrigation systems. Journal of Pharmacy and Pharmacology. 2018(6):380-94.

What patients with an injury above the T6 level will recognize is that the catheter with the balloon could trigger autonomic dysreflexia; however, if they have lived with a spinal cord injury for a while, they will have learned to recognize the symptoms and would most likely not overinflate the balloon. It is interesting to note that just the balloon per se might be enough of a stimulus to trigger a gastrocolic reflex. After this procedure, the patient should press the button on the Navina Smart device to set it into the other mode and to start injecting the lukewarm water. He or she can start with a lesser volume, roughly 300 to 400 mL. There is a grading scale on the plastic compartment that indicates how much water has been injected. There is always a risk that if a patient uses this method every day and if he or she has a tendency to increase the volume of water over time, the patient may become caught in a vicious circle where he or she has to inject more and more water every time without a proper result. Therefore, the patient should be a little careful and start with 300 to 400 mL. When the patient uses the Navina Smart device, he or she can also control the speed of the water being infused, which may in itself trigger the rectocolic reflex. If the patient is extremely sensitive for autonomic dysreflexia, he or she might want to have a very slow infusion rate. In general, 300, 400, 500, or 600 mL for 1 minute should be infused.

A personal reflection concerning the electronic TAI device: with this device, I know exactly what volume I shall have on the balloon and how much water I shall introduce into the bowel and I also know with what speed I shall introduce that water to get the optimal effect trying to acquire a rectocolic reflex. It took me about 6 weeks before I could adjust the various variables to suit my needs. It is definitely a technique that can diminish the time the people living with paraplegia and tetraplegia spend on the toilet seat.[10]

What Happens Then?

Will the patient just sit on the toilet seat waiting for the rectocolic reflex to start? Yes; that is kind of true. What he or she can do is to keep the catheter with the inflated balloon in place, waiting for the water to do its work for up to 5 minutes. After that, you can give it a little extra push (add an additional 100–200 mL if the reflex is not triggered) after 2 to 3 minutes and thereafter deflate the air balloon leading to the catheter falling out or the catheter is pulled out nice and gently.

How do we know that the full ampulla content is out? Well, we do not (unless a digital rectal examination is performed). There is always a risk that there is something left, but the risk is dramatically decreased by this procedure.

If the patient has a lower motor neuron injury with the complications of flaccid sphincter and less reactive colon around the ampulla, the patient is more likely to leak. This is of course always a problem because the patient must then wear a plug or diapers. I think that the advantages of TAI might be even greater for patients with lower motor neuron injury, because they are the most afraid of leaking and most likely to leak. For a patient with a lower motor neuron injury, there is a risk that even if the patient has evacuated their ampulla thoroughly, there will be some mucus coming through the anus between procedures. This factor needs to be managed through the use of diapers and unfortunately a plug. However, by using TAI, the patient will at least have much fewer bowel accidents than before.

The devices are delivered with many rectal catheters and the patient is supposed to use a new catheter every time he or she embarks on to a TAI procedure. The TAI equipment is quite easy to carry along and the best thing is that, even if the patient does not have access to a shower next to the toilet seat, he or she can still perform a proper defecation maneuver, which would put them into a much better mood when embarking onto a busy day.

ANTEGRADE COLONIC IRRIGATION/ENEMA

The reasons for the antegrade colonic enema surgery include problems such as constipation and fecal incontinence, where other methods (diet, fluid, bowel care techniques, medications) have not been successful.[11] The procedure allows the emptying of the bowel by using fluid (similar to an enema) that is inserted into a small opening (nipple) into the colon at the right colon flexure at the lateral side of the abdomen. It has proven to be effective and has been used mostly by children born with a spina bifida; however, it requires surgery.

SACRAL ANTERIOR ROOT STIMULATOR

In the early 1980s, a distinguished English neurophysiologist Giles Brindley started to experiment with electrical stimulation of the sacral roots S2, S3, and S4 to see whether that would be an opportunity to trigger defecation, micturition, ejaculation, and erection.[12] He was quite successful, and a small number of spinal cord injury units tried this device.[13] Our spinal cord injury unit was among the first to purchase 6 units and tried it on patients during the early 1990s. Unfortunately, in 1998 a big American company took over the operations and bought the rights for the sacral anterior root stimulator. The expectations by the company were not met and after trying to introduce the technique on a more worldwide basis, they decided to pull out and the production of the unit ceased. It reflects the dilemma with trying to introduce new medical device. If venture capital comes in and if the return on investment does not meet the expectations of the investors, they usually do not have enough endurance to continue with development. The result is that a large number of people, in this case spinal cord injured patients, do not have the opportunity to try a device or therapy, in this case, a bladder emptying technique and bowel emptying technique that could have been much more effective and easier than the other alternatives. The future will tell if there will be a new possibility for this technique.

FUTURE DIRECTIONS

When addressing the problems with neurogenic bowel for paraplegics and tetraplegics, the profession needs to be more focused on this matter, which, in my opinion, has been neglected or given too little attention for decades. The reason for this has been mentioned elsewhere in this issue, being repeated and stressed. Going to the toilet emptying your bowel has been a less attractive subject among scientists, researchers, and clinicians. Other areas have drawn more attention, which highlights that sometimes the medical profession does not pay attention to areas of major concern expressed by patients. Entering into an area where empowerment is a virtue, I strongly believe that this area will be prioritized. TAI is definitely a step forward and, when this technique has been more established and becomes well-known, a large number of paraplegics and tetraplegics will spend less time on the toilet and bowel program days will become a memory from the past and obsolete.

Sacral anterior root stimulation and sacral anterior root modulation have a great potential and there will be opportunities to explore those techniques much further. A handful of scientists have been addressing sacral anterior root stimulation for the last 10 years, but the matter is still pending, for a number of reasons, such as lower priority and less funding. I strongly believe that the future for solving the problem with constipation and evacuating your bowel for spinal cord injury persons lies within the area of next generation electronic devices.

ACKNOWLEDGMENTS

The author has been supported by the Spinalis Foundation since it was constituted back in 1991. The Spinalis out-patient cohort constitutes today 1437 spinal cord injured patients. That group comes from catchment area of 2.5 million people representing the greater Stockholm area. The author has been fortunate to work with these patients for more than 35 years and is indebted to all patients for their contribution to training and clinical research conducted over time. The author would also like to thank the late Jan Stenbeck and Kinnevik, who were indispensable in the startup of Spinalis Foundation in 1990.

DISCLOSURE

The author has participated in advisory boards for the companies Wellspect Healthcare/Dentsply IH AB and Coloplast UK.

REFERENCES

1. Glickman S, Kamm MA. Bowel dysfunction in spinal-cord-injury patients. Lancet 1996;347(9016):1651–3.
2. Guttmann L. Spinal cord injuries. Comprehensive management and research. Oxford: Blackwell Scientific Publications; 1973.
3. Bedbrook GM. The care and management of spinal cord injuries. Berlin: Springer-Verlag; 1981.

4. RYK (Danish Spinal Cord Injuries Association) internal report. 2019. "Ny viden om tarmproblemer blandt mennesker med rygmarvsskade." (New knowledge on bowel problems in persons with spinal cord injury).

5. Kellogg JH. Subject Files (primarily medical missionary materials)—Legal Papers and Patents, 1896-1936. Available at: https://deepblue.lib.umich.edu/handle/2027.42/102939. Accessed January 9, 2020.

6. Friedenwald J, Morrison S. The history of the enema with some notes on related procedures (part II). In: Bulletin of the history of medicine, vol. 8. Baltimore: The Johns Hopkins University; 1940. p. 239–76. No. 2.

7. Shandling B, Gilmour RF. The enema continence catheter in spina bifida: successful bowel management. J Pediatr Surg 1987;22(3):271–3.

8. Navina TM Smart control unit – Instillation. Available at: https://www.youtube.com/watch?v=IvNQIVs8t1E. Accessed January 9, 2020.

9. Peristeen Product Demo FINAL. Available at: https://www.youtube.com/watch?v=jmyLXEDYb-4. Accessed January 9, 2020.

10. Christensen P, Andreasen J, Ehlers L. Cost-effectiveness of transanal irrigation versus conservative bowel management for spinal cord injury patients. Spinal Cord 2009;47:138–43.

11. Kokoska ER, Keller MS, Weber TR. Outcome of the antegrade colonic enema procedure in children with chronic constipation. Am J Surg 2001;182(6):625–9.

12. Brindley GS, Polkey CE, Rushton DN. Sacral anterior root stimulators for bladder control in paraplegia. Paraplegia 1982;20(6):365–81.

13. Rasmussen MM, Kutzenberger J, Krogh K, et al. Sacral anterior root stimulation improves bowel function in subjects with spinal cord injury. Spinal Cord 2015;53:297–301.

Updates of the International Standards for Neurologic Classification of Spinal Cord Injury: 2015 and 2019

Steven Kirshblum, MD[a,b,c],*, Brittany Snider, DO[a,b],
Rüdiger Rupp, PhD[d], Mary Schmidt Read, PT, DPT, MS[e],
International Standards Committee of ASIA and ISCoS[1]

KEYWORDS

• Spinal cord injury • International standards • Classification • Neurologic examination

KEY POINTS

• The latest changes to the International Standards for Neurologic Classification of Spinal Cord Injury (ISNCSCI) were published in 2015 and 2019.
• The ISNCSCI continues to evolve with advances in SCI medicine.
• All ISNCSCI updates are implemented with the goal of increasing examination and classification accuracy.

INTRODUCTION

The International Standards for Neurologic Classification of Spinal Cord Injury (ISNCSCI) are the most widely accepted system for the examination and classification of sensorimotor impairments in patients with spinal cord injury (SCI). The ISNCSCI facilitates accurate and consistent communication among clinicians, researchers, and patients. Information obtained from the ISNCSCI is used to guide the development of individualized rehabilitation programs, predict outcomes, document neurologic recovery, and evaluate the effectiveness of interventions.

[a] Kessler Institute for Rehabilitation, 1199 Pleasant Valley Way, West Orange, NJ 07052, USA; [b] Rutgers New Jersey Medical School, Newark, NJ 07103, USA; [c] Kessler Foundation, West Orange, NJ 07052, USA; [d] Spinal Cord Injury Center, Heidelberg University Hospital, Schlierbacher Landstrasse 200a, Heidelberg 69118, Germany; [e] Magee Rehabilitation Hospital, Jefferson Health, 1513 Race Street, Philadelphia, PA 19102, USA
[1] International Standards Committee of the American Spinal Injury Association (ASIA) and International Spinal Cord Society (ISCoS). A list of members can be found before the Reference section.
* Corresponding author. Kessler Institute for Rehabilitation, Rutgers New Jersey Medical School, 1199 Pleasant Valley Way, West Orange, NJ 07052.
E-mail address: skirshblum@kessler-rehab.com

Phys Med Rehabil Clin N Am 31 (2020) 319–330
https://doi.org/10.1016/j.pmr.2020.03.005
1047-9651/20/© 2020 Elsevier Inc. All rights reserved.

The first edition, *Standards for the Neurologic Classification of Spinal Cord Injury*, was published by the American Spinal Injury Association (ASIA) in 1982.[1] Since then, the ISNCSCI has continued to evolve with the changing landscape of SCI medicine. The ISNCSCI is maintained and updated by the International Standards Committee of ASIA and the International Spinal Cord Society. Each revision assimilates input from SCI professionals and is implemented with the purpose of increasing accuracy and utility of the classification system. Historical background and ISNCSCI changes before 2015 are found in an earlier publication of this journal.[2] This article details the ISNCSCI update from 2015[3] and revision in 2019.[4]

2015 UPDATES TO THE INTERNATIONAL STANDARDS FOR NEUROLOGIC CLASSIFICATION OF SPINAL CORD INJURY

The 2015 publication[3] represented an update to the seventh edition[5,6] of the ISNCSCI. Although there were no specific changes to the examination or classification schema, the 2015 update incorporated a new worksheet and provided additional clarification on the revisions made in 2011. The following sections discuss items clarified in this version.

Use of Not Determinable

"Not determinable" (ND) was to be documented for any component of the classification that could not be defined based on the examination results. For example, if a motor or sensory score of "not testable" (NT) precluded the ability to determine the motor or sensory level, total motor or sensory scores, neurologic level of injury (NLI), zone of partial preservation (ZPP), and/or ASIA Impairment Scale (AIS) grade, ND would be recorded on the worksheet for each component that was impacted. It was strongly recommended that the reason for the NT grade be documented in the comments box. The introduction of ND helped to indicate completeness of a worksheet and ensure that no variable had been missed (**Fig. 1**).

Use of Nonkey Muscle Functions

Nonkey muscle functions and corresponding myotomes, and the rules for their use, were included in the 2015 booklet (**Table 1**).[3] The examination of nonkey muscles

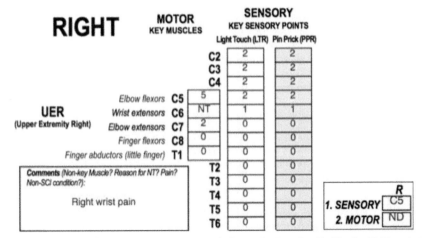

Fig. 1. Case scenario demonstrating recommended use of ND as detailed in the 2015 update.[3] NT is present in a level that impacts the ability to define the right motor level, resulting in a designation of ND. (© 2020 American Spinal Injury Association. Reprinted with permission.)

Table 1
Nonkey muscle functions

Movement	Root Level
Shoulder: Flexion, extension, abduction, adduction, internal and external rotation Elbow: Supination	C5
Elbow: Pronation Wrist: Flexion	C6
Finger: Flexion at proximal joint, extension Thumb: Flexion, extension and abduction in plane of thumb	C7
Finger: Flexion at MCP joint Thumb: Opposition, adduction and abduction perpendicular to palm	C8
Finger: Abduction of the index finger	T1
Hip: Adduction	L2
Hip: External rotation	L3
Hip: Extension, abduction, internal rotation Knee: Flexion Ankle: Inversion and eversion Toe: MP and IP extension	L4
Hallux and Toe: DIP and PIP Flexion and abduction	L5
Hallux: Adduction	S1

Abbreviation DIP, distal interphalangeal; IP, interphalangeal; MCP, metacarpophalangeal; MP, metatarsophalangeal; PIP, proximal interphalangeal

© 2020 American Spinal Injury Association. Reprinted with permission.

more than three levels below the motor level on each side of the body was recommended "to rule out or rule in a motor incomplete status"[3] when voluntary anal contraction (VAC) and all key muscle functions more than three levels below the ipsilateral motor level were absent in patients with a sensory incomplete injury (sacral sparing of light touch [LT] or pin prick [PP] sensation, or presence of deep anal pressure [DAP]). In such cases, the injury was classified as AIS B if there was no motor function in nonkey muscles more than three segments below the motor level on each side and was classified as AIS C if motor function was present in a nonkey muscle more than three segments below the ipsilateral motor level. When relevant for classification of the AIS and the motor ZPPs, nonkey muscle functions were to be recorded in the comments box.

Definition of Motor Incomplete

The definition of a motor incomplete injury was refined. The 2011 definition described, "Motor function is preserved below the neurologic level** and more than half of key muscle functions below the NLI have a muscle grade less than 3 (Grades 0–2)."[6] The footnote specified, "** For an individual to receive a motor incomplete status they must have either (1) VAC or (2) sacral sensory sparing with sparing of motor function more than three levels below the motor level for that side of the body."[6]

The 2015 definition was updated to "Motor function is preserved at the most caudal sacral segments on VAC OR the patient meets the criteria for sensory incomplete status (sensory function preserved at the most caudal sacral segments [S4-S5] by LT, PP or DAP), and has some sparing of motor function more than three levels below the ipsilateral motor level on either side of the body."[3]

Terminology Added

Additional terms were added to the glossary including "key muscle functions," "non-key muscle functions," "sacral sparing," "complete injury," and "not determinable," because these were not included in previous booklets.

2015 Worksheet Changes

Two minor adjustments to the worksheet were made:

1. On page 1, the dermatomal map of key sensory points C6-C8 (of the hand) was repositioned in the middle of the page.
2. On page 2, the section "When to Test Nonkey Muscles" was added for further clarification. This rule stated, "In a patient with an apparent AIS B classification, nonkey muscle functions more than 3 levels below the motor level on each side should be tested to most accurately classify the injury (differentiate between AIS B and C)."[3]

2019 REVISIONS OF THE INTERNATIONAL STANDARDS FOR NEUROLOGIC CLASSIFICATION OF SPINAL CORD INJURY

The eighth edition of the ISNCSCI and an editorial summarizing the changes were published in 2019.[4,7] Two main concepts were introduced, including a new taxonomy for the documentation of non-SCI-related conditions and a revised definition of the applicability of ZPP. The updates were incorporated into the 2019 ISNCSCI worksheet and booklet[4] and the International Standards Training e-Learning Program.[8]

Documentation of Non–Spinal Cord Injury–Related Conditions

Persons with SCI may have preexisting or concomitant non-SCI-related conditions that influence performance and documentation of the ISNCSCI examination. Conditions may include, but are not limited to, burns, general weakness, peripheral nerve injuries, musculoskeletal injuries, casts/limb immobilization, amputations, and pain. Non-SCI-related conditions may be present above, at, or below the level of the spinal cord lesion and may impact the ability to examine or grade certain myotomes and dermatomes. In these cases, accurate classification of the SCI relies on clinical judgment. Before the 2019 ISNCSCI revision, the motor grade "5*" was used when full muscle strength was not achieved because of identified inhibiting factors (ie, pain, disuse) and the examiner believed that full muscle function would have been achieved in the absence of that inhibiting factor.

The "5*" designation resulted in some important limitations. First, use of the asterisk (score tagged with the asterisk) was restricted to the motor examination with no standardized method for denoting impaired sensation because of a non-SCI condition. Second, record of the actual motor function grade obtained was lost unless the examined score was documented in the comments box. This prevented comparisons of muscle strength on serial examinations or the ability to later reclassify ISNCSCI datasets over time. Recognizing these limitations, the International Standards Committee developed a new taxonomy for the documentation of non-SCI-related conditions as detailed next.

1. The concept of the asterisk includes all components of the examination, motor and sensory, and is used to denote classification that is impacted by a non-SCI condition.
2. If motor function is impaired because of a non-SCI condition, the actual examined score is recorded and tagged with an asterisk. The asterisk is applied to motor grades 0 to 4 and NT (0*, 1*, 2*, 3*, 4*, NT*). The "5*" is no longer used when grading

muscle strength because the asterisk, when applied to motor scores, indicates full muscle strength was not initially achieved.

3. If sensory function is impaired because of a non-SCI condition, the actual examined score is recorded and tagged with an asterisk. The asterisk is applied to sensory grades 0 to 1 and NT (0*, 1*, NT*). There is no "2*" because the asterisk, when applied to sensory scores, indicates normal sensation was not initially achieved.

4. All asterisk-tagged scores should be explained in the comments box.

5. The examiner should specify in the comments box how the tagged scores should be rated during classification. In most cases "normal/not normal for classification" is stipulated. However, in a chronic injury, prior examination results might be considered.

6. Assumed scores (based on the asterisk) are not used to calculate sum scores. Instead, sum motor and sensory scores are calculated using the actual examined scores. If NT or NT* is present, the sum score is ND.

7. Any classification variable (eg, motor or sensory level, NLI, AIS grade, and ZPP) requires an asterisk if a clinical assumption impacted its designation.

8. The following approach is used to determine if any classification variable (sensory/motor level, NLI, ZPP, and/or AIS grade) requires the asterisk in the presence of a non-SCI-related condition.

   A. First, replace the asterisk-tagged scores with the assumed ones (based on whether these scores were considered "normal" or "not normal" for classification as documented in the comments box), and write down the classification results in the respective boxes.

   B. Then determine the classification (motor and sensory levels) using the examined scores (without consideration of the asterisk-tagged scores) and reclassify.

   C. Any classification variable (sensory, motor and/or NLI, ZPP, or AIS grade) that is, different because of the asterisk-tagged scores should then also be tagged with an asterisk.

See **Figs. 2** and **3** for examples of changes in the documentation of non-SCI-related conditions.

Definition of the Zone of Partial Preservation

ZPPs were previously used only for complete lesions (AIS A) as the most caudal myotome and dermatome below the defined motor or sensory levels on each side with partially preserved functions.[3,6] They have been used to characterize neurologic impairment and predict recovery.[9–14] However, there were limitations to restricting the ZPP to complete injuries alone. To increase clinical value, the use of ZPP was expanded,[4] as detailed next.

1. ZPP is used to describe the extent of preserved sensory and motor function in complete (AIS A) or incomplete injuries (AIS B, C, or D).

2. In complete (AIS A) injuries, the rules for classification of motor and sensory sparing are consistent with the previous ZPP definition.[3,5]

3. Sensory ZPP may be applicable in incomplete injuries and is determined independently for each side of the body. A sensory ZPP is documented in cases where DAP is absent and S4-5 dermatome LT and PP sensation are also absent on that side of the body. Sensory ZPP represents the most caudal dermatome on each side with at least partial innervation.

4. A sensory ZPP is not applicable (NA) in lesions with preserved DAP (represents both sides of the body), or LT or PP sensation in the S4-5 dermatome on each side of the body. In cases where DAP sensation is present, NA is recorded in the

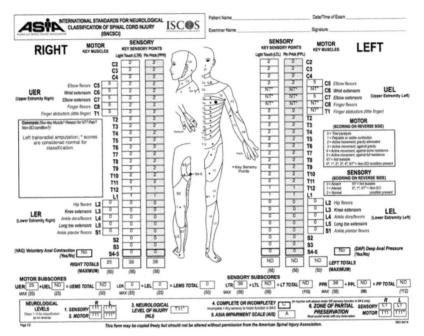

Fig. 2. Case scenario demonstrating classification of AIS A paraplegia in the presence of a concomitant left transradial (below elbow) amputation. Motor and sensory scores impacted by the presence of a left transradial amputation are recorded as NT* because these myotomes and dermatomes are unable to be examined. Based on clinical judgment, these asterisk-tagged scores are considered "normal for classification" because the non-SCI-related condition is present above the level of the spinal cord lesion. This clinical assumption, and the non-SCI condition, are recorded in the comments box. All classification variables impacted by the clinical assumption, including left motor and sensory levels, NLI, and left motor ZPP, are also tagged with the asterisk. Actual examination scores are used to calculate sum motor and sensory scores; as demonstrated in this case, sum scores are recorded as ND if NT* is present. (© 2020 American Spinal Injury Association. Reprinted with permission.)

right and left sensory ZPP boxes on the ISNCSCI worksheet. With DAP absent, if S4-5 LT and/or PP sensation is preserved only on one side, sensory ZPP is recorded as NA for that side. With S4-5 LT and PP absent only on one side, it is possible to have a unilateral sensory ZPP as long as DAP is also absent.

5. Motor ZPP is documented in incomplete injuries and represents the most caudal myotome on each side with at least partial innervation. Motor ZPP is determined individually for each side and is applicable in all injuries with absent VAC.

6. Motor ZPP is NA in lesions with preserved VAC. In these cases, NA is recorded in the right and left motor ZPP boxes on the ISNCSCI worksheet.

7. Nonkey muscles are generally not considered in the determination of motor ZPP. The only exception to this rule is in cases where the AIS designation is based on the presence of nonkey muscles. In such cases, the most caudal nonkey muscle with motor sparing should be considered for the motor ZPP. Preserved function in a nonkey muscle must be documented in the comments box. For example, in a case where the motor/sensory levels and NLI are T6 and there is preserved DAP sensation, absent VAC, and 1/5 strength in bilateral hip adduction (L2

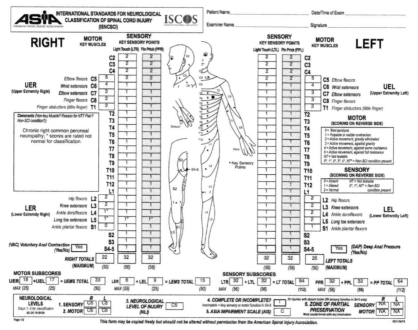

Fig. 3. Case scenario demonstrating classification of AIS C tetraplegia in the setting of an old, right common peroneal neuropathy. Motor and sensory scores impacted by the presence of a right common peroneal neuropathy are tagged with an asterisk to indicate normal function was not initially achieved. Based on clinical judgment, these asterisk-tagged scores are rated "not normal for classification" because the non-SCI-related condition is present below the level of the spinal cord lesion. In this case, there are no classification variables impacted by a clinical assumption. Motor ZPP is NA bilaterally because VAC is preserved. Sensory ZPP is NA bilaterally because of preserved DAP and PP/LT sensation in the S4-5 dermatomes. Sum motor and sensory scores are calculated using the actual examination scores. NA, not applicable. (© 2020 American Spinal Injury Association. Reprinted with permission.)

myotome), the injury is classified as T6 AIS C (because there is nonkey voluntary muscle function more than three levels below the motor level). The sensory ZPPs are NA bilaterally (discussed previously) because of the preserved DAP, and motor ZPP on each side is L2. The information regarding presence of bilateral hip adduction is documented in the comments box.

8. ZPPs can usually be determined in cases with asterisk-tagged scores. A ZPP may also be tagged with an asterisk if its designation is impacted by a non-SCI-related condition. In rare cases, an asterisk-tagged score precludes ZPP designation. An example of this includes a case classified as L1 AIS B with a right motor level of L2, right L3 motor function graded as 1/5, and right L4 motor function graded 0* in the setting of an old common peroneal neuropathy with no presumption of what the strength would be in this case if the non-SCI issue was absent. In this situation, the right motor ZPP is documented as ND*.

See **Figs. 4** and **5** for examples of how to determine the ZPP in cases with incomplete injuries.

A quantitative comparison between the 2011 and 2019 ZPP definitions was performed using the European Multicenter Study about Spinal Cord Injury database.[15] ISNCSCI examinations of 665 adult patients with traumatic SCI were reviewed and

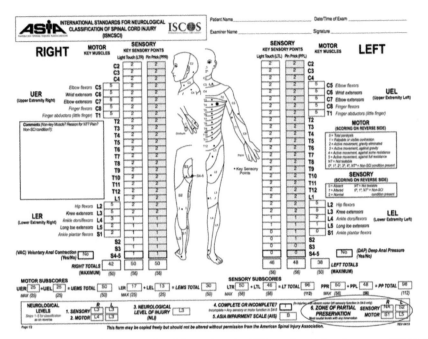

Fig. 4. Case scenario demonstrating bilateral motor ZPPs and unilateral sensory ZPP in an AIS B injury. In this case, motor ZPPs reveal meaningful information about the caudal extent of preserved motor function in the absence of VAC. Likewise, the left sensory ZPP provides important information about the caudal extent of sensory innervation in the absence of DAP and LT/PP sensation in the left S4-5 dermatomes. When DAP is present, both sensory ZPPs would be designated as NA. (© 2020 American Spinal Injury Association. Reprinted with permission.)

reclassified using the 2019 ZPP rules. Approximately one-third of patients with incomplete injuries were found to have a meaningful ZPP. As expected, ZPP remained unchanged for AIS A injuries. Further analysis also revealed increased prognostic value in motor recovery 1 year after injury using the new ZPP definition.[15]

2019 Worksheet Changes

The following are changes incorporated into the 2019 worksheet (**Fig. 6**).
 On page 1 of the worksheet:

1. The words "Non-SCI condition" were added to the comments box to serve as a reminder that non-SCI-related impairments should be described and documented as "normal/not normal for classification" when present.
2. In the motor scoring key on the right side of the page, "5* = normal corrected for pain/disuse" was removed, and the asterisk was extended to "0*, 1*, 2*, 3*, 4*, NT*" as possible motor scores for non-SCI-related conditions.
3. In the sensory scoring key on the right side of the page, the asterisk was extended to "0*, 1*, NT*" as potential sensory scores for non-SCI-related conditions.
4. In accordance with the changed applicability of ZPP, wording above "Zone of Partial Preservation" was changed from "In complete injuries only" to "In injuries with absent motor OR sensory function in S4-5 only."
5. ZPP was included in the "Steps 1 to 6 for classification" and numbered 6, corresponding to directions on page 2 of the worksheet.

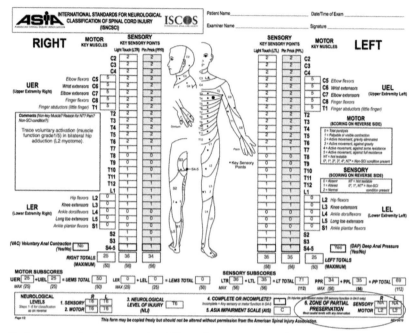

Fig. 5. Case scenario demonstrating bilateral motor ZPPs and use of nonkey muscle functions in an AIS C injury. This injury is classified as AIS C because there is nonkey voluntary muscle function at L2, which is more than three levels below the motor level of T6. Hip adductors represent the most caudal extent of preserved motor function, so L2 is recorded for each motor ZPP. Nonkey muscle function is documented in the comments box. In this case, sensory ZPP is NA bilaterally because there is preserved DAP and preserved LT/PP sensation in the S4-5 dermatomes on each side. (© 2020 American Spinal Injury Association. Reprinted with permission.)

6. To differentiate the updated worksheet from previous versions, the revision date of 2019 was replaced in the bottom right corner.
7. To indicate that the ISNCSCI worksheet consists of a front and back page, "Page 1/2" has been added to the bottom left corner.

On page 2 of the worksheet:

1. Under the section, "Muscle Function Grading," the "5*" was removed as a possible motor score, and "0*, 1*, 2*, 3*, 4*, NT*" were added.
2. Under the section, "Sensory Grading," scores "0*, 1*, NT*" were added.
3. An annotation ("a") further clarified use of the asterisk. This note stated, "Abnormal motor and sensory scores should be tagged with an '*' to indicate an impairment caused by a non-SCI condition. The non-SCI condition should be explained in the 'Comments box' together with information about how the score is rated for classification purposes (at least normal/not normal for classification)."
4. Under the section, "Steps in Classification," for item #5 "Determine ASIA Impairment Scale (AIS) Grade," wording was adjusted to be consistent with the expanded use of ZPP. For grade AIS A, the words, "...and can record ZPP (lowest dermatome or myotome on each side with some preservation)" were removed because ZPP can now also be used for incomplete lesions.

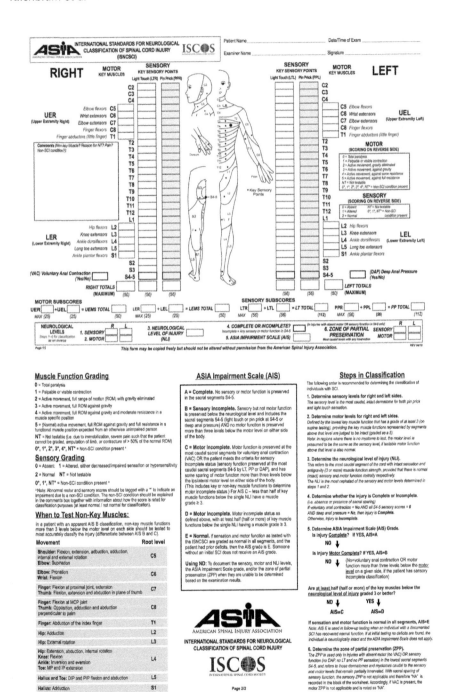

Fig. 6. Worksheet for ISNCSCI, 2019. (© 2020 American Spinal Injury Association. Reprinted with permission.)

5. A sixth step, "Determine the zone of partial preservation (ZPP)," was added to the "Steps in Classification." This section of the worksheet explains the expanded use of ZPP and its relevance in injuries without sacral sparing of sensory or motor function.
6. To indicate that this is the back side of the ISNCSCI worksheet, "Page 2/2" was added in the bottom center.

INTERNATIONAL STANDARDS FOR NEUROLOGIC CLASSIFICATION OF SPINAL CORD INJURY REVISIONS IN THE RESEARCH SETTING

For clinical studies where the previous version (2015) of the ISNCSCI is being used (eg, the use of 5* as a motor grade and ZPP only for complete injuries), it is not recommended that changes be made to the documentation. The recommendation, as outlined in a recent editorial from the International Standards Committee,[7] is that the research study should continue with the ISNCSCI edition in use, and the resultant publication should specify the ISNCSCI edition that was used in the study.

SUMMARY

The ISNCSCI is an evolving classification system. Updates incorporate feedback from SCI professionals and assimilate empirical evidence as it becomes available. This article and the previous publication[2] provide a summary of ISNCSCI changes since its inception in 1982. Historical background and awareness of earlier versions, including the reasons for each revision, may increase understanding, appreciation, and use of the newest changes and help guide future updates.

DISCLOSURE

Members of the International Standards Committee of American Spinal Injury Association and International Spinal Cord Society: Randal Betz (Institute for Spine and Scoliosis, Lawrenceville, NJ); Fin Biering-Soerensen (Clinic for Spinal Cord Injuries, Rigshospitalet, University of Copenhagen, Copenhagen, Denmark); Stephen P. Burns (Department of Rehabilitation Medicine, University of Washington School of Medicine, Seattle, WA); William H. Donovan (Institute for Rehabilitation and Research, Houston, TX); Daniel E. Graves (Thomas Jefferson University, Philadelphia, PA); James Guest (Department of Neurologic Surgery, University of Miami Miller School of Medicine, Miami, FL); Linda Jones (University of Colorado, Denver, CO); Steven Kirshblum (Kessler Institute for Rehabilitation, Rutgers New Jersey Medical School, West Orange, NJ); Andrei Krassioukov (International Collaboration On Repair Discovery, Vancouver, Canada); Mary-Jane Mulcahey (Thomas Jefferson University, Philadelphia, PA); Gianna Rodriguez (Michigan Medicine, University of Michigan, Ann Arbor, MI); Rüdiger Rupp (Spinal Cord Injury Center, Heidelberg University Hospital, Heidelberg, Germany); Mary Schmidt Read (Magee Rehabilitation Hospital - Jefferson Health, Philadelphia, PA); Christian Schuld (Spinal Cord Injury Center, Heidelberg University Hospital, Heidelberg, Germany); Keith Tansey (Departments of Neurosurgery and Neurobiology, University of Mississippi Medical Center, Jackson, MS); and Kristen Walden (Rick Hansen Institute, Vancouver, Canada).

FUNDING STATEMENT

The authors received Funding in part by the National Institute on Disability, Independent Living, and Rehabilitation Research (NIDILRR grant no. 90SI5026).

REFERENCES

1. American Spinal Injury Association. Standards for neurological classification of spinal injury patients. Chicago: ASIA; 1982.
2. Kirshblum SC, Waring WP III. Updates for the International Standards for Neurological Classification of Spinal Cord Injury. Phys Med Rehabil Clin N Am 2014; 25(3):505–17.
3. American Spinal Injury Association. International Standards for Neurological Classification of Spinal Cord Injury. Revised 2011; Atlanta (GA). Updated 2015.
4. American Spinal Injury Association. International Standards for Neurological Classification of Spinal Cord Injury. Richmond (VA): ASIA; 2019.
5. American Spinal Injury Association. International Standards for Neurological Classification of Spinal Cord Injury. Revised 2011; Atlanta (GA).
6. Kirshblum SC, Waring W, Beiring-Sorensen F, et al. Reference for the 2011 revision of the International Standards for Neurological Classification of Spinal Cord Injury. J Spinal Cord Med 2011;34(6):547–54.
7. ASIA, ISCoS International Standards Committee. The 2019 revision of the International Standards for Neurological Classification of Spinal Cord Injury (ISNCSCI) – What's new? Spinal Cord 2019. https://doi.org/10.1038/s41393-019-0350-9.
8. Available at: https://asia-spinalinjury.org/learning/. Accessed October 3, 2019.
9. Browne BJ, Jacobs SR, Herbison GJ, et al. Pin sensation as a predictor of extensor carpi radialis recovery in spinal cord injury. Arch Phys Med Rehabil 1993;74(1):14–8.
10. Ditunno JF Jr, Stover SL, Freed MM, et al. Motor recovery of the upper extremities in traumatic quadriplegia: a multicenter study. Arch Phys Med Rehabil 1992; 73(5):431–6.
11. Mange KC, Marino RJ, Gregory PC, et al. Course of motor recovery in the zone of partial preservation in spinal cord injury. Arch Phys Med Rehabil 1992;73(5): 437–41.
12. Waters RL, Adkins RH, Yahura JS, et al. Motor and sensory recovery following complete tetraplegia. Arch Phys Med Rehabil 1993;74(3):242–7.
13. Wilson JR, Cadotte DW, Fehlings MG. Clinical predictors of neurological outcome, functional status, and survival after traumatic spinal cord injury: a systematic review. J Neurosurg Spine 2012;17(Suppl):11–26.
14. Wu L, Marino RJ, Herbison GJ, et al. Recovery of zero-grade muscles in the zone of partial preservation in motor complete quadriplegia. Arch Phys Med Rehabil 1992;73(1):40–3.
15. Schuld C, Franz S, Weidner N, et al. Increasing the clinical value of the zones of partial preservation: a quantitative comparison of a new definition rule applicable also in incomplete lesions. Top Spinal Cord Inj Rehabil 2018;24(Suppl 1):120–1.

Predicting Outcomes After Spinal Cord Injury

Wesley Chay, MD[a,b,*], Steven Kirshblum, MD[c,d]

KEYWORDS

- Spinal cord injury • Neurologic recovery • Prognosis of recovery
- Predicting outcome • Complete SCI • Incomplete SCI • Paraplegia • Quadriplegia

KEY POINTS

- In order to establish reasonable goals in therapy and plan for postdischarge care, patients, families, and health care providers need accurate information about prognosis of recovery.
- The most important determinant of long-term prognosis is the neurologic completeness of the spinal cord injury (SCI) based on the sacral sparing definition.
- Age, timing of surgical decompression, and penetrating injuries are special factors that have an impact on functional/neurologic recovery.
- Early improvement in neurologic status is associated with greater recovery than slow improvement.
- After SCI, a majority of walking determinants relate to injury severity, in particular the extent of lower extremity motor function. Other common impairments include spasticity, balance, proprioception, and truncal control, with cognition also playing a role in walking.

CASE 1

John Doe is a 22-year-old man who sustained a C5 fracture while diving into the ocean when on spring break with friends. He describes immediately being unable to move his arms or legs, but he could feel "all over." After undergoing emergent C4-6 laminectomy and posterior spinal fusion, he reports that over the next few days he started moving some muscles in his arms and feet. He is now 2 weeks post-injury and admitted for inpatient rehabilitation. Comprehensive examination performed is consistent with a diagnosis of C5 American Spinal Injury Association Impairment Scale (AIS) D spinal cord injury (SCI). He inquires if he will be able to return to college and drive.

[a] Physical Medicine and Rehabilitation, Shepherd Center, 2020 Peachtree Road, NW, Atlanta, GA 30309, USA; [b] Emory University School of Medicine, Atlanta, Georgia, USA; [c] Kessler Institute for Rehabilitation, 1199 Pleasant Valley Way, West Orange, NJ 07052, USA; [d] Rutgers New Jersey Medical School, Newark, NJ, USA
* Corresponding author.
E-mail address: wes.chay@shepherd.org

Phys Med Rehabil Clin N Am 31 (2020) 331–343
https://doi.org/10.1016/j.pmr.2020.03.003
1047-9651/20/© 2020 Elsevier Inc. All rights reserved.

CASE 2

Jane Doe is a 66-year-old woman who was involved in a motor vehicle crash where she sustained a T6 burst fracture. She underwent T5-7 laminectomy and posterior spinal fusion. She notes that immediately after the accident, she could not feel below her chest or move any muscles in her legs and has not noticed any neurologic change since then. She now is admitted for inpatient rehabilitation at 1 week postinjury. Comprehensive examination performed is consistent with a diagnosis of T4 AIS A. She inquires if she will ever be able to walk again.

INTRODUCTION

One of the central questions fielded by clinicians working with individuals who have sustained a traumatic SCI is "Will I be able to get back to my life?" This may be presented through different questions about the chance of walking, working, caring for oneself, achieving sexual intimacy, or having children. In order to establish reasonable goals in therapy and plan for postdischarge care, patients, families, and health care providers need accurate information about prognosis of recovery. The aim of this article is to provide a broad overview of prognosis and outcomes after SCI, including reviewing variables that have an impact on neurologic assessment, describing the extent and time frame of natural recovery after traumatic SCI, clarifying specific factors having an impact on prognosis of ambulation, reviewing the role of imaging and modalities for assessing the injured spinal cord, and discussing some strategies on presenting information to patients and families in the context of some cases.

ASSESSING SEVERITY OF INJURY AFTER TRAUMATIC SPINAL CORD INJURY

Discussing prognosis and expected outcomes with patients and families, necessitates an accurate picture of the neurologic impact of the SCI. This requires the recommended neurologic examination be performed in accordance to the International Standards for Neurological Classification of Spinal Cord Injury (ISNCSCI).[1] The most important determinant of long-term prognosis is the neurologic completeness of the SCI based on the sacral sparing definition.[2] The ISNCSCI defines SCI as neurologically complete when there is no evidence of sacral sparing or sensory and/or motor function at the lowest sacral level (sensory function in dermatome S4-5, presence of deep anal pressure [DAP], or voluntary anal contraction [VAC]).[1] If there is any sparing in these areas, then the individual is classified as having an incomplete injury. After it has been determined whether the injury is neurologically complete or incomplete, the severity of the SCI is classified using the AIS, with grades of A to E.

RELATIONSHIP BETWEEN TIMING OF ASSESSMENT AND PROGNOSIS

It is important to perform an examination as soon as possible in order to establish a baseline for monitoring improvement or decline in neurologic status. This may be in the emergency department trauma bay, postoperatively, or after admission to inpatient SCI rehabilitation.

Burns and colleagues[3] described factors having an impact on the reliability of the initial assessment within the first 2 days of injury based on higher conversion rates (complete to incomplete) at both 1 week and 1 year postinjury time points. These factors include mechanical ventilation; intoxication, chemical sedation, or paralysis; concomitant closed head injury; psychiatric illness; language barrier; severe pain; and cerebral palsy.[3]

The 72-hour examination has been suggested as having superior accuracy due to the presence of postinjury swelling and cord edema that may increase between 24 hours and 72 hours after injury.[4] Although historically the 1-month time point had been a common baseline interval for predicting recovery,[5–8] because this time point corresponded closely with the timing of admission to a rehabilitation facility, transfer to rehabilitation is now earlier and prognostication data are available from multiple sources based on earlier examination time points.[9–12]

SPECIAL FACTORS THAT HAVE AN IMPACT ON FUNCTIONAL/NEUROLOGIC RECOVERY

Age has been demonstrated as a significant factor in functional recovery after SCI.[13–15] Wilson and colleagues[13] found that Functional Independence Measure scores were significantly lower (particularly in AIS B and AIS C) in individuals ages 65 years and older compared with those less than 65 years of age. Lee and colleagues[14] also reported less improvement for persons older than age 50 years in thoracic-level injuries. Oleson and colleagues[15] and Penrod and colleagues[16] found that overall patients ages greater than 50 years had a decreased likelihood of recovering walking ability 1 year postinjury relative to patients under age 50 years. Burns and colleagues[17] reported increased likelihood of achieving community ambulation in persons with incomplete tetraplegia and paraplegia on discharge from rehabilitation. Specifically, individuals with AIS C aged less than 50 years (91%) were more likely to achieve community ambulation compared with those aged greater than or equal to 50 years (42%). Of note, for individuals presenting with an initial AIS D, age was not a factor in ambulation because all were able to ambulate 3 months to 6 months postinjury.[17]

Varying opinions exist on whether timing of surgical decompression and stabilization affect neurological recovery. Early surgery, however, defined as within 24 hours after SCI, seems to offer neurologic advantage for recovery, most especially for cervical patients with complete and incomplete injuries. The Surgical Treatment for Acute Spinal Cord Injury Study (STASCIS) was a prospective cohort study in persons with cervical SCI.[18] The early decompression group (<24 hours after SCI) had a 2.8-times chance to improve at least a 2-grade improvement in AIS grade at 6 months relative to a late decompression group (≥24 hours after SCI). Reanalysis of the raw data of the STASCIS study by van Middendorp and colleagues[19] demonstrated a tendency toward the efficacy of early decompression but no statistical significant difference. Other studies reported improvements post–early surgery,[20–22] although some studies have not shown significant benefit in persons with thoracic or thoracolumbar injuries.[22,23]

Most recent studies support the effectiveness of early surgery, especially with a cervical-level injury.[24,25] In regard to surgery even earlier than 24 hours, there are differences of opinion, with some studies showing effectiveness if decompression with 8 hours to 12 hours,[26–29] although some have shown no benefit if within 12 hours[30] or within 4 hours to 5 hours.[31,32] Further study may be needed, especially in the elderly, cases of central cord syndrome, and thoracic-level injuries.

Penetrating injury is more likely to lead to a neurologic complete injury compared with blunt trauma. The prognosis for recovery of patients with complete injury from a penetrating injury also is worse compared with those with blunt trauma, although not necessarily for incomplete injuries.[33]

GENERAL TRENDS IN NATURAL RECOVERY AFTER TRAUMATIC SPINAL CORD INJURY

After traumatic SCI, the most rapid rate of neurologic recovery occurs in the first 3 months. The majority of neurologic recovery occurs within the first 6 months to

9 months. Although some late neurologic recovery has been reported 2 years to 5 years postinjury,[34] for most individuals with traumatic SCI, neurologic recovery plateaus at approximately 12 months to 18 months postinjury.[5–8] Early improvement in neurologic status is associated with greater recovery than slow improvement.

As a general rule, the amount of neurologic recovery based on change of motor recovery is significantly different between the initial AIS grades of SCI in the following order: AIS C > B > D > A.[33] Overall, patients with complete SCI (tetraplegia and paraplegia combined) have the least amount of motor score change in 1 year, with averages of 6.6 (4.7–8.5) versus 24.0 (20.3–27.8) for incomplete injuries. This has been further defined by initial severity of injury; 25.6 (19.7–31.5) for AIS B, 36.5 (25.1–47.8) for AIS C, and 14.7 for AIS D. Persons with AIS D experience less motor recovery compared with AIS C or B most likely because of a ceiling effect.

COMPLETE SPINAL CORD INJURY: CONVERSION OF COMPLETE TO INCOMPLETE

There have been analyses and reviews of different databases to determine prognosis after an acute SCI.[5–12,35–39] Following is a summary of these studies. Overall, approximately 20% to 30% of individuals classified with an initial AIS A convert to incomplete status, with approximately half converting to AIS B and the other half to motor incomplete status. There has been a trend over the years of increasing conversion to incomplete status, especially for persons with tetraplegia.[14,39,40] Data from multiple sources show that complete high thoracic SCI is associated with the lowest (approximately 10%) rate of conversion to incomplete status, with complete lumbar SCI associated with the highest (approximately 35%) rate of neurologic recovery, followed by cervical level (25%–30%) and low paraplegia levels (approximately 17%).[12,30,33] Zariffa and colleagues[12] described the differences in conversion between levels of thoracic injury with 9.46% of T2-5 AIS A, 15.56% of T6-9 AIS A, and 29.17% of persons with an initial classification of T10-12 AIS A converting to incomplete SCI. There are multiple factors that can explain why persons with complete paraplegia (thoracic levels of injury) have the poorest prognosis, including the inherent stability of the thoracic spine; thereby, trauma leading to an initial complete SCI would most likely cause severe damage, decreased vascular supply to the thoracic cord, and a narrower thoracic canal. Lumbar injuries most likely have the greatest prognosis due to the presence of nerve root injuries that have an improved ability for healing relative to upper motor neuron cord damage.[33]

SPECIAL FEATURES OF RECOVERY IN COMPLETE TETRAPLEGIA

Recovery of functional strength (defined as motor score ≥3/5) is minimal in muscles with grade 0/5 at 1 month.[5,41] Most patients (67%–80%) with complete tetraplegia regain at least 1 level of motor function.[5,11,42,43] Fischer and colleagues[42] found 67% of subjects regained function in 1 motor level, 16% of subjects regained function in 2 motor levels, and 3% of subjects regained function in 3 motor levels. Steeves and colleagues[11] reported that for individuals with complete SCI and motor levels of C4-7, 16.7% to 46.2% gained 1 level, and 15.4% to 50% gained 2 or more levels. Approximately 90% of muscles presenting with initial strength grade of 1/5 or 2/5, 1 week to 1 month after injury, recover to greater than or equal to 3/5 by 1 year. The chance of motor recovery in the lower extremities (LEs) is low (<10%) if a patient remains motor and sensory complete for more than 1 month postinjury.[5]

SPECIAL FEATURES OF RECOVERY IN COMPLETE PARAPLEGIA

In comparison to tetraplegia, neurologic status after complete paraplegia is relatively static. A majority of individuals with complete paraplegia at 1-month postinjury remain complete. Recovery of motor function in paraplegia is related to level of injury. Waters and colleagues[6] reported that in 73% of individuals with paraplegia, the neurologic level of injury (NLI) did not change at 1 year postinjury. No subjects with NLI above T9 regained any motor function below 1 year postinjury, whereas at more caudal levels of injury, greater recovery of motor function was observed. Lee and colleagues[14] reported individuals with low thoracic paraplegia (T10-12) demonstrated greater LE motor scores and higher 1-year Functional Independence Measure scores than those with high paraplegia (T2-9). Similar results were reported in a meta-analysis of studies, with the lowest rates of neurologic recovery in persons with complete thoracic SCI (10%) and the highest in lumbar SCI (35.3%).[33] Aimetti and colleagues[44] also observed that AIS conversion were related to level of injury with rates of 13.3% for T2-5, 16.0% for T6-9, and 29.3% for T10-12.

SENSORY INCOMPLETE, MOTOR COMPLETE (AMERICAN SPINAL INJURY ASSOCIATION IMPAIRMENT SCALE B) SPINAL CORD INJURY

Approximately 11% of initial SCI cases are classified as sensory incomplete but motor complete. Multiple studies report varying percentages of conversions: AIS B regressing to AIS A (10.0%–20.6%), AIS B staying AIS B (20.6%–35.7%), AIS B to AIS C (26.5%–35%), and AIS B to AIS D (21.4%–32.5%).[10,14,37] Kirshblum and colleagues[37] found that in individuals with AIS B injuries, those with sacral sparing with a combination of modalities light touch [LT], pin prick [PP], and DAP spared were more likely to gain motor recovery than with less modalities spared.

Crozier and colleagues[45] in a small study reported that PP sparing below the level of injury (not using the sacral sparing definition of a complete injury) at 72 hours had a positive prognostication for community ambulation. In a study using the sacral sparing definition, Oleson and colleagues[46] in analysis of data from the Sygen (GM-1 ganglioside) multicenter clinical trial, reported that although a higher percentage of subjects with sacral PP sparing (39.4% vs 28.3%) were ambulating at 26 weeks, the results did not reach significance. Walking outcomes available at 1 year also were not significantly different in subjects with and without initial PP sparing (53.6% vs 41.5%; $P = .31$). Therefore, although ambulation was improved for persons with PP preservation in the lowest sacral segments 4 weeks pos-, it was not based on S4-5 PP preservation at the 72-hour examination. Additionally, LE PP preservation in greater than 50% of LE dermatomes L2-S1, at 72 hours, was predictive of future ambulation.

MOTOR INCOMPLETE (AMERICAN SPINAL INJURY ASSOCIATION IMPAIRMENT SCALE C AND D) SPINAL CORD INJURY

The prognosis for persons with an initial motor incomplete injury for further neurologic recovery is greater than for those with a motor complete injury. The modality and extent of sacral sparing, however, may play a role. Kirshblum and colleagues[37] reported that at admission to inpatient rehabilitation, 44% of individuals admitted with a classification of AIS C remained AIS C and 52% improved to AIS D. Individuals with an initial AIS C with VAC as the only measure of motor function below the NLI had the poorest prognosis for improvement to AIS D (no patients progressed to AIS D at discharge from rehab or 1 year postinjury). In contrast, those individuals with an initial AIS classification with VAC, DAP, and either LT or PP at S4-5 progressed at 1 year to AIS D 60% to 67% of the time and those with VAC, DAP, LT, and PP at S4-5 progressed at 1 year to AIS D 87% of the time.

Although the specific NLI does not necessarily correlate with walking ability,[47,48] not surprisingly, those with incomplete paraplegia are more likely to achieve higher ambulatory rates at 1 year and 2 years postinjury than those with incomplete tetraplegia (76% vs 46%) and, in order to achieve comparable walking function, individuals with tetraplegia require greater LE motor scores compared with those with paraplegia.[7,8,48] For those with incomplete tetraplegia, motor recovery of the LEs is more favorable than motor recovery of upper extremities, and many individuals with both AIS C and AIS D SCI demonstrate residual upper extremity weakness that leaves them dependent on others for aspects of activities of daily living/self-care.[16]

DETERMINANTS OF WALKING AFTER SPINAL CORD INJURY

The overall rate of ambulation after SCI depends on the initial level and severity of the injury, the extent of LE motor function, and the age of the individual. Other common impairments include spasticity, balance, proprioception, and truncal control, with cognition also playing a role in walking.

In 1968, Stauffer[49] described ambulatory status in 4 categories: community ambulatory, household ambulatory, exercise ambulatory, and nonambulatory. Community ambulators were defined as those who are able to walk a "reasonable" distance (later estimated at >150 feet), in and out of the home without assistance from another person, who ambulate as their primary means of mobility in the community. Household ambulators are able to ambulate in the home with relative independence but are unable to ambulate outside of the home for any significant distance. Exercise ambulators are able to ambulate only under closely controlled conditions and attains functional mobility with a wheelchair. Nonambulators rely exclusively on a wheelchair for mobility.

In 1973, Hussey and Stauffer[50] reported that a reciprocal gait pattern could be utilized when there was pelvic control with at least 3/5 strength bilateral hip flexors and 1 quadriceps (knee extensor) with greater than or equal to 3/5 in at least 1 leg. This was not, however, a predictor of future recovery but rather described the strength required for ambulation. More recently, several clinical prediction rules have been described for predicting independence in walking at 1-year postinjury based on an examination within 15 days postinjury based on motor and sensory status.[51,52] van Middendorp and colleagues'[51] prediction rule is based on ability to walk independently indoors (Spinal Cord Independence Measure scores 4–8) based on 5 variables, including age (<65 years vs ≥65 years), L3 and S1 motor and LT scores. Hicks and colleagues'[52] prediction rule, "independent walking" was defined based on a Functional Independence Measure score of 6 or 7 based on 3 variables, including age at injury (<65 years vs ≥65 years), L3 motor score, and S1 dermatome LT sensory score. Phan and colleagues,[53] however, reported that these models were less accurate for persons with AIS B + C as opposed to AIS A + D. Recovery of ambulation is reportedly at approximately 5% of persons with complete paraplegia, 46% for incomplete tetraplegia, and 76% for incomplete paraplegia. There are several identifiable incomplete syndromes that may be seen with traumatic SCI, of which some have a favorable prognosis for ambulation. Central cord syndrome, believed to result from an injury that primarily affects the center of the spinal cord, and Brown-Sequard syndrome (BSS), classically described from a spinal hemisection, both have been reported as having a favorable outcome for ambulation.[54–57] The prognosis for functional recovery in acute traumatic central cord syndrome is less optimistic in older patients relative to younger patients,[16] with younger patients (less than 50 years old) more successful in becoming independent ambulators than older patients (97% vs 41%). These percentages are similar to other reports.[54,55] Roth and colleagues[56] reported 75% of individuals with BSS were ambulating independently at discharge from rehabilitation, and Bosch and colleagues[57] reported 100% of individuals with BSS were able to ambulate at discharge from rehabilitation.

ROLE OF IMAGING FOR PROGNOSIS AND FUNCTIONAL RECOVERY

Magnetic resonance imaging (MRI) intramedullary signal characteristics early (hours to days) after SCI provides important clinical information for predicting recovery SCI.[58–60] The patterns described most commonly include hemorrhage, edema, and no abnormal findings.[61,62] In some cases, the degree of compression as well as transection is used. The T2 sagittal images are considered the most useful for prognostic purposes.

Certain generalizations can be made based on these studies. Lack of MRI signal abnormality is associated with less severe grades of injury and the greatest amount of recovery. Patients with no abnormal signals almost always have incomplete injuries. Hemorrhage is seen more consistently with a neurologic complete injury based on physical examination, especially if exceeding a single segment[63–65] and associated with the least amount of neurologic recovery. Hemorrhage size/length has been associated with a more severe injury and poorer prognosis for neurologic recovery. The upper boundary of the anatomic location of the hemorrhage seems to best correspond to the NLI.[66]

The presence of spinal cord edema on MRI is associated more commonly with a neurologic incomplete injury on examination and an improved predictor of neurologic recovery. A greater extent of cord edema, however, is a predictor of a poorer neurologic recovery.[67] If edema involves multiple levels, there is a worse prognosis and greater chance of correlating with a complete lesion based on neurologic examination and if limited to single level or less than 3 segments, the injury tends to have a better prognosis and to be incomplete.

Although some studies have shown that spinal cord compression correlated with neurologic outcome in cervical SCI[68,69] and thoracolumbar SCI,[70] others did not.[71]

The recently described Brain and Spinal Injury Center (BASIC) classification for SCI strongly correlates with potential neurologic recovery after cervical and thoracolumbar injury. Talbott and colleagues[72] developed a 5-point ordinal BASIC score system on MRI based on the extent of axial T2-weighted images: 0—no signal abnormality; 1—T2 hyperintensity confined to central gray matter; 2—T2 hyperintensity extends beyond gray matter, margins to involve spinal white matter but does not involve entire transverse extent of the spinal cord; 3—T2 hyperintensity involves entire transverse extent of spinal cord; and 4—grade 3 plus T2 hypointense consistent with macrohemorrhage. They found a strong correlation between BASIC score and admission AIS grades and AIS conversion rates prior to discharge (range 4–128 days, performed at the time of discharge from the acute care hospital).[72] They demonstrated that patients with BASIC score of 2 experienced better recovery than those with a BASIC score of 3, with 88% of BASIC score 2 patients achieving an AIS C or D classification and no AIS A classification at discharge whereas 67% of BASIC score 3 patients discharged with AIS A or B classifications. All of the patients with BASIC score of 4 discharged with classifications of AIS A.[72] Farhadi and colleagues[73] studied multiple radiological findings and concluded that BASIC score is the best predictor of both neurologic severity and AIS conversion.

DISCUSSING PROGNOSIS

Discussing prognosis for recovery after an SCI, especially for a neurologically complete injury, is a difficult task for the spinal cord medicine specialist. If delivered poorly, families and patients may experience confusion, long lasting distress, and resentment; if done well, families and patients may find comfort through understanding, adjusting, and accepting their situation.[74]

The 4 ethical principles that guide prognosis discussions include respecting autonomy, which encompasses the concepts of disclosure and informed consent; beneficence, providing the best care for patients; nonmaleficence, obligation to do no harm; and justice, the principle of social obligation that encompasses being fair.[75] These ethical principles in conjunction with person-centered care (eg, patient values and psychosocial issues) can result in positive results, such as increased engagement in rehabilitation.[76–78]

Kirshblum and colleagues[79] reported findings from their study on when, by whom, and in what setting individuals with neurologically complete SCI wanted to hear of their prognosis. A majority of patients surveyed indicated they wanted to know their prognosis early after injury and to hear the information by the physician in a clear and sensitive manner.[79]

Although there may be no ideal method of breaking the news, and differences in approach is appropriate based on setting, patient background, education, culture, age, and life situations, certain recommendations to facilitate communication have been made.[74,79,80] These include that an experienced clinician in SCI should lead the conversation; utilizing a trained health interpreter if a language barriers exist (not a patient family member); sitting close to the patient, speaking slowly, deliberately, and clearly; providing information in simple language and honestly; providing information in small doses (at a pace the patient can follow); using eye contact and body language to convey warmth, sympathy, encouragement, and/or reassurance to the patient; discussing treatment options; avoiding the notion "that nothing can be done"; and providing information about support services.

CASE REVIEW

Looking back to the 2 cases presented initially, for the first case, where it appears that in a relative short period of time, John Doe initially had a sensory incomplete injury, followed by fairly rapid onset of motor recovery, given his age and trajectory of recovery, his likelihood of walking is favorable. Depending on the recovery of his upper extremities, however, he may have to look into some adaptive equipment, assistive technology, or accommodations for him to be able to return to college, take notes, complete assignments, and take tests. Driving also is not necessarily out of the question, but depending on his upper extremity strength/dexterity, he may require the use of some adaptive equipment to drive safely.

Regarding Jane Doe in case 2, she has a higher paraplegia and is over 65 years of age. She has some factors that are associated with poorer prognosis/recovery, but she should be able to achieve a fair amount of functional independence in light of her upper extremity strength. It also may be helpful to discuss varying levels of walking (community vs household vs exercise) and that, as she progresses with her rehabilitation program, she may be able to work on walking in therapy.

SUMMARY

The ability to predict outcome after SCI is extremely important not only for individuals who sustained a traumatic SCI and their families but also for the rehabilitation professionals charged with developing an appropriate plan of care and the researchers investigating the role of natural recovery in future therapeutic investigations.

DISCLOSURE

The authors have nothing to disclose.

REFERENCES

1. American Spinal Injury Association. International standards for neurological classification of spinal cord injury. Richmond (VA): ASIA; 2019.
2. Kirshblum SC, O'Connor KC. Levels of spinal cord injury and predictors of neurologic recovery. Phys Med Rehabil Clin N Am 2000;11(1):1–27.
3. Burns AS, Lee BS, Ditunno JF, et al. Patient selection for clinical trials: the reliability of the early spinal cord injury examination. J Neurotrauma 2003;20:477–82.
4. Brown PJ, Marino RJ, Herbison GJ, et al. The 72-hour examination as a predictor of recovery in motor complete quadriplegia. Arch Phys Med Rehabil 1991;72:546–8.
5. Waters RL, Yakura JS, Adkins RH, et al. Motor and sensory recovery following complete tetraplegia. Arch Phys Med Rehabil 1993;74:242–7.
6. Waters RL, Yakura JS, Adkins RH, et al. Recovery following complete paraplegia. Arch Phys Med Rehabil 1992;73:784–9.
7. Waters RL, Adkins RH, Yakura JS, et al. Motor and sensory recovery following incomplete tetraplegia. Arch Phys Med Rehabil 1994;75:306–11.
8. Waters RL, Adkins RH, Yakura JS, et al. Motor and sensory recovery following incomplete paraplegia. Arch Phys Med Rehabil 1994;75:67–72.
9. Marino RJ, Burns S, Graves DE, et al. Upper- and lower-extremity motor recovery after traumatic cervical spinal cord injury: an update from the National Spinal Cord Injury Database. Arch Phys Med Rehabil 2011;92:369–75.
10. Spiess MR, Mueller RM, Rupp R, et al. Conversion in ASIA Impairment Scale during the first year after traumatic spinal cord injury. J Neurotrauma 2009;26:2027–36.
11. Steeves JD, Kramer JK, Fawcett JW, et al. Extent of spontaneous motor recovery after traumatic cervical sensorimotor complete spinal cord injury. Spinal Cord 2011;49(2):257–65.
12. Zariffa J, Kramer JL, Fawcett JW, et al. Characterization of neurological recovery following traumatic sensorimotor complete thoracic spinal cord injury. Spinal Cord 2011;49:463–547.
13. Wilson JR, Davis AM, Kulkarni AV, et al. Defining age-related differences in outcome after traumatic spinal cord injury: analysis of a combined, multicenter dataset. Spine J 2014;14(7):1192–8.
14. Lee BA, Leiby BE, Marino RJ. Neurological and functional recovery after thoracic spinal cord injury. J Spinal Cord Med 2016;39(1):67–76.
15. Oleson CV, Marino RJ, Leiby BE, et al. Influence of age alone, and age combined with pinprick, on recovery of walking function in motor complete, sensory incomplete spinal cord injury. Arch Phys Med Rehabil 2016;97:1635–41.
16. Penrod LE, Hegde SK, Ditunno JF Jr. Age effect on prognosis for functional recovery in acute, traumatic central cord syndrome. Arch Phys Med Rehabil 1990;71(12):963–8.
17. Burns SP, Golding DG, Rolle WA, et al. Recovery of ambulation in motor-incompelte tetraplegia. Arch Phys Med Rehabil 1997;78:1169–72.

18. Fehlings MG, Vaccaro A, Wilson JR, et al. Early versus delayed decompression for traumatic cervical spinal cord injury: results of the Surgical Timing in Acute Spinal Cord Injury Study (STASCIS). PLoS One 2012;7:e32037.

19. van Middendorp JJ. Letter to the editor regarding: "Early versus delayed decompression for traumatic cervical spinal cord injury: results of the Surgical Timing in Acute Spinal Cord Injury Study (STASCIS)". Spine J 2012;12:540 [author reply: 1-2].

20. Wilson JR, Singh A, Craven C, et al. Early versus late surgery for traumatic spinal cord injury: the results of a prospective Canadian cohort study. Spinal Cord 2012; 50:840–3.

21. Dvorak MF, Noonan VK, Fallah N, et al. The influence of time from injury to surgery on motor recovery and length of hospital stay in acute traumatic spinal cord injury: an observational Canadian cohort study. J Neurotrauma 2015;32:645–54.

22. Bourassa-Moreau E, Mac-Thiong JM, Li A, et al. Do patients with complete spinal cord injury benefit from early surgical decompression? Analysis of neurological improvement in a prospective cohort study. J Neurotrauma 2016;33:301–6.

23. Ter Wengel PV, Martin E, De Witt Hamer PC, et al. Impact of early (<24 h) surgical decompression on neurological recovery in thoracic spinal cord injury: a meta-analysis. J Neurotrauma 2019;36(18):2609–17.

24. Wilson JR, Tetreault LA, Kwon BK, et al. Timing of decompression in patients with acute spinal cord injury: a systematic review. Glob Spine J 2017;7(3_suppl): 95S–115S.

25. Ter Wengel PV, De Witt Hamer PC, Pauptit JC, et al. Early surgical decompression improves neurological outcome after complete traumatic cervical spinal cord injury: a meta-analysis. J Neurotrauma 2019;36(6):835–44.

26. Lee DY, Park YJ, Kim HJ, et al. Early surgical decompression within 8 hours for traumatic spinal cord injury: Is it beneficial? A meta-analysis. Acta Orthop Traumatol Turc 2018;52(2):101–8.

27. Grassner L, Wutte C, Klein B, et al. Early decompression (< 8 h) after traumatic cervical spinal cord injury improves functional outcome as assessed by spinal cord independence measure after one year. J Neurotrauma 2016;33(18): 1658–66.

28. Wutte C, Becker J, Klein B, et al. Early decompression (< 8 hours) improves the functional bladder outcome and mobility after traumatic thoracic spinal cord injury. World Neurosurg 2020;134:e847–54.

29. Burke JF, Yue JK, Ngwenya LB, et al. Ultra-early (<12 Hours) surgery correlates with higher rate of American Spinal Injury Association impairment scale conversion after cervical spinal cord injury. Neurosurgery 2019;85(2):199–203.

30. Aarabi B, Akhtar-Danesh N, Chryssikos T, et al. Efficacy of ultra-early (< 12 h), early (12-24 h), and late (>24-138.5 h) surgery with magnetic resonance imaging-confirmed decompression in American Spinal Injury Association impairment scale grades A, B, and C cervical spinal cord injury. J Neurotrauma 2019. https://doi.org/10.1089/neu.2019.6606.

31. Biglari B, Child C, Yildirim TM, et al. Does surgical treatment within 4 hours after trauma have an influence on neurological remission in patients with acute spinal cord injury? Ther Clin Risk Manag 2016;12:1339–46.

32. Mattiassich G, Gollwitzer M, Gaderer F, et al. Functional outcomes in individuals undergoing very early (< 5 h) and early (5-24 h) surgical decompression in traumatic cervical spinal cord injury: analysis of neurological improvement from the Austrian Spinal Cord Injury Study. J Neurotrauma 2017;34(24):3362–71.

33. Khorasanizadeh M, Yousefifard M, Eskian M, et al. Neurological recovery following traumatic spinal cord injury: a systematic review and meta-analysis. J Neurosurg Spine 2019;30:683–99.
34. Kirshblum S, Millis S, McKinley W, et al. Late recovery after traumatic spinal cord injury. Arch Phys Med Rehabil 2004;85:1811–7.
35. Marino RJ, Ditunno JF, Donovan WH, et al. Neurologic recovery after traumatic spinal cord injury: Data from model spinal cord injury systems. Arch Phys Med Rehabil 1999;80:1391–6.
36. Fawcett JW, Curt LA, Steeves JD, et al. Guidelines for the conduct of clinical trials for spinal cord injury as developed by the ICCP panel: Spontaneous recovery after spinal cord injury and statistical power needed for therapeutic clinical trials. Spinal Cord 2007;45:190–205.
37. Kirshblum SC, Botticello AL, Dyson-Hudson TA, et al. Patterns of sacral sparing components on neurological recovery in newly injured persons with traumatic spinal cord injury. Arch Phys Med Rehabil 2016;97(10):1647–55.
38. Marino RJ, Schmidt-Read M, Kirshblum SC, et al. Reliability and validity of S3 pressure sensation as an alternative to deep anal pressure in neurologic classification of persons with spinal cord injury. Arch Phys Med Rehabil 2016;97(10): 1642–6.
39. El Teche NE, Dahdaleh NS, Bydon M, et al. The natural history of complete spinal cord injury: a pooled analysis of 1162 patients and a meta-analysis of modern data. J Neurosurg Spine 2018;28:436–43.
40. Marino R, Leff M, Cardenas D, et al. Trends in rates of ASIA Impairment Scale conversion in traumatic spinal cord injury. Poster Presentation at ASIA 45th Annual Scientific Meeting. Waikiki, HI; April 4, 2019. Top Spinal Cord Inj Rehabil 2019; 25(S1):126–7.
41. Ditunno JF, Cohen ME, Hauck WW, et al. Recovery of upper-extremity strength in complete and incomplete tetraplegia: a multicenter study. Arch Phys Med Rehabil 2000;81:389–93.
42. Fischer CG, Noonan VK, Smith DE, et al. Motor recovery, functional status, and health related quality of life in patients with complete spinal cord injuries. Spine 2005;30:2200–7.
43. Ditunno JF, Stover SL, Freed MM, et al. Motor recovery of the upper extremities in traumatic quadriplegia: a multicenter study. Arch Phys Med Rehabil 1992;73: 431–6.
44. Aimetti AA, Kirshblum S, Curt A, et al. Natural history of neurological improvement following complete (AIS A) thoracic spinal cord injury across three registries to guide acute clinical trial design and interpretation. Spinal Cord 2019;57(9): 753–62.
45. Crozier KS, Graziani V, Ditunno JF, et al. Spinal cord injury: prognosis for ambulation based on sensory examination in patients who are initially motor complete. Arch Phys Med Rehabil 1991;72:119–21.
46. Oleson CV, Burns AS, Ditunno JF, et al. Prognostic value of pinprick preservation in motor complete, sensory incomplete spinal cord injury. Arch Phys Med Rehabil 2005;86:988–92.
47. Kay ED, Deutsch A, Wuermser LA. Predicting walking at discharge from inpatient rehabilitation after a traumatic spinal cord injury. Arch Phys Med Rehabil 2008;88: 745–50.
48. Wirz M, van Hedel HJ, Rupp R, et al. Muscle force and gait performance: relationships after spinal cord injury. Arch Phys Med Rehabil 2006;87:1218–22.
49. Stauffer ES. Study of 100 paraplegics. Rancho Los Amigos Papers; 1968.

50. Hussey RW, Stauffer ES. Spinal cord injury: requirements for ambulation. Arch Phys Med Rehabil 1973;54:544–7.

51. Van Middendorp JJ, Hosman AJ, Donders ART, et al. A clinical prediction rule for ambulation outcomes after traumatic spinal cord injury: a longitudinal cohort study. Lancet 2011;377(9770):1004–10.

52. Hicks KE, Zhao Y, Fallah N, et al. A simplified clinical prediction rule for prognosticating independent walking after spinal cord injury: a prospective study from a Canadian multicenter spinal cord injury registry. Spine J 2017;17(10):1383–92.

53. Phan P, Budhram B, Zhang Q, et al. Highlighting discrepancies in walking prediction accuracy for patients with traumatic spinal cord injury: an evaluation of validated prediction models using a Canadian Multicenter Spinal Cord Injury Registry. Spine J 2019;19(4):703–10.

54. Merriam WF, Taylor TKF, Ruff SJ, et al. A reappraisal of acute traumatic central cord syndrome. J Bone Joint Surg Am 1986;68(5):708–13.

55. Foo D. Spinal cord injury in fort-four patients with cervical spondylosis. Paraplegia 1986;24:301–6.

56. Roth EJ, Park T, Pang T, et al. Traumatic cervical Brown-Sequard and Brown-Sequard plus syndromes: the spectrum of presentations and outcomes. Paraplegia 1991;29:582–9.

57. Bosch A, Stauffer ES, Nickel VL. Incomplete traumatic quadriplegia. A ten-year review. JAMA 1971;216(3):473–8.

58. Takahashi M, Harada Y, Inoue H, et al. Traumatic cervical cord injury at C3-4 without radiographic abnormalities: correlation of magnetic resonance findings with clinical features and outcome. J Orthop Surg 2002;10(2):129–35.

59. Bozzo A, Marcoux J, Radhakrishna M, et al. The role of magnetic resonance imaging in the management of acute spinal cord injury. J Neurotrauma 2010;28(8):1401–11.

60. Silberstein M, Tress BM, Hennessy O. Prediction of neurologic outcome in acute spinal cord injury: the role of CT and MR. AJNR Am J Neuroradiol 1992;13(6):1597–608.

61. Bondurant FJ, Cotler HB, Kulkarni MV, et al. Acute spinal cord injury. A study using physical examination and magnetic resonance imaging. Spine (Phila Pa 1976) 1990;15(3):161–8.

62. Andreoli C, Colaiacomo MC, Rojas Beccaglia M, et al. MRI in the acute phase of spinal cord traumatic lesions: Relationship between MRI findings and neurological outcome. Radiol Med 2005;110(5–6):636–45.

63. Flanders AE, Schaefer DM, Doan HT, et al. Acute cervical spine trauma: correlation of MR imaging findings with degree of neurologic deficit. Radiology 1990;177(1):25–33.

64. Miyanji F, Furlan JC, Aarabi B, et al. Acute cervical traumatic spinal cord injury: MR imaging findings correlated with neurologic outcome–prospective study with 100 consecutive patients. Radiology 2007;243(3):820–7.

65. Le E, Aarabi B, Hersh DS, et al. Predictors of intramedullary lesion expansion rate on MR images of patients with subaxial spinal cord injury. J Neurosurg Spine 2015;22(6):611–21.

66. Zohrabian VM, Parker L, Harrop JS, et al. Can anatomic level of injury on MRI predict neurological level in acute cervical spinal cord injury? Br J Neurosurg 2016;30(2):204–10.

67. Martinez-Perez R, Cepeda S, Paredes I, et al. MRI prognostication factors in the setting of cervical spinal cord injury secondary to trauma. World Neurosurg 2017;101:623–32.

68. Wilson JR, Grossman RG, Frankowski RF, et al. A clinical prediction model for long-term functional outcome after traumatic spinal cord injury based on acute clinical and imaging factors. J Neurotrauma 2012;29(13):2263–71.
69. Haefeli J, Mabray MC, Whetstone WD, et al. Multivariate analysis of MRI biomarkers for predicting neurologic impairment in cervical spinal cord injury. AJNR Am J Neuroradiol 2017;38(3):648–55.
70. Skeers P, Battistuzzo CR, Clark JM, et al. Acute thoracolumbar spinal cord injury: relationship of cord compression to neurological outcome. J Bone Joint Surg Am 2018;100(4):305–15.
71. Mabray MC, Talbott JF, Whetstone WD, et al. Multidimensional analysis of magnetic resonance imaging predicts early impairment in thoracic and thoracolumbar spinal cord injury. J Neurotrauma 2016;33(10):954–62.
72. Talbott JF, Whetstone WD, Readdy WJ, et al. The Brain and Spinal Injury Center score: a novel, simple, and reproducible method for assessing the severity of acute cervical spinal cord injury with axial T2-weighted MRI findings. J Neurosurg Spine 2015;23(4):495–504.
73. Farhadi HF, Kukreja S, Minnema A, et al. Impact of admission imaging findings on neurological outcomes in acute cervical traumatic spinal cord injury. J Neurotrauma 2018;35(12):1398–406.
74. Kirshblum S, Fichtenbaum J. Breaking the news in spinal cord injury. J Spinal Cord Med 2008;31(1):7–12.
75. Post LF, Blustein J, Dubler NN. Handbook for health care ethics committees. Baltimore (MD): John Hopkins University Press; 2007. p. 15.
76. Heinemann AW, Sherri LL, Etinger B, et al. Perceptions of person-centered care following spinal cord injury. Arch Phys Med Rehabil 2016;97:1338–44.
77. Kogan AC, Wilber K, Mosqueda L. Person-centered care for older adults with chronic conditions and functional impairment: A systematic literature review. J Am Geriatr Soc 2016;64:e1–7.
78. Papadimitriou C, Carpenter C. Client-centered practice in Spinal Cord injury rehabilitation: a field guide. CARF International; 2013. Available at: http://www.carf.org/ClientCenteredPracticeinSCIRehab/.
79. Kirshblum S, Botticello A, Benaquista DeSipio G, et al. Breaking the news: a pilot study on patient perspectives of discussing prognosis after traumatic spinal cord injury. J Spinal Cord Med 2016;39(2):155–6.
80. Donovan J, Kirshblum S, Didesch M, et al. Spinal cord rehabilitation. In: Kirshblum S, Lin V, editors. Spinal cord medicine. 2019. p. 688–706.

Cognitive Dysfunction in Persons with Chronic Spinal Cord Injuries

Donald F. Distel, MD[a], Matthew Amodeo, MD[a], Shawn Joshi, BS[b], Benjamin A. Abramoff, MD, MS[a],*

KEYWORDS

- Cognitive dysfunction • Spinal cord injury • Cognitive impairment
- Neuroinflammation • Cortical reorganization • Rehabilitation

KEY POINTS

- Cognitive dysfunction (CD) is pervasive in individuals with spinal cord injury (SCI) from the acute to chronic stages.
- There are many proposed causes for the development of CD in those with SCI, although traumatic brain injuries likely contribute.
- Individuals with SCI should be routinely screened for CD, particularly if they are having difficulty with progressing in rehabilitation or community functioning.
- Treatment strategies explicitly focused toward individuals with CD may be needed to optimize rehabilitation and functional outcome.

INTRODUCTION

Since the initial descriptions of spinal cord injury (SCI) dating back to antiquity, SCIs have been known to have profound effects on the relationship between the mind and the body.[1] What has become clear only over the last century is the profound effect SCIs have on the mind itself, with cognitive dysfunction (CD) occurring in a large subset (and potentially the majority) of individuals with SCIs. This article reviews some potential causes, consequences, and management of CD in individuals with SCI.

COGNITIVE DYSFUNCTION IN INDIVIDUALS WITH CHRONIC SPINAL CORD INJURY

Although it had been established since the 1960s that acute SCI was associated with traumatic brain injuries (TBIs) and CD in the acute phases, the focus of CD in individuals with chronic SCI started to emerge in the 1990s.[2] In 1995, Dowler and colleagues[3]

[a] Department of Physical Medicine and Rehabilitation, University of Pennsylvania–Perelman School of Medicine, 1800 Lombard Street, Philadelphia, PA 19146, USA; [b] Drexel School of Medicine, 2900 W. Queen Lane, Philadelphia, PA 19129, USA
* Corresponding author.
E-mail address: Benjamin.Abramoff@pennmedicine.upenn.edu

Phys Med Rehabil Clin N Am 31 (2020) 345–368
https://doi.org/10.1016/j.pmr.2020.04.001
1047-9651/20/© 2020 Elsevier Inc. All rights reserved.

completed one of the first studies looking specifically at rates of CD in individuals with chronic SCIs (averaging 17 years after injury). Their findings were dramatic, with 41% of individuals with SCI showing significant delays in processing speed in comparison to matched controls. There were no delays noted in memory, visuospatial skills, and attention/executive functioning.

This finding was followed by another study by Dowler and colleagues[4] that demonstrated 6 distinct profiles (groups 1–6 in later discussion) of cognitive performance in individuals with chronic SCI (**Fig. 1**). Group 1 was found to demonstrate normal cognitive functioning, and group 2 demonstrated mild deficits in memory, which were not thought to be clinically meaningful. The remaining 4 groups (60% of those tested) demonstrated significant deficits in one or more cognitive domains. Group 3 demonstrated deficits in attention and processing speed. Group 4 had limited processing speed. Group 5 only had deficits in cognitive flexibility. Finally, group 6 showed significant decreased memory performance. Overall, these impaired cognitive profiles were thought to be due to a history of concomitant TBI at the time of the individual sustaining their SCI.

Tun and colleagues[5] investigated age-related differences in cognitive function in individuals with chronic SCI (**Fig. 2**). Their study demonstrated impaired memory (short term, working, and prose recall) in elderly individuals, which was attributed to age-related differences. Interestingly, there was no relationship found between the degree of CD and duration nor the level of SCI. Individuals also generally felt comfortable with their own cognitive performance. Of note, this study did not compare the populations to a control group without SCIs.

Moving into the twenty-first century, Gordon and colleagues[6] evaluated self-reported symptoms of CD in individuals with SCI who were, on average, 7 years after injury. Individuals with SCI self-reported an average of 4.2 ongoing cognitive symptoms compared with 2.0 symptoms in control subjects.

Recently, Cohen and colleagues[7] completed a matched study looking at cognitive function in 156 individuals with SCI at least 1 year after injury compared with 156 individuals without SCI. Their study used a standardized, National Institutes of Health (NIH) toolbox cognitive battery and high-quality normative data. They found significantly worse performance in those with SCI in fluid composite scores (a measure of executive function), psychomotor speed, and episodic memory (**Table 1**).

Unlike most previous studies,[8] which did not demonstrate differences by level of SCI, Cohen and colleagues[7] found that fluid composite scores were significantly worse in individuals with tetraplegia compared with individuals with paraplegia. They also found that the scores of crystallized cognition composite (a measure of past learning experiences) were similar, which suggested similar premorbid functioning (**Table 2**).

Craig and colleagues[9] recently investigated cognition in 150 individuals with SCI who were a mean of 3.4 years after injury and compared them to 45 controls. Using the neuropsychiatry unit cognitive assessment tool (NUCOG), they found that individuals with SCI had significantly worse cognitive function across a wide range of domains, including attention, visoconstructional skills, memory, executive functioning, and language. Of individuals, 28.6% were 1 standard deviation (SD) below the NUCOG norm score and classified as cognitively impaired, whereas 16.6% were 2 SD below, suggesting more severe impairment. It was calculated that the odds of cognitive impairment was 17.7 times greater for someone with SCI compared with controls (and relative risk 12.9 times greater). No differences again were noted based on level of injury (or sex). Interestingly, individuals with SCI who scored within the normal range (which represented most of the sample) did not score significantly worse than individuals without SCI who scored within the normal range.

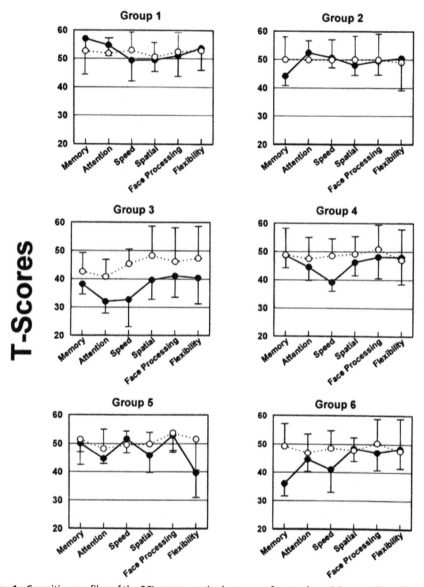

Fig. 1. Cognitive profiles of the SCI groups and subgroups of control participants. The 6 figures display the means (standard deviations) for each cognitive domain. Closed circles designate the means for each of the 6 SCI groups, which were derived from the cluster analysis. Open circles designate the means for subgroups of control participants who were of similar age and premorbid level of functioning related to their respective SCI group. (*From* Dowler RN, Harrington DL, Haaland KY, et al. Profiles of cognitive functioning in chronic spinal cord injury and the role of moderating variables. J Int Neuropsychol Soc. 1997;3(5):464–72; with permission.)

In their systematic review of CD at all stages following SCI, Sachdeva and colleagues[8] found that significant impairment was found in 38 of 70 studies that reported cognitive functioning after SCI (at all stages). In controlled studies, 15 of 21 showed significant CD in individuals with SCI (as opposed to 23 of 49 in noncontrolled studies).

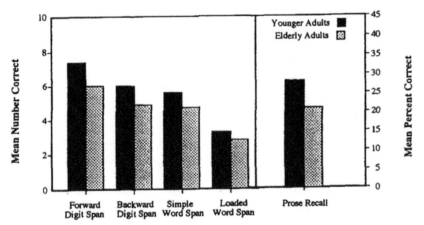

Fig. 2. Cognitive performance in young and elderly adults with chronic SCI. (*From* Tun CG, Tun PA, Wingfield A. Cognitive function following long-term spinal cord injury. Rehabil Psychol. 1997;42(3):163–82; with permission.)

These studies strongly suggest a relationship between CD and chronic SCIs. It is important to investigate potential causes of this relationship in order to better prevent and treat this potential complication of SCI.

PROPOSED MECHANISMS OF COGNITIVE DYSFUNCTION IN INDIVIDUALS WITH SPINAL CORD INJURY

This section will review some of the proposed mechanisms that lead to cognitive dysfunction in individuals with SCI (**Box 1**).

Traumatic Brain Injury

Before the recognition of CD in chronic SCI, it was well appreciated that there were significant associations between having an SCI and a TBI, particularly in the acute and subacute stages. Guttmann[10] noted that among 396 patients with acute traumatic paraplegia/tetraplegia, seven died of associated head injuries. Harris[11] found that among 114 cervical SCI, 31 had initially suffered serious injuries to the head or face, noting, "head injury is the commonest severe associated injury with a cervical cord lesion."

Wilmot and colleagues[12] performed one of the first studies using objective cognitive testing in individuals with acute and subacute SCIs. Their study noted that, despite cognitive impairment being common following SCI (64% of patients tested), these were often missed. The investigators suspected that CD owing to TBI at the time of injury was present in approximately 36% of patients.

Davidoff and colleagues[13] used the Halstead Categorical Test to evaluate cognition in patients in rehabilitation for SCIs. They found that 57% of their subjects, 8 to 12 weeks from obtaining their SCI, had evidence of higher-level CD. This CD was thought likely to be due to closed head injury. The investigators of this study also took the additional step of suggesting that unrecognized closed head injuries could lead to loss of ability to learn new skills and ultimately impede rehabilitation. At this point, the long-term effects of TBI on cognition in those with SCI had not been addressed.

Table 1
Comparison of National Institutes of Health toolbox cognitive battery results between individuals with chronic SCI and age-matched controls

Score	SCI Mean (SD)	Control Mean (SD)	F	P	d	% <1 SD SCI	% <1 SD Control	% <2 SD SCI	% <2 SD Control
Composite scores									
Fluid	46.3 (8.6)	50.8(10.0)	17.45	<.001	0.50	25.0	15.4	4.5	1.9
Crystallized	50.7 (10.1)	50.8 (9.7)	0.01	.92	0.01	15.4	12.8	0.0	0.6
Subtest scores									
Picture vocabulary	51.3 (10.2)	50.4 (9.6)	0.56	.45	0.09	16.0	13.5	1.3	1.9
Oral reading recognition	50.1 (10.2)	51.2(10.3)	0.96	.34	0.11	16.0	14.8	0.6	1.3
Picture sequence memory	47.4 (9.5)	50.5(10.1)	7.35	<.01	0.32	21.8	15.5	3.2	0.6
Pattern comparison	48.6 (8.4)	51.4 (9.7)	7.14	<.01	0.31	14.1	11.0	1.3	1.3
List sorting	49.5 (9.3)	50.7(10.0)	1.33	.25	0.12	13.5	18.1	1.9	1.9
Flanker	46.4 (9.2)	50.2 (9.7)	12.91	<.001	0.40	24.4	16.1	4.5	2.6
Dimensional change card sort	46.5 (9.1)	50.6 (9.5)	15.00	<.001	0.44	26.3	10.3	1.9	3.2

Note. % < x SD indicates the percentage of each group that produced scores below x SD ($T < 40$) of the entire NIHTB-CB normative sample.
Abbreviation: NIHTB-CB, National Institutes of Health toolbox cognitive battery.
Cohen ML, Tulsky DS, Holdnack JA, et al. Cognition among community-dwelling individuals with spinal cord injury. Rehabil Psychol. 2017;62(4):425–34; with permission.

Table 2
Comparison of National Institutes of Health toolbox cognitive battery results between individuals with individuals with paraplegia and tetraplegia

Variables	Tetra (n = 64)	Para (n = 92)	F	P	d
Composite scores					
Fluid	43.0 (8.8)	48.6 (7.8)	17.3	<.001	0.67
Crystallized	51.9(10.0)	50.5(10.2)	0.1	.78	0.14
Subtest scores					
Picture vocabulary	51.2(10.0)	51.3(10.4)	<0.01	.95	0.01
Oral reading recognition	50.7 (10.4)	49.7(10.1)	0.36	.55	0.09
Picture sequence memory	47.0(10.6)	47.8 (8.6)	0.26	.61	0.08
Pattern comparison	45.5 (7.8)	50.8(8.1)	16.53	<.001	0.67
List sorting	49.3(10.1)	49.6 (8.7)	0.04	.85	0.03
Flanker	42.3 (8.9)	49.2 (8.4)	24.15	<.001	0.80
Dimensional change card sorting	43.6 (8.9)	48.5 (8.8)	11.61	<.01	0.55

Cohen ML, Tulsky DS, Holdnack JA, et al. Cognition among community-dwelling individuals with spinal cord injury. Rehabil Psychol. 2017;62(4):425–34; with permission.

Richards and colleagues[14] expanded upon previous studies by longitudinally investigating cognitive deficits in 150 patients with SCI. Their subjects completed a battery of neuropsychological testing on average 7 weeks and 38 weeks after their SCIs. They found that over time, neuropsychological performance did improve, with a pattern thought to be consistent with mild to moderate TBI. Therefore, many of these SCI patients were hypothesized to have concomitant TBI and needed to have rehabilitation modalities directed toward both TBI and SCI.

Roth and colleagues[15] performed cognitive testing in 81 individuals with acute SCI matched with 61 noninjured controls. Their study found that 44% of the individuals with SCI had some interval of posttraumatic amnesia. They found significantly more cognitive abnormalities in the individuals with SCI among a wide variety of domains representing impairment in concentration/attention, initial learning, and poor problem solving (**Fig. 3**). This study is also one of the earliest to bring attention to other possible causes of CD, including mood disorders and substance abuse.

Since these early studies, rates of reporting the coexistence of TBI and SCI have been corroborated in numerous studies, with between 16% and 74% of individuals with traumatic SCI having concomitant TBI (mild 30%–44%, moderate 10%–11%, or severe 5%–10%).[16–21] In contrast, in a cohort of individuals with chronic SCI, Craig and colleagues[9] did not find an association between concomitant TBI and reduced cognitive performance.

Unfortunately, TBI is often underdiagnosed in patients with SCI, indicating the need for more consistent evaluation.[13,22] A study by Sharma and colleagues[20] found that 58.5% of individuals with traumatic SCI had a missed diagnosis of TBI. Missed diagnosis of TBI was more likely to occur outside of motor vehicle accidents (75.0% missed in individuals not involved in motor vehicle accidents vs. 42.9% missed in individuals involved in motor vehicle accidents).

It should also be noted that history of previous TBI can lead to impulsivity, risk-taking behavior, and CD.[23] These factors increase one's risk of obtaining an SCI. More research is needed to investigate if prior history of TBI, in addition to concomitant TBI, may be contributing to CD in the chronic phase of SCI.

Box 1
Potential causes of cognitive dysfunction in individuals with spinal cord injury

Traumatic brain injury
   Premorbid neuropsychological conditions
- Attention-deficit/hyperactivity disorder
- Impulsivity/risk taking
- Personality type
- Learning disabilities

Mood and psychiatric disorders

Substance abuse
   Polypharmacy
- Benzodiazepines and nonbenzodiazepine hypnotic
- Baclofen
- Opioids
- Antipsychotics
- Antiepileptics (calcium channel alpha 2-delta ligands)
- Anticholinergics

Chronic pain

Chronic fatigue

Chronic respiratory changes

Sleep-disordered breathing
   Autonomic dysregulation
- Hypotension
- Autonomic dysreflexia
- Metabolic syndrome

Postintensive care syndrome

Cortical reorganization

Neuroinflammation

Combination of factors

Premorbid Neuropsychological Conditions

Another potential mechanism for the CD noted in individuals with chronic SCI is a history of premorbid neuropsychological conditions. These factors may be associated with CD (and possibly have led their initial SCI).

Attention-Deficit/Hyperactivity Disorder

Multiple retrospective studies have identified psychiatric illnesses such as attention-deficit disorder/attention-deficit/hyperactivity disorder (ADHD) as predisposing adolescents to bodily injury including SCI.[24] Merrill and colleagues[25] found the rate of "severe injury" (fracture of skull, neck, and trunk; intracranial injury; and injuries to nerves and spinal cord) to be 3 times higher in a population with ADHD when compared with a population without ADHD. Although these studies were not sufficiently powered to provide data on SCI specifically, they both included SCI in their outcomes.

Impulsivity/Risk Taking Behavior

Mawson and colleagues[26] attempted to draw direct associations between sensation-seeking, criminality, and SCI, and matched 140 patients with SCI to a similar

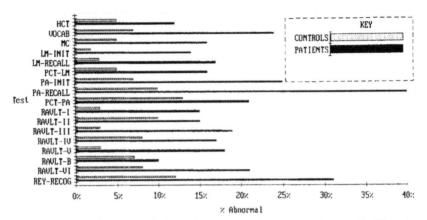

Fig. 3. Comparison of neuropsychological test results between patients with SCI and controls. HCT, Halstead Category Test; LM, Logical Memory Subtest of the WMS Russell Adaptation (has Initial (INIT) and 30-minute Recall (RECALL) trials; MC, Mental Control Subtest (MC) of the Wechsler Memory Scale; PA, Paired Association Subtest of the WMS Russell Adaptation (has Initial (INIT) and 30-minute Recall (RECALL) trials; PCT-LM, Percent retention of stored information for the LM; PCT-PA, Percent retention of stored information for the PA; RAVLT, Rey Auditory Verbal Learning Test (this test is made up of eight trials, I, II, III, IV, V, interference (B), and recognition (Recog); VOCAB, Vocabulary Subtest of the Wechsler Adult Intelligence Scale-Revised. (*From* Roth E, Davidoff G, Thomas P, et al. A controlled study of neuropsychological deficits in acute spinal cord injury patients. Paraplegia. 1989;27(6):480–9; with permission.)

population without SCI. They found that those with SCI were significantly more likely to have criminal history, disinhibition, boredom susceptibility, and sensation seeking than matched controls before their SCI. Both criminality and sensation seeking were suggested as independent and statistically significant predictors of SCI.

Personality Type

Personality type may also be related to sustaining an SCI. A previous study performed the NEO Five-Factor Inventory (a description of the "Big Five" personality types: neuroticism, extraversion, openness, agreeableness, and conscientiousness). This study found that, in comparison to community adult samples, patients with SCI had significantly lower levels of resilient prototypes, and more "undercontrolled" and "overcontrolled" personality types. It is unclear if these changes resulted from their injuries or were possibly risk factors to obtaining their SCI.[27] In contrast, a small pilot study found that externalizing/impulsive personality disorders (such as histrionic, narcissistic, antisocial aggressive, and borderline) were not higher in patients with SCIs than controls. Instead, the investigators did note a high level of avoidant and depressive disorders in the SCI population.[28]

Learning Difficulties

In some of the earliest studies of CD in individuals with SCI, it was recognized that patients had poor premorbid academic performance.[12] A metaanalysis by Macciocchi and colleagues[29] found that those who obtained traumatic SCI did not have significantly worse cognitive performance than those who obtained traumatic SCI and a mild TBI. Instead, sociodemographic factors, education level, and self-reported preinjury history of learning disability were more predictive of performance on cognitive testing. A total of

13.7% of spinal cord–injured patients had self-reported history of learning problems. If these factors were proven to be more common in those with SCI, it may play a large role in explaining some of the CD following SCI. It is possible that the learning difficulties may be the common denominator of both the SCI and the CD.

Mood and Psychiatric Disorders

In addition to the premorbid psychiatric and psychological disorders that are discussed above, there are increased rates of psychological and psychiatric disorders following SCI. In an Australian population following SCI, psychological disorders were found in 17% at discharge from rehabilitation and 25% 6 months following discharge. This finding is significantly higher than the rates of mood disorders in the general population (8.5%). Depression was seen in 14.1% of patients 6 months after discharge. Less common disorders, including bipolar disorder (4.2%), suicidality (7.0%), posttraumatic stress disorder (PTSD; 1.4%), and general anxiety (4.2%), were also found. Of note, no significant improvement was seen in this set of patients in the 6 months after discharge (**Table 3**).[30] This study is supported by Perkes and colleagues,[31] who found high rates of depression in those with SCI: 40% during rehabilitation, 30% upon discharge, 20% at 1 year after injury.

Marvel and Paradiso[32] found that depression, bipolar disorder, and anxiety are associated with CD (**Table 4**). Furthermore, mood disorders were found to be associated with structural and functional abnormalities in the prefrontal cortex, hippocampus, and anterior cingulate cortex. Differences were also noted in emotion-related brain activity via functional MRI (fMRI). Interestingly, these investigators noted that neurologic testing in this population remained affected despite a current state of euthymia; the investigators suggest that current treatment of mood disorders may not improve cognitive deficits caused by mood disorders.

In contrast to the above studies, Davidoff and colleagues[33] found no effect of depression on cognition in those with SCI and stated that "depression (or depressed affect) and impaired cognitive performance in the acute SCI patient are two separate problems which are casually but not causally related."

Craig and colleagues[9] found that levels of depression and anxiety were not different between spinal cord–injured individuals with and without CD in the inpatient rehabilitation stage. In contrast, depression anxiety was increased significantly after living for 6 months in the community in individuals with CD compared with individuals without CD, suggesting that mood disorders may be a consequence of CD instead of a cause of CD.

Substance Abuse

Another possible contributor to CD in those with SCI is substance abuse. Substance abuse is common both before and after an individual suffers an SCI and is often a contributor to the initial SCI, with estimates of alcohol being a contributor in 35% to 40% of traumatic SCIs and more than 30% of individuals with new SCIs having positive tests for illicit drugs.[34] Tate and colleagues[35] used a retrospective cross-sectional design investigating alcohol and substance use in more than 3 thousand subjects with traumatic SCI between 1975 and 2002. They found that alcohol abuse was prevalent in 14.2% of individuals with SCI. Furthermore, drug use was present in 11% of the population (mostly consisting of marijuana).

Similarly, Craig and colleagues[15] found that 8.6% and 7.0% of individuals with SCI had evidence of alcohol dependence or abuse 6 months after injury. Rates of overall substance abuse in 1 study has been as high as 32% in those suffering an SCI.[15]

It is clear that alcohol and drug abuse have widespread cognitive effects, with dysfunction being noted in attention, memory, planning, behavior, and decision

Table 3
Frequency of psychological disorders following spinal cord injury

Psychological Disorder	Initial (N = 87)[a]	Discharge (N = 81)[b]	6-mo Postdischarge (N = 71)[c]
Major depressive disorders	10.3 (9; 4.0–16.6)	8.6 (7; 2.6–14.6)	14.1 (10; 6.1–22.1)
Bipolar disorders	4.6 (4; 0.7–8.5)	1.2 (1; 0–3.5)	4.2 (3; 0–8.9)
Suicidality	8.0 (7; 2.1–13.9)	4.9 (4; 0.2–9.6)	7.0 (5; 1.1–12.9)
PTSD	1.1 (1; 0–3.2)	0	1.4 (1; 0–4.1)
Generalized anxiety disorder	3.4 (3; 0–7.1)	4.9 (4; 0.2–9.6)	4.2 (3; 0–8.9)
Alcohol dependence and abuse disorder	10.3 (9; 3.8–16.8)	7.4 (6; 1.7–13.1)	8.6 (6; 2.1–15.1)
Drug dependence and abuse disorder	2.3 (2; 0.8–5.4)	1.2 (1; 0–3.5)	7.0 (5; 1.1–12.9)
Psychoses	1.1 (1; 0–2.9)	0	0
Proportion with mental disorders	21.8 (19; 13.2–30.4)	17.3 (14; 9.1–25.5)	25.3 (18; 20.1–30.5)

NOTE. Values are % of participants, with actual frequencies (n) and 95% confidence intervals in parentheses.
[a] One participant did not wish to complete the Mini International Neuropsychiatric Interview.
[b] Seven were not able to be interviewed.
[c] Ten were not able to be located, and 7 refused to be interviewed.
From Craig A, Nicholson Perry K, Guest R, et al. Prospective Study of the Occurrence of Psychological Disorders and Comorbidities after Spinal Cord Injury. Arch Phys Med Rehabil. 2015;96(8):1426–34; with permission.

making.[34] Marijuana, in particular, is becoming more widely accepted and used in the SCI community for the treatment of pain and spasticity. The predominance of evidence suggests cannabis intake is harmful to cognitive functioning (including verbal memory, processing speed, and complex executive function).[36]

Table 4
Relationships between cognitive deficits and mood states

Cognitive Domain	Cognitive Task	Euthymic State	Depressed State	Manic State	Deficits Increase with Symptom Severity
Attention	Continuous Performance Test (CPT)	X	Yes	Yes	Yes
	Trails Making Test Part A (TMT-A)	Yes	Yes	X	
	Digit Symbol Substitution (DSST)	Yes	Yes	?	
Executive function	Wisconsin Card Sort Test (WCST)	Yes	?	Yes	Yes
	Stroop test	Yes	?	Yes	
	Trail Making Test, Part B (TMT-B)	Yes	Yes	?	
Memory	Verbal recall	Yes	Yes	Yes	Yes
	Nonverbal recall	?	Yes	?	?
	Implicit memory	?	X	?	?

From Marvel CL, Paradiso S. Cognitive and neurological impairment in mood disorders. Psychiatr Clin North Am. 2004;27(1):19–36, vii–viii; with permission.

Substance abuse may directly or indirectly (possibly because of its effect on cognitive functioning) lead to worse rehabilitation outcomes. Heavy preinjury alcohol users were noted to have limited participation in acute rehabilitation, which was found to be a significant barrier to transition to home after acute injury. Alcohol and substance abuse, both preinjury and postinjury, are associated with increased incidence of urinary tract infections and pressure injuries. Among persons undergoing acute SCI rehabilitation, those with histories of severe alcoholism before SCI were 2.5 times more likely to develop a deep tissue injury than their peers.[37]

Polypharmacy

Many pharmacologic agents interfere with neurotransmission in areas of the brain that control cognitive function, and this effect is compounded the more agents a patient is prescribed.[38] Kitzman and colleagues[39] looked at 13,160 individuals with SCI and compared them with able-bodied controls and found that individuals with SCI were prescribed multiple medications significantly more frequently than those without SCI. Specifically, the study found that 56% of the SCI population were prescribed 5 or more medications, compared with 27% in the control population. Of the SCI population, 23% were taking 10 or more medications, compared with only 7% of the control population (**Table 5**).

In addition, high-risk medications (defined as sedative-hypnotics [nonbarbiturate], anxiolytics, antispasmodics, serotoninergic agents, narcotics, anticonvulsants, tricyclic antidepressants, and skeletal muscle relaxants) were prescribed more often in those with SCIs compared with controls, 92% versus 44%[39] (**Table 6**).

Benzodiazepines and Nonbenzodiazepine Hypnotics

Benzodiazepines and nonbenzodiazepine hypnotics are commonly associated with CD. Benzodiazepines act by enhancing gamma-aminobutyric acid-A (GABA-A), the primary inhibitory neurotransmitter. These medications have been shown to have amnestic and nonamnestic cognitive effects in patients with SCI, with these impairments increasing in a dose-related manner. Similarly, nonbenzodiazepine hypnotics also act by enhancing GABA-A; however, studies of their effects on cognition have

Table 5
Incidence of polypharmacy in a population with spinal cord injury compared with a control population

| | SCI | | | Control | |
Number of Drugs Prescribed	Number of Patients	% of Total SCI Population	Number of Drugs Prescribed	Number of Patients	% of Total Control Population
5–9	4401	33	5–9	2607	20
10–14	1962	15	10–14	725	5.5
15–19	754	6	15–19	155	1.2
20 or more	282	2	20 or more	50	0.3
Total	7399	56		3537	27

This table demonstrates a significantly higher number of individuals with SCI were on 5 or more medications compared with the non-SCI group (11.07 ± 3.58 vs 7.88 ± 2.95; $X \pm$ SD, $P<.001$). Twenty-three percent of the total SCI population was on 10 or more medications compared with only 7% in the control group.

From Kitzman P, Cecil D, Kolpek JH. The risks of polypharmacy following spinal cord injury. J Spinal Cord Med. 2016;40(2):1–7; with permission.

Table 6
Incidence of high-risk medications prescriptions between a population with spinal cord injury compared with a control population

	SCI			Control		
Number of Distinct High-Risk Classes	Number of Subjects	% of Total SCI Group with Polypharmacy ($n = 7399$)	Number of Distinct High-Risk Classes	Number of Subjects	% of Total Control Group with Polypharmacy ($n = 5761$)
1	1738	24	1	1129	20
2	1881	25	2	790	14
3	1692	23	3	358	6
4	841	11	4	157	3
5	520	7	5	58	1
6	147	2	6	15	<1
7	12	<1	7	0	0
Total	6831	92		2507	44

This table demonstrated a significantly higher percentage of individuals with SCI, who were classified as being on polypharmacy and were prescribed medications from more than one or more of the high-risk classes of medications (5.49 ± 4.33 vs 3 ± 2.51; $X \pm SD$, $P < .0001$). Sixty-eight percent of the SCI polypharmacy group was on 2 or more high-risk medications compared with 24% of controls.

From Kitzman P, Cecil D, Kolpek JH. The risks of polypharmacy following spinal cord injury. J Spinal Cord Med. 2016;40(2):1–7; with permission.

yielded mixed effects in the SCI population, demonstrating the need for further research with these drugs.[40]

Baclofen

Baclofen is a commonly used agent in the SCI population and is often the first choice for spasticity management. However, the effects of baclofen on cognition remain unclear. Baclofen acts as an agonist at GABA-B receptors. Multiple studies in the mouse model have showed evidence that baclofen leads to CD, although there have not been studies examining these effects in humans.[41–44] Interestingly, outside of the SCI model, baclofen use has recently been shown to alleviate cognitive effects in animal models of Alzheimer disease, the most common genetic deletion seen in intellectual disability.[45,46]

Opioid

Although there is a concentrated effort to decrease the amount of opiate medications prescribed, they are still used for analgesia in individuals with SCI. Opioids work by binding to opioid receptors in the central nervous system. Opioids have been shown to cause both amnestic and nonamnestic impairments. These cognitive effects include difficulties with sustained attention, reaction time, complex executive functioning, response inhibition, and set shifting. Importantly, studies have shown that only a small amount of opioid is required to cause cognitive impairment, with adverse effects occurring with as low as a single dose of 10 mg oxycodone in 1 study.[40,47]

Antipsychotics

Antipsychotics, which act by increasing dopamine in the central nervous system, are often used in those hospitalized with SCI who have delirium, in those with SCI who have coexistent TBI, and for sleep. There is evidence that these medications impair recall and reaction time.[40]

Antiepileptics

Antiepileptics act in a variety of ways to suppress neuronal excitability or enhance inhibitory neurotransmitters. These medications are often used in those with SCI for neuropathic pain management or for seizures (often in the setting of a concomitant TBI). Potential adverse cognitive effects include impaired concentration, memory, processing speed, verbal fluency, complex cognitive processing, and mental flexibility.[48] In addition, a 2018 study showed that most antiepileptics exhibit a dose-response effect in terms of cognitive side effects, further demonstrating the need for clinicians to be mindful of this potential side effect when prescribing these agents.[49]

Two medications that demand particular scrutiny in individuals with SCI are gabapentin and pregabalin. Both of these medications are calcium channel alpha 2-delta ligands and affect the release of neurotransmitters. Pregabalin has been shown to have extensive cognitive effects both in rat models and in humans.[50] Salimzade and colleagues[38] administered pregabalin to rats for 21 days and then administered an object recognition (memory) task. The study found that rats given pregabalin or a pregabalin/baclofen combination performed worse than controls that were not given the drug. Similarly, in the human population, Salinsky and colleagues[51] administered pregabalin to healthy volunteers for 12 weeks and found significant cognitive impairment in objective measures of memory as well as in participant self-reporting.

Literature on gabapentin has shown the agent to be sedating, but multiple studies have failed to show clear cognitive effects of the drug.[50,52–55] A recent study by Shem and colleagues[56] demonstrated that gabapentin use was associated with a decline in memory, executive function, and attention in individuals with an SCI.

Anticholinergic Medications

Medications with anticholinergic properties are also frequently prescribed to patients with SCI for clinical issues, such as bladder overactivity (for example, bladder antimuscarinics) and mood/pain management (for example, tricyclic antidepressants). The cholinergic system projects into the cortex and hippocampus and is involved with memory storage, retrieval, arousal, perception, and attention. Antimuscarinic drugs are the most studied agent in this category, but results examining cognitive impairment are mixed, with oxybutynin showing the greatest negative effect on cognition.[40,57] However, a recent 2018 study that monitored antimuscarinic use for lower urinary tract dysfunction failed to show a significant deterioration in cognition, although none of these patients used oxybutynin and only 10 subjects were enrolled.[58] Tricyclic antidepressants consistently show cognitive impairment predominantly with attention and reaction time.[40]

Chronic Pain

Chronic pain is another possible contributor to alterations in cognition in patients with SCI, especially given the frequency of pain in this population. A 2013 study of patients with chronic SCI found that 30% experienced visceral pain, whereas 40% to 50% experienced neuropathic pain.[59] Pain has been shown in the literature to interfere with cognitive processing, most commonly affecting memory (both working and short term) and concentration, and this may be due to the brain plasticity associated with chronic pain resulting in functional and structural changes to the brain.[60]

Chronic Fatigue

Chronic fatigue may also contribute to impaired cognition following SCI. Patients with chronic SCI have been shown to have higher levels of chronic fatigue compared with controls, with 1 study finding that 56% of patients with SCI reported chronic fatigue compared with 29% of controls. In this study, patients with SCI also reported an increased feeling of "tiredness" after completing a 2-hour cognitive task. Chronic fatigue has also been associated with increased depression and lower self-efficacy, factors that may further negatively impact cognition.[61]

Respiratory Disorders

Respiratory disorders are common in both the acute and the chronic phases of SCI. Although a well-known contributor to hospitalizations, morbidity, and mortality following SCIs, respiratory dysfunction to CD in individuals with SCI has not garnered much attention.[62] Although individuals with high cervical tetraplegia are at risk of chronic respiratory failure with hypercapnia and hypoxemia, there are respiratory physiologic effects of SCIs even at thoracic level injuries. Some of the respiratory physiologic changes include decreased chest wall compliance, inefficient ventilation, reduced vital capacity, reduced forced expiratory volume in the first second, and reduced peak expiratory and inspiratory pressure.[63] Chronic hypoxemia and hypercapnia along with severity of respiratory impairment have both been associated with CD in other pulmonary disorders.[64–67] There is also evidence of respiratory changes in response to cognitive load.[68] How the respiratory impairment related to SCI affects cognition and response to cognitive load is unknown.

Sleep-Disordered Breathing

Sleep-disordered breathing is common following SCI, especially with more severe injuries, approaching nearly 60% in complete tetraplegics.[69] A 2017 systematic review and metaanalysis study found that sleep-disordered breathing was associated with impaired executive functioning, although there was no impairment found in global cognition or executive functioning.[70] Sajkov and colleagues[71] found that CD was correlated with sleep hypoxia. Schembri and colleagues[72] also found significant correlation between degree of sleep apnea and CD in individuals with tetraplegia.

Autonomic Dysregulation

Autonomic dysfunctions, such as hypotension and autonomic dysreflexia, are other common sequelae of SCIs that may impact cognition.

Hypotension

Hypotension has been shown to have adverse cognitive effects on non-SCI populations, such as in the elderly with heart failure, individuals with pure autonomic failure, and the otherwise healthy (both young and old) with hypotension. These impairments stretch across multiple domains and include attention, memory, calculation, processing speed, and global impairment.[73–75]

These effects have been further validated in the SCI population. Jegede and colleagues[76] found that SCI patients with hypotension had significantly worse memory, with a trend toward slower processing speed and impaired attentions, compared with SCI patients without hypotension. Wecht and Bauman[75] demonstrated that SCI individuals had decreased cerebral blood flow in response to cognitive testing compared with non-SCI individuals, which demonstrated an increase in cerebral blood flow (**Fig. 4**).

A recent study analyzed the effects of chronic hypotension and hypertension in those with SCI. The study found that those with upper-thoracic and cervical SCI exhibited significantly lower cerebral blood flow at rest, which correlated with reduced cognitive performance, compared with controls.[77] In addition, a study investigating athletes at the 2015 ParaPan American Games found that SCI was associated with significant cerebrovascular dysfunction (with cerebral hypoperfusion, impaired neurovascular coupling, and impaired cerebral blood flow regulation), which was thought to likely lead to CD.[78] Phillips and colleagues[79] found that midodrine, an alpha-1 agonist, increased cerebral blood flow in response to cognitive tasks and led to improved performance on cognitive testing in individuals with tetraplegia.

Autonomic Dysreflexia

Wide fluctuations in blood pressure, such as those seen in autonomic dysreflexia, may also be detrimental to cerebral microvasculature and lead to CD; this has been postulated to be due to the presence of chronic silent infarcts occurring.[75]

Metabolic Syndrome

Disorders of carbohydrate and lipid metabolism are more common in SCI individuals and occur at a younger age. It is well understood that diabetes and dyslipidemia may lead to vascular disease that limits tissue perfusion; this, particularly in association with other autonomic factors mentioned above, may also adversely affect cognition.

Post–Intensive Care Unit Syndrome

Almost universally after an acute SCI, treatment begins in the intensive care unit (ICU). It is being increasingly recognized that individuals who are hospitalized with critical illness and are in the ICU develop significant CD both acutely and chronically. This CD is known as post–intensive care syndrome (PICS) and constitutes the physical and psychological sequelae related to injuries upon discharge of critical care.

Previous studies have found that acute brain dysfunction occurs in 20% to 80% of patients admitted to the ICU.[80] Even after discharge from the ICU, cognitive impairment occurs in 30% to 80% of patients; psychiatric illnesses, such as anxiety,

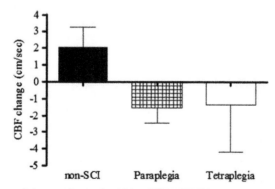

Fig. 4. Comparison of changes in cerebral blood flow (CBF) in response to cognitive testing. (*From* Wecht JM, Bauman WA. Decentralized cardiovascular autonomic control and cognitive deficits in persons with spinal cord injury. J Spinal Cord Med. 2013;36(2):74–81; with permission.)

depression, and PTSD, occur in 8% to 57% of patients, and new physical impairment occurs in 25% to 80% of patients. Risk factors that have been associated with PICS include hypotension, sedation, hypoxemia, prolonged mechanical ventilation, multiorgan failure, systemic corticosteroids, and younger age.[81] These same factors are often present in individuals with SCI during the acute stages.

Cortical Reorganization

One of the most interesting possible causes of CD in individuals with SCI is cortical reorganization. Several studies have demonstrated that "trauma-induced spinal degenerative process spreads toward the brain."[82] In both animal and human studies, significant functional reorganization occurs after SCI, not only in the spinal cord but also within higher-order structures, including sensory and motor cortices. Cortical reorganization has been demonstrated involving numerous differing methodologies, including transcranial magnetic stimulation, stimulated motor-evoked potentials, PET, electroencephalography, MRI, fMRI, voxel-based morphometry, and diffusion tensor imaging. Potential mechanisms of cortical reorganization after SCI include the slowing of spontaneous cortical activity, cortical atrophy, and neuronal loss (apoptosis) in the sensorimotor cortex, changes to large cortical networks, and changes in synaptic spine density and neuronal morphology.[83]

Although most studies focus on cortical atrophy/plasticity after SCI in directly associated regions (for example, the sensorimotor cortex), larger global effects are also noted in the brain that are not directly connected to the injury site. Nicotra and colleagues[84] used fMRI in 7 participants with SCI and 7 controls in tasks involving aversive fear conditioning. SCI patients differed from control in conditioning-related brain activity, showing enhancement of activity within dorsal anterior cingulate cortex, periaqueductal gray matter and superior temporoparietal gyrus, and attenuation of activity in subgenual cingulate, ventromedial prefrontal, and posterior cingulate cortices. This finding suggests that SCI patients have significant differences in experiencing and evoking emotion-related brain activity and information related to high-level cognitive function and may account for motivation and affective sequelae of SCI in some individuals.

Wrigley and colleagues[85] support that many SCI subjects develop additional sequelae beyond the typical motor/sensory impairments and that central processes may be involved in somatosensory cortex reorganization and pain intensity. They conducted fMRI of 20 subjects with complete thoracic SCI (10 subjects experiencing persistent neuropathic pain immediately before scanning) and 21 healthy controls. SCI participants witnessed decreased gray-matter volume in the primary motor cortex, superior cerebellar cortex, medial prefrontal cortex (involved with emotional responses, memory, decision making), and anterior cingulate cortex (involved with error detection, conflicts in information processing, evaluation of decisions, and emotion regulation) (**Fig. 5**). Participants with SCI also experienced fiber loss/demyelination of the corticospinal and corticopontine tracts. It is important to note that the corticopontine tract is not directly interrupted by SCIs.

Neuroinflammation

Finally, neuroinflammation is another potential cause of CD in individuals with SCI. SCI has been shown to lead to chronic inflammation of the brain and progressive neurodegeneration in animal models. Neuroinflammation pathologic mechanisms through glial activation are important causes of posttraumatic neurodegeneration (**Fig. 6**).[86]

Wu and colleagues[87] examined the broad effects of SCI among the cognitive and affective function, brain inflammation, and neuropathology in mice. They found that SCI caused the upregulation of neurotoxic reactive phenotype (M1) of microglia. These microglia have increased expression of proinflammatory cytokines, reactive oxygen species, and nitric oxide, which likely leads to tissue inflammation. This neuroinflammation in the cortex, thalamus, and hippocampus (which plays role in memory) leads to neuronal loss, a pathway similar to rodents with TBI. Interleukin-6 was also increased after SCI, which acts as a microglial activator and neuromodulator. These findings suggest that isolated SCI may lead to central neuroinflammatory sequelae and cognitive deficits. Similar to rodents, humans have been shown to have increased low-level systematic inflammation both acutely and chronically after SCI.[88,89]

Combination of Mechanisms

It is important to note that there is unlikely to be 1 sole cause of the CD noted after SCI. In fact, the mechanisms above are highly interrelated, and their effects may be exponential. For example, chronic pain may lead to polypharmacy, which may lead to

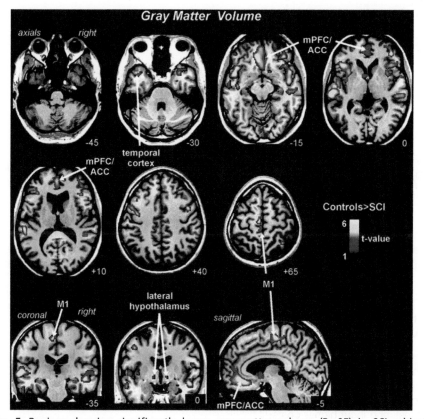

Fig. 5. Regions showing significantly lower gray-matter volume (P<.05) in SCI subjects compared with controls overlaid on a single subject's T1-weighted anatomic scan. ACC, anterior cingulate cortex; M1, primary motor cortex; mPFC, medial prefrontal cortex. (*From* Wrigley PJ, Gustin SM, Macey PM, et al. Anatomical changes in human motor cortex and motor pathways following complete thoracic spinal cord injury. Cereb Cortex. 2009;19(1):224–32; with permission.)

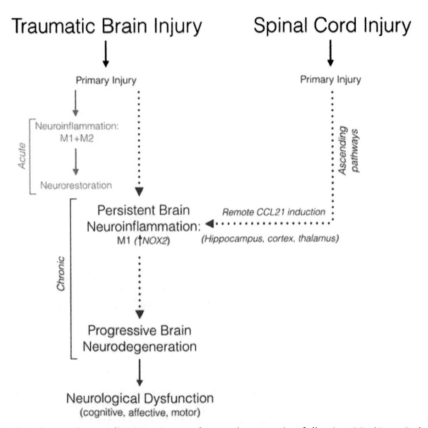

Fig. 6. Inflammation mediated pathway of neurodegeneration following SCI. (*From* Faden AI, Wu J, Stoica BA, et al. Progressive inflammation-mediated neurodegeneration after traumatic brain or spinal cord injury. Br J Pharmacol. 2016:681–91; with permission.)

sleep-disordered breathing, which may lead to fatigue. It will be likely to address many of these areas in order to get a full understanding of, and potentially treat or prevent, CD in SCI.

SIGNIFICANCE OF COGNITIVE DYSFUNCTION FOR INDIVIDUALS WITH SPINAL CORD INJURY

There are several potential adverse effects of CD for individuals with SCI. Individuals with TBI history and SCI are more likely to have behavioral incidents while in rehabilitation, have higher levels of psychopathology, require increased nursing care, have longer length of stay (with lower or similar functional independence measure outcomes), and incur higher costs.[19,90,91]

Rehospitalization in the first year after an SCI is common with 36.2% of individuals being hospitalized at least once and 12.5% being hospitalized at least twice. Common causes of rehospitalization include urinary tract infections, pneumonia, and pressure ulcers.[92] This rehospitalization may be in part due to CD impairing the ability of individuals in rehabilitation to acquire the vital new skills they need following discharge to stay healthy.[2] Similar to those with CD, individuals with less education are more likely to have readmission in the first year.[93] Elliott and colleagues[94] found that impaired problem solving predicted pressure ulcer development in the 3 years following SCI.

Besides direct health-related issues, CD may impair the learning of important mobility, self-care, community, and vocational skills. CD may lead to less social integration and occupational success.[2] It has also been shown that CD is predictive of social participation following discharge from rehabilitation.[95] Those with CD are also likely to have higher rates of the development of mental health problems.[9]

TREATMENT OF COGNITIVE DYSFUNCTION IN INDIVIDUALS WITH SPINAL CORD INJURY

Although no standard guidelines exist for evaluating CD in individuals with SCI, several recommendations can be considered[90,96]:

- Approach with higher suspicion all patients with SCI independent of mechanism of injury.
- Screen patients admitted to SCI rehabilitation and over the course of their lifetime.
- Do not assume cognitive changes are situational or reactive.
- Consider neuropsychological testing, particularly if the individual is thinking about returning to school or work.
- Realize that difficulty in learning new skills may be due to comorbid CD.
- Consider having rehabilitation programs focused on employment and community integration.
- Limit environmental stimuli to improve attention on the given task.
- Repeat frequently teaching/instruction(s).
- Use simplified directions.
- Have early involvement of caregivers and family.
- Have memory books and aids (timers), which may be helpful.
- Consider "learning approaches that are most effective for people with explicit memory deficits, such as procedural learning and errorless learning. For the learning of self-care routines, these approaches might prove more effective for acquisition in the short term, and more resistant to decay in the longer term."[90]

SUMMARY

CD is a significant sequela of SCIs. Although various mechanisms have been suggested to cause CD in those with SCI, no specific cause has been identified, and it is likely a combination of factors. Despite the various causes and adverse effects of CD, preventive and treatment mechanisms have not been clearly elucidated. In order to best treat patients, it may be time to "considerably revise concepts about the nature of SCI as a focal acute neurodegenerative disorder" affecting the spinal cord.[87] More focus and sustained attention are needed in this critical area.

ACKNOWLEDGMENTS

The authors thank Dr Elliot Roth for his advice and review in writing this article.

DISCLOSURE

The authors have nothing to disclose.

REFERENCES

1. Van Middendorp JJ, Sanchez GM, Burridge AL. The Edwin Smith papyrus: a clinical reappraisal of the oldest known document on spinal injuries. Eur Spine J 2010;1815–23. https://doi.org/10.1007/s00586-010-1523-6.
2. Davidoff GN, Roth EJ, Richards JS. Cognitive deficits in spinal cord injury: epidemiology and outcome. Arch Phys Med Rehabil 1992;73:275–84.
3. Dowler RN, O'Brien SA, Haaland KY, et al. Neuropsychological functioning following a spinal cord injury. Appl Neuropsychol 1995;2(3–4):124–9.
4. Dowler RN, Harrington DL, Haaland KY, et al. Profiles of cognitive functioning in chronic spinal cord injury and the role of moderating variables. J Int Neuropsychol Soc 1997;3(5):464–72.
5. Tun CG, Tun PA, Wingfield A. Cognitive function following long-term spinal cord injury. Rehabil Psychol 1997;42(3):163–82.
6. Gordon WA, Haddad L, Brown M, et al. The sensitivity and specificity of self-reported symptoms in individuals with traumatic brain injury. Brain Inj 2000; 14(1):21–33.
7. Cohen ML, Tulsky DS, Holdnack JA, et al. Cognition among community-dwelling individuals with spinal cord injury. Rehabil Psychol 2017;62(4):425–34.
8. Sachdeva R, Gao F, Chan CCH, et al. Cognitive function after spinal cord injury: a systematic review. Neurology 2018;611–21. https://doi.org/10.1212/WNL. 0000000000006244.
9. Craig A, Guest R, Tran Y, et al. Cognitive impairment and mood states after spinal cord injury. J Neurotrauma 2017;34(6):1156–63.
10. Guttmann L. Spinal injuries. Edinburgh: Royal College of Surgeons; 1963.
11. Harris P. Associated injuries in traumatic paraplegia and tetraplegia. Spinal Cord 1968;5(4):215–20.
12. Wilmot CB, Cope DN, Hall KM, et al. Occult head injury: its incidence in spinal cord injury. Arch Phys Med Rehabil 1985;66(4):227–31.
13. Davidoff G, Morris J, Roth E, et al. Closed head injury in spinal cord injured patients: retrospective study of loss of consciousness and post-traumatic amnesia. Arch Phys Med Rehabil 1985;66(1):41–3.
14. Richards JS, Brown L, Hagglund K, et al. Spinal cord injury and concomitant traumatic brain injury. Results of a longitudinal investigation. Am J Phys Med Rehabil 1988;67(5):211–6.
15. Roth E, Davidoff G, Thomas P, et al. A controlled study of neuropsychological deficits in acute spinal cord injury patients. Paraplegia 1989;27(6):480–9.
16. Hagen EM, Eide GE, Rekand T, et al. Traumatic spinal cord injury and concomitant brain injury: a cohort study. Acta Neurol Scand 2010;122(Suppl. 190):51–7.
17. Davidoff G, Thomas P, Johnson M, et al. Closed head injury in acute traumatic spinal cord injury: incidence and risk factors. Arch Phys Med Rehabil 1988; 69(10):869–72.
18. Macciocchi S, Seel RT, Thompson N, et al. Spinal cord injury and co-occurring traumatic brain injury: assessment and incidence. Arch Phys Med Rehabil 2008;89(7):1350–7.
19. Macciocchi S, Seel RT, Warshowsky A, et al. Co-occurring traumatic brain injury and acute spinal cord injury rehabilitation outcomes. Arch Phys Med Rehabil 2012;93(10):1788–94.
20. Sharma B, Bradbury C, Mikulis D, et al. Missed diagnosis of traumatic brain injury in patients with traumatic spinal cord injury. J Rehabil Med 2014;46(4):370–3.

21. Strubreither W, Hackbusch B, Hermann-Gruber M, et al. Neuropsychological aspects of the rehabilitation of patients with paralysis from a spinal injury who also have a brain injury. Spinal Cord 1997;35(8):487–92.
22. Tolonen A, Turkka J, Salonen O, et al. Traumatic brain injury is under-diagnosed in patients with spinal cord injury. J Rehabil Med 2007;39(8):622–6.
23. Fleminger S. Long-term psychiatric disorders after traumatic brain injury. Eur J Anaesthesiol 2008;123–30. https://doi.org/10.1017/S0265021507003250.
24. Kang J-H, Lin H-C, Chung S-D. Attention-deficit/hyperactivity disorder increased the risk of injury: a population-based follow-up study. Acta Paediatr 2013;102(6): 640–3.
25. Merrill RM, Lyon JL, Baker RK, et al. Attention deficit hyperactivity disorder and increased risk of injury. Adv Med Sci 2009;54(1):20–6.
26. Mawson AR, Biundo JJ, Clemmer DI, et al. Sensation-seeking, criminality, and spinal cord injury: a case-control study. Am J Epidemiol 1996;144(5):463–72.
27. Berry JW, Elliott TR, Rivera P. Resilient, undercontrolled, and overcontrolled personality prototypes among persons with spinal cord injury. J Pers Assess 2007; 89(3):292–302.
28. Bockian NR, Lee A, Fidanque CS. Personality disorders and spinal cord injury: a pilot study. J Clin Psychol Med Settings 2003;10(4):307–13.
29. Macciocchi SN, Seel RT, Thompson N. The impact of mild traumatic brain injury on cognitive functioning following co-occurring spinal cord injury. Arch Clin Neuropsychol 2013;28(7):684–91.
30. Craig A, Nicholson Perry K, Guest R, et al. Prospective study of the occurrence of psychological disorders and comorbidities after spinal cord injury. Arch Phys Med Rehabil 2015;96(8):1426–34.
31. Perkes SJ, Bowman J, Penkala S. Psychological therapies for the management of co-morbid depression following a spinal cord injury: a systematic review. J Health Psychol 2014;19(12):1597–612.
32. Marvel CL, Paradiso S. Cognitive and neurological impairment in mood disorders. Psychiatr Clin North Am 2004;27(1):19–36, vii–viii.
33. Davidoff G, Roth E, Thomas P, et al. Depression and neuropsychological test performance in acute spinal cord injury patients: lack of correlation. Arch Clin Neuropsychol 1990;5(1):77–88.
34. Warren AN, Pullins J, Elliott TR. Concomitant cognitive impairment in persons with spinal cord injuries in rehabilitation settings. In: Gontovsky ST, Golden CJ, editors. Europsychology within the inpatient rehabilitation environment. Hauppauge (NY): Nova Science Publishers, Inc; 2008. p. 79–98.
35. Tate DG, Forchheimer MB, Krause JS, et al. Patterns of alcohol and substance use and abuse in persons with spinal cord injury: risk factors and correlates. Arch Phys Med Rehabil 2004;85(11):1837–47.
36. Hall W, Lynskey M. Long-term marijuana use and cognitive impairment in middle age. JAMA Intern Med 2016;362–3. https://doi.org/10.1001/jamainternmed.2015. 7850.
37. Hawkins DA, Heinemann AW. Substance abuse and medical complications following spinal cord injury. Rehabil Psychol 1998;43(3):219–31.
38. Salimzade A, Hosseini-Sharifabad A, Rabbani M. Comparative effects of chronic administrations of gabapentin, pregabalin and baclofen on rat memory using object recognition test. Res Pharm Sci 2017;12(3):204–10.
39. Kitzman P, Cecil D, Kolpek JH. The risks of polypharmacy following spinal cord injury. J Spinal Cord Med 2016;40(2):1–7.

40. Tannenbaum C, Paquette A, Hilmer S, et al. A systematic review of amnestic and non-amnestic mild cognitive impairment induced by anticholinergic, antihistamine, GABAergic and opioid drugs. Drugs Aging 2012;29(8):639–58.

41. Levin ED, Weber E, Icenogle L. Baclofen interactions with nicotine in rats: effects on memory. Pharmacol Biochem Behav 2004;79(2):343–8.

42. Zarrindast MR, Khodjastehfar E, Oryan S, et al. Baclofen-impairment of memory retention in rats: possible interaction with adrenoceptor mechanism(s). Eur J Pharmacol 2001;411(3):283–8.

43. Tang AC, Hasselmo ME. Effect of long term baclofen treatment on recognition memory and novelty detection. Behav Brain Res 1996;74(1–2):145–52.

44. Pujol CN, Paasche C, Laprevote V, et al. Cognitive effects of labeled addictolytic medications. Prog Neuropsychopharmacol Biol Psychiatry 2018;306–32. https://doi.org/10.1016/j.pnpbp.2017.09.008.

45. Stoppel LJ, Kazdoba TM, Schaffler MD, et al. R-Baclofen reverses cognitive deficits and improves social interactions in two lines of 16p11.2 deletion mice. Neuropsychopharmacology 2018;43(3):513–24.

46. Pilipenko V, Narbute K, Beitnere U, et al. Very low doses of muscimol and baclofen ameliorate cognitive deficits and regulate protein expression in the brain of a rat model of streptozocin-induced Alzheimer's disease. Eur J Pharmacol 2018; 818:381–99.

47. Berryman C, Stanton TR, Bowering KJ, et al. Do people with chronic pain have impaired executive function? A meta-analytical review. Clin Psychol Rev 2014;563–79. https://doi.org/10.1016/j.cpr.2014.08.003.

48. Eddy CM, Rickards HE, Cavanna AE. The cognitive impact of antiepileptic drugs. Ther Adv Neurol Disord 2011;4(6):385–407.

49. Sarkis RA, Goksen Y, Mu Y, et al. Cognitive and fatigue side effects of antiepileptic drugs: an analysis of phase III add-on trials. J Neurol 2018;265(9): 2137–42.

50. Chavant F, Favrelière S, Lafay-Chebassier C, et al. Memory disorders associated with consumption of drugs: updating through a case/noncase study in the French PharmacoVigilance Database. Br J Clin Pharmacol 2011;72(6):898–904.

51. Salinsky M, Storzbach D, Munoz S. Cognitive effects of pregabalin in healthy volunteers: a double-blind, placebo-controlled trial. Neurology 2010;74(9):755–61.

52. Leach JP, Girvan J, Paul A, et al. Gabapentin and cognition: a double blind, dose ranging, placebo controlled study in refractory epilepsy. J Neurol Neurosurg Psychiatry 1997;62(4):372–6.

53. Mortimore C, Trimble M, Emmers E. Effects of gabapentin on cognition and quality of life in patients with epilepsy. Seizure 1998;7(5):359–64.

54. Dodrill CB, Arnett JL, Hayes AG, et al. Cognitive abilities and adjustment with gabapentin: results of a multisite study. Epilepsy Res 1999;35(2):109–21.

55. Salinsky MC, Storzbach D, Spencer DC, et al. Effects of topiramate and gabapentin on cognitive abilities in healthy volunteers. Neurology 2005;64(5):792–8.

56. Shem K, Barncord S, Flavin K, et al. Adverse cognitive effect of gabapentin in individuals with spinal cord injury: preliminary findings. Spinal Cord Ser Cases 2018;4(1):9.

57. Scheife R, Takeda M. Central nervous system safety of anticholinergic drugs for the treatment of overactive bladder in the elderly. Clin Ther 2005;144–53. https://doi.org/10.1016/j.clinthera.2005.02.014.

58. Krebs J, Scheel-Sailer A, Oertli R, et al. The effects of antimuscarinic treatment on the cognition of spinal cord injured individuals with neurogenic lower urinary tract

dysfunction: a prospective controlled before-and-after study. Spinal Cord 2018; 56(1):22–7.

59. Finnerup NB. Pain in patients with spinal cord injury. Pain 2013;154:S71–6.

60. Mazza S, Frot M, Rey AE. A comprehensive literature review of chronic pain and memory. Prog Neuropsychopharmacol Biol Psychiatry 2018;183–92. https://doi.org/10.1016/j.pnpbp.2017.08.006.

61. Craig A, Tran Y, Wijesuriya N, et al. Fatigue and tiredness in people with spinal cord injury. J Psychosom Res 2012;73(3):205–10.

62. Berlowitz DJ, Wadsworth B, Ross J. Respiratory problems and management in people with spinal cord injury. Breathe (Sheff) 2016;12(4):328–40.

63. Brown R, DiMarco AF, Hoit JD, et al. Respiratory dysfunction and management in spinal cord injury. Respir Care 2006;51(8):853–68.

64. Areza-Fegyveres R, Kairalla RA, Carvalho CRR, et al. Cognition and chronic hypoxia in pulmonary diseases. Dement Neuropsychol 2010;4(1):14–22.

65. Cleutjens FAHM, Janssen DJA, Ponds RWHM, et al. COgnitive-pulmonary disease. Biomed Res Int 2014;1–8. https://doi.org/10.1155/2014/697825.

66. Bors M, Tomic R, Perlman DM, et al. Cognitive function in idiopathic pulmonary fibrosis. Chron Respir Dis 2015;12(4):365–72.

67. Caldera-Alvarado G, Khan DA, Defina LF, et al. Relationship between asthma and cognition: the Cooper Center Longitudinal Study. Allergy 2013;68(4):545–8.

68. Grassmann M, Vlemincx E, Von Leupoldt A, et al. Respiratory changes in response to cognitive load: a systematic review. Neural Plast 2016;1–16. https://doi.org/10.1155/2016/8146809.

69. Chiodo AE, Sitrin RG, Bauman KA. Sleep disordered breathing in spinal cord injury: a systematic review. J Spinal Cord Med 2016;374–82. https://doi.org/10.1080/10790268.2015.1126449.

70. Leng Y, McEvoy CT, Allen IE, et al. Association of sleep-disordered breathing with cognitive function and risk of cognitive impairment: a systematic review and meta-analysis. JAMA Neurol 2017;74(10):1237–45.

71. Sajkov D, Marshall R, Walker P, et al. Sleep apnoea related hypoxia is associated with cognitive disturbances in patients with tetraplegia. Spinal Cord 1998;36(4):231–9.

72. Schembri R, Spong J, Graco M, et al. Neuropsychological function in patients with acute tetraplegia and sleep disordered breathing. Sleep 2017;40(2). https://doi.org/10.1093/sleep/zsw037.

73. Zuccalà G, Onder G, Pedone C, et al. Hypotension and cognitive impairment: selective association in patients with heart failure. Neurology 2001;57(11):1986–92.

74. Heims HC, Critchley HD, Martin NH, et al. Cognitive functioning in orthostatic hypotension due to pure autonomic failure. Clin Auton Res 2006;16(2):113–20.

75. Wecht JM, Bauman WA. Decentralized cardiovascular autonomic control and cognitive deficits in persons with spinal cord injury. J Spinal Cord Med 2013; 36(2):74–81.

76. Jegede AB, Rosado-Rivera D, Bauman WA, et al. Cognitive performance in hypotensive persons with spinal cord injury. Clin Auton Res 2010;20(1):3–9.

77. Sachdeva R, Nightingale TE, Krassioukov AV. The blood pressure pendulum following spinal cord injury: implications for vascular cognitive impairment. Int J Mol Sci 2019. https://doi.org/10.3390/ijms20102464.

78. Phillips AA, Squair JR, Currie KD, et al. 2015 ParaPan American Games: autonomic function, but not physical activity, is associated with vascular-cognitive impairment in spinal cord injury. J Neurotrauma 2017;34(6):1283–8.

79. Phillips AA, Warburton DER, Ainslie PN, et al. Regional neurovascular coupling and cognitive performance in those with low blood pressure secondary to high-level spinal cord injury: improved by alpha-1 agonist midodrine hydrochloride. J Cereb Blood Flow Metab 2014;34(5):794–801.

80. Girard TD, Pandharipande PP, Ely EW. Delirium in the intensive care unit. Crit Care 2008;12(Suppl 3):S3.

81. Colbenson GA, Johnson A, Wilson ME. Post-intensive care syndrome: impact, prevention, and management. Breathe (Sheff) 2019;98–101. https://doi.org/10.1183/20734735.0013-2019.

82. Jure I, Labombarda F. Spinal cord injury drives chronic brain changes. Neural Regen Res 2017;1044–7. https://doi.org/10.4103/1673-5374.211177.

83. Nardone R, Höller Y, Brigo F, et al. Functional brain reorganization after spinal cord injury: systematic review of animal and human studies. Brain Res 2013;58–73. https://doi.org/10.1016/j.brainres.2012.12.034.

84. Nicotra A, Critchley HD, Mathias CJ, et al. Emotional and autonomic consequences of spinal cord injury explored using functional brain imaging. Brain 2006;129(3):718–28.

85. Wrigley PJ, Gustin SM, Macey PM, et al. Anatomical changes in human motor cortex and motor pathways following complete thoracic spinal cord injury. Cereb Cortex 2009;19(1):224–32.

86. Faden AI, Wu J, Stoica BA, et al. Progressive inflammation-mediated neurodegeneration after traumatic brain or spinal cord injury. Br J Pharmacol 2016;681–91. https://doi.org/10.1111/bph.13179.

87. Wu J, Zhao Z, Sabirzhanov B, et al. Spinal cord injury causes brain inflammation associated with cognitive and affective changes: role of cell cycle pathways. J Neurosci 2014;34(33):10989–1006.

88. Gris D, Hamilton EF, Weaver LC. The systemic inflammatory response after spinal cord injury damages lungs and kidneys. Exp Neurol 2008;211(1):259–70.

89. Allison DJ, Ditor DS. Immune dysfunction and chronic inflammation following spinal cord injury. Spinal Cord 2015;53(1):14–8.

90. Bradbury CL, Wodchis WP, Mikulis DJ, et al. Traumatic brain injury in patients with traumatic spinal cord injury: clinical and economic consequences. Arch Phys Med Rehabil 2008;89(12 Suppl):S77–84.

91. Macciocchi SN, Bowman B, Coker J, et al. Effect of co-morbid traumatic brain injury on functional outcome of persons with spinal cord injuries. Am J Phys Med Rehabil 2004;83(1):22–6.

92. DeJong G, Tian W, Hsieh C-H, et al. Rehospitalization in the first year of traumatic spinal cord injury after discharge from medical rehabilitation. Arch Phys Med Rehabil 2013;94(4):S87–97.

93. Davidoff G, Schultz JS, Lieb T, et al. Rehospitalization after initial rehabilitation for acute spinal cord injury: incidence and risk factors. Arch Phys Med Rehabil 1990; 71(2):121–4.

94. Elliott TR, Bush BA, Chen Y. Social problem-solving abilities predict pressure sore occurrence in the first 3 years of spinal cord injury. Rehabil Psychol 2006;51(1): 69–77.

95. Craig A, Nicholson Perry K, Guest R, et al. Adjustment following chronic spinal cord injury: determining factors that contribute to social participation. Br J Health Psychol 2015;20(4):807–23.

96. Lombard L, Kwasnika C, Brooks M. Spinal cord medicine. In: Kirshblum SC, Lin VW, editors. Spinal cord medicine. 3rd edition. New York: Springer; 2019. p. 573.

Management Strategies for Spinal Cord Injury Pain Updated for the Twenty-First Century

Erik Shaw, DO[a],*, Michael Saulino, MD, PhD[b]

KEYWORDS

- Spinal cord injury • Traumatic myelopathy • Chronic pain • Neuropathic pain

KEY POINTS

- Chronic neuropathic pain is a common, yet vexing, condition following traumatic spinal cord injury with numerous treatment modalities available to the managing physiatrist.
- Oral medication strategies include antiepileptics, antidepressants, spasmolytics, and other pharmacologic interventions.
- Interventional approaches include spinal cord stimulator, peripheral nerve stimulation, and intrathecal drug delivery.

INTRODUCTION

Traumatic spinal cord injury (SCI) often results in several life-altering impairments, including paralysis, sensory loss, and neurogenic bowel/bladder dysfunction. Some of these SCI-related conditions can be accommodated with compensatory strategies. Perhaps no SCI-associated condition is more troublesome and recalcitrant to the treating physiatrist than chronic neuropathic pain. In addition to the expected challenges in treating any chronic pain condition, treatment of SCI-related pain has the added difficulty of disruption of normal neural pathways that subserve pain transmission and attenuation. This article reviews selected treatment strategies for SCI-associated neuropathic pain.

PHARMACOLOGIC
Antiepileptic Drugs

At present, pregabalin (brand-name Lyrica, Pfizer) is the only medication that currently has Food and Drug Administration (FDA) indication for SCI-associated pain. This agent

[a] Shepherd Spine and Pain Institute, 2020 Peachtree Street Northwest, Atlanta, GA 30309, USA;
[b] Sidney Kimmel Medical College, MossRehab, 60 Township Line Road, Elkins Park, PA 19027, USA
* Corresponding author.
E-mail address: Erik.Shaw@shepherd.org

Phys Med Rehabil Clin N Am 31 (2020) 369–378
https://doi.org/10.1016/j.pmr.2020.03.004
1047-9651/20/© 2020 Elsevier Inc. All rights reserved.

received approval in 2004 for treatment of seizures, postherpetic neuralgia, and diabetic neuropathy. It was subsequently approved for treatment of fibromyalgia (in 2007), and last, for pain associated with SCI (in 2012). The medication now has approval in more than 100 countries. Pregabalin is a structural derivative of the inhibitory neurotransmitter gamma-aminobutyric acid. It is an alpha 2-delta ligand that has analgesic, anticonvulsant, anxiolytic, and sleep-modulating properties. Pregabalin binds potently to the alpha 2-delta subunit of voltage-gated calcium channels. It is hypothesized that this binding reduces the influx of calcium into hyperexcited neurons, which in turn results in a reduction in the release of several neurotransmitters, including glutamate, noradrenaline, serotonin, dopamine, and substance P.[1] This purported mechanism supports the use of pregabalin in numerous neuropathic pain conditions, including SCI-neuropathic pain. There is some concern that use of pregabalin for off-label use is excessively ubiquitous.[2]

A recent metaanalysis of randomized controlled trials examined the safety and effectiveness of pregabalin in SCI-associated neuropathic pain. This analysis identified 5 high-level studies, including 3 randomized controlled trials, 1 open-label trial, and 1 crossover trial. Study duration varied from 4 to 53 weeks. Most pregabalin-treated patients demonstrated a 30% to 50% reduction in pain compared with placebo-treated subjects. The pain relief appeared to be well sustained. The dosing ranged from 150 to 600 mg/d in 2 or 3 divided doses. The most common adverse events were mild or moderate, typically transient, somnolence and dizziness. Edema was reported in 15% to 20% of the pregabalin patients across all trials.[3] There is some suggestion that the emergence of pregabalin-related adverse effects may be a dose-dependent phenomenon.[4]

Similar to pregabalin, gabapentin is also active at voltage-gated calcium channels. Gabapentin and pregabalin (along with several other experimental agents, such as mirogablin, phenibut, and atagabalin) are collectively known as gabapentinoids.[5] Gabapentin has been considered effective in SCI-associated neuropathic pain in several smaller studies. Levendoglu and colleagues[6] reported that gabapentin was more effective than placebo in a crossover study involving 20 paraplegics with neuropathic pain that had been present for more than 6 months. Tai and colleagues[7] executed a prospective, randomized, double-blind, crossover study on 7 patients when they were more than 30 days after their injury with SCI-related pain. To and associates[8] did a retrospective chart review of 44 patients with SCI-related neuropathic pain examining the effectiveness of gabapentin. Seventy-six percent of these subjects reported a reduction in pain intensity. Last, Putzke and colleagues[9] examined the use of gabapentin in this population with a longitudinal observational study on 27 patients. This group observed a relatively high discontinuance rate (6/27 or 22%). Of the remaining 21 patients, 14 (67%) reported a greater than 2 point reduction in visual analogue scale (VAS) at 6 months. There is some concern that gabapentin use in the SCI patient is associated with cognitive dysfunction.[10] It is reasonable to conclude that gabapentin can be effective in neuropathic pain in SCI-associated neuropathic pain. One important collateral effect of gabapentinoid therapy early in the course of SCI is the potential linkage to improved motor recovery.[11,12] This effect was not seen in non–gabapentinoid anticonvulsants.[5] Of interest, a study of intrathecal gabapentin failed to demonstrate any benefit in an unselected chronic pain population despite promising results from animal data, particularly with neuropathic pain.[13]

The use of antidepressants for below-level neuropathic SCI pain has a long-standing tradition. The substantial benefit of tricyclic antidepressants (TCAs) in neuropathic pain has led to this use.[14] Perhaps the most commonly used agent is amitriptyline. There are conflicting results in the medical literature with some studies demonstrating efficacy[15] and other studies descriptive of minimal efficacy[16] in SCI-associated pain. One comparison trial described a therapeutic benefit of amitriptyline over gabapentin.[15] The so-called second-generation TCAs (ie, secondary amines, such as nortriptyline, desipramine, and protriptyline) are preferred because analgesic efficacy is equivalent, and tolerability is better compared with first-generation TCAs (ie, tertiary amines such as amitriptyline, clomipramine, and doxepin). All TCAs are considered to have a ceiling effect. Thus, once a therapeutic effect is achieved, further dosing increases should be avoided in order to minimize adverse effects.[17] Although polypharmacy is a common approach in many chronic pain patients, a small study failed to demonstrate improved effectiveness of combining anticonvulsant and antidepressant therapy compared with individual therapy.[18]

A most recent addition to the armamentarium of antidepressant use for chronic pain is the dual serotonin and norepinephrine reuptake inhibitors (SNRIs). Medications in this class include duloxetine, milnacipran, levomilnacipran, venlafaxine, and desvenlafaxine. Pain modulation appears to be independent of their antidepressant properties. Duloxetine, the first medication approved for use in the United States within this class, has FDA indication for chronic musculoskeletal pain, fibromyalgia, and diabetic neuropathy. A small trial of duloxetine for central neuropathic pain caused by either stroke or SCI failed to show a reduction in pain intensity but did demonstrate changes in other aspects of these chronic pain syndromes, including allodynia.[19] A randomized trial of extended venlafaxine for depression associated with SCI suggested benefit of this medication for non–neuropathic pain but not neuropathic pain.[20] There are no reports of using of either milnacipran or levomilnacipran for chronic SCI-associated pain. There are several SNRIs in various stages of clinical development for a wide variety of indications.[21]

Opioid medications have been suggested as a reasonable option for chronic nociceptive and perhaps neuropathic pain. Perhaps no other decision in medicine causes more anxiety than prescribing opiates for patients with chronic, non–cancer pain. Concerns over diversion, misuse, dependence, addiction, monitoring, and cost can make the analysis of using chronic opiate therapy troublesome for even experienced clinicians.[22] The SCI patient may be at great risk for substance abuse disorder compared with non-SCI individuals.[23] The potential exacerbation of neurogenic bowel dysfunction owing to opioid-related constipation makes this decision even more challenging. There are several new strategies for management of opioid-related constipation, including peripheral opioid receptor antagonists and prokinetic agents.[24] In addition, there is some suggestion that opioid use in acute SCI might decrease locomotor recovery as well as increase the propensity for development of neuropathic pain.[25] A review of the use of opioids in neuropathic pain suggested clinical efficacy of this medication class for long-term use. It is relevant to note that this review has a large preponderance of peripheral-based neuropathic pain (diabetic neuropathy or postherpetic neuropathy), but some SCI subjects were included.[26] One retrospective review reported that opioids were the most commonly used oral pain agent in a Veterans Administration population of SCI/spinal cord disorders.[27]

There are several developments within the opioid class of medications that may be of specific interest to physiatrists treating SCI-related pain. Tapentadol is a centrally acting analgesic with dual mechanisms of action, agonist activity at the mu-opioid receptor and inhibition of norepinephrine reuptake. A potential therapeutic advantage of this agent is its utility in neuropathic pain.[28] One small randomized trial of tapentadol in SCI patients with neuropathic pain suggested a positive therapeutic benefit with the recognition of significant adverse-effect profile.[29] Another dual-acting product is tramadol, which is a combination of an SNRI and a mu-opioid agonist. This medication is noteworthy because its mechanism of action is distinct from those of other opioids. Tramadol has been shown to demonstrate benefit in osteoarthritis, fibromyalgia, and neuropathic pain; however, there is insufficient evidence to definitely define tramadol as more effective compared with other opioids.[30] A small, randomized controlled trial in SCI-related neuropathic pain demonstrated a positive response to this medication.[29] Tramadol does not appear to influence neurologic outcomes after SCI.[31]

The relationship between pain and spasticity is complex. Reduction of spasticity may reduce the pain associated with biomechanical pain. Modulation of spasticity may not be effective in reducing neuropathic pain.[32] There are several oral medications that can accomplish spasticity reduction, including baclofen, tizanidine, diazepam, and dantrolene. Of particular interest, tizanidine has a dual mechanism of action, an alpha-2 adrenergic agonist at the spinal level and an influence on descending noradrenergic pathways. It is this latter mechanism that may be of particular interest in the management of SCI-related pain.[33] There is some suggestion that tizanidine can improve ambulatory capacity when combined with locomotor training.[34] Similarly, botulinum toxins have the potential to reduce muscle overactivity in a focally directed manner.[35] Over and above their antispasticity activities, botulinum toxins have the capacity to be antinociceptive.[36,37] One randomized trial suggested benefit of botulinum toxin injections into painful areas.[38]

Although unknown to many providers, lithium has shown promise in treating neuropathic pain in persons with chronic SCI. Yang and colleagues[39] demonstrated that lithium reduced pain in C4 through T10 in American Spinal Injury Association impairment scale A-C patients after 6 weeks of treatment. The target laboratory level of 0.6 to 1.2 nmol was observed, and dramatic reductions were seen. Some patients even had complete elimination of their pain. Shimizu and colleagues[40] showed that in a rat model of SCI, intrathecal lithium reduced heat hyperalgesia and cold and mechanical allodynia but did not affect mechanical hyperalgesia. Shaw reviewed results of a consecutive series of 27 patients treated with oral lithium.[41] Characteristics of the patients included tetraplegia and paraplegia as well as complete and incomplete patients, and there is a statistically significant reduction in pain in all categories. Almost half had a 50% or greater reduction in pain, whereas 2 patients had an increase in pain. There are no significant safety issues during the treatment. Treatment was for 12 weeks, and laboratory values were assessed every 2 to 3 weeks. In this case series, there was a tendency for those with incomplete injuries and tetraplegics to have better improvement in pain.

Medicinal marijuana and synthetic cannabinoids represent intriguing pharmacologic choices for the management of SCI-associated pain. *Cannabis* contains 60 or more cannabinoids, the most abundant of which are delta-9-tetrahydrocannabinol (THC) and cannabidiol (CBD). Rintala and colleagues[42] executed a small study with dronabinol on SCI-related neuropathic pain. This agent is a pure isomer of THC. This investigation failed to demonstrate a significant difference in pain intensity compared with an active control. Sativex (GW Pharma Ltd) is a cannabis extract that contains THC + CBD at a fixed ratio, delivered as an oromucosal spray. It has indication for multiple sclerosis–related spasticity in several countries but not as of yet in the United States.[43] A study of neuropathic pain associated with multiple sclerosis failed to demonstrate significant differences during the double-blind phase of this trial.[44] There are no specific reports on the use of this agent in SCI-associated pain. One randomized trial suggested benefit of vaporized cannabis over placebo for SCI neuropathic pain.[34]

Nicotine has been reported to exacerbate SCI-related pain with abstinence resulting in relief. One recent study examined the effect of nicotine in a randomized, placebo-controlled crossover design on the subtypes of SCI-related pain (neuropathic, musculoskeletal, and mixed pain) among smokers and nonsmokers. This study involved 42 subjects of which two-thirds were paraplegic. Nonsmokers with SCI showed a reduction in mixed forms of pain following nicotine exposure, whereas smokers with SCI reported an increase in pain for both mixed and neuropathic pain. This study suggests differential effects on SCI-related pain for smokers and nonsmokers. This observation potentially offers some insight into the mechanisms of SCI-associated pain as well as supporting the suggestion of smoking cessation in some spinal cord–injured patients.[45]

Interventional

Intrathecal drug delivery provides direct administration of therapeutic agents to the subarachnoid space where they have enhanced access to receptor sites. Intrathecal baclofen is a well-established technique for reduction of spasticity associated with SCI.[46,47] To the extent that spasticity is related to musculoskeletal pain, this technique has the capacity to attenuate pain in this population. However, the use of intrathecal baclofen as a pure pain-modulating agent is limited.[48] Intrathecal opioids in combination with baclofen, bupivacaine, and clonidine show promise. According to the Polyanalgesic Consensus Guidelines, morphine and ziconotide are first-line medications along with hydromorphone.[49] Combination therapy, although off label, is the standard of practice according to a survey of active pump patients, and the overwhelming majority were combination therapy.[50] Although this study was not specific to SCI, the investigators have considerable clinical experience treating SCI in a combination manner with success.

Ziconotide is an N-type calcium channel blocker approved in 2004 by the FDA to treat severe chronic pain of both nociceptive and neuropathic type.[51] Given the refractory nature of SCI neuropathic pain, some researchers have shown that ziconotide is helpful in this clinical situation. Saulino[52] reported a case report of a patient with severe at and below-level neuropathic pain. Previously on hydromorphone, the patient had been titrated up to hydromorphone at 8 mg/d over 15 months. The below-level pain was not improved. Ziconotide was added, after weaning hydromorphone, at 2.4 μg/d and titrated up to 10 μg/d. No side effects were noted. Hydromorphone was added back in at 1.32 mg/d, and ziconotide was added back in at 11 μg/d. At and below-level pain was improved by 80%. In another study, Brinzeu and colleagues[53] trialed ziconotide in a prospective manner. Patients received 0.5-, 1.0-, or 1.5-μg bolus doses in 2 mL every 72 hours. If successful, as noted by improved pain of 40% or more, the pump was implanted. If the bolus trial was not successful, a catheter was placed with larger boluses over 3 to 5 days. Fourteen out of 20 patients were responders, although 2 patients had side effects, including elevated creatine phosphokinase levels, which precluded implantation of the pump. Long-term follow-up pain demonstrated an improvement in pain of 50% or better in the 11 subjects who had been implanted. Shaw[54] found that in patients with multiple sclerosis and SCI, a combination of ziconotide with baclofen reduced the need for baclofen by roughly 25% to 30% in patients who were on more than 800 μg/d of intrathecal baclofen. This reduced the need for more frequent pump refill as well as reduced side effects and increased overall control of spasticity.

Spinal cord stimulation (SCS) is defined as posterior epidural stimulation of the dorsal columns. The concept of sensory spasticity has been presented, and the treatment of pain will also improve spasticity.[55] In fact, SCS has been used to treat spasticity since the 1980s, with good results.[56] Shaw has presented a meeting abstract in which 12 spinal cord–injured patients received dorsal column stimulation for treatment of pain.[57] Placement of the electrodes was above the injury in most cases. The patients with complete injuries had variable success; however, none of them experienced paresthesia at stimulation below their injury. In the incompletely injured patients, paresthesias were experienced at varying levels of stimulation intensity. The incomplete spinal cord–injured patients had a higher degree of pain relief than did the complete patients; although 1 complete patient, who had been injured less than 2 years, had complete relief of pain.[57] Lagauche and colleagues[58] executed a review of this modality in SCI-related pain and failed to find a consistently positive therapeutic effect.

A particularly interesting, albeit experimental, neuromodulation approach to SCI-associated pain is oscillating field stimulation. To assess the possibility of this therapy, a human trial of a low-voltage, alternating polarity device caused substantive neurologic recovery, as was suspected from animal studies. Pain was assessed during this trial to ensure that this device did not cause pain. Somewhat surprisingly, use of this device was associated with a rather dramatic reduction in pain. Following the 15-week treatment phase, VAS scores improved from a mean of 8 to a mean of 2 at 6 months after treatment had been discontinued. No neuropathic pain was reported in any patient. The status of this device is uncertain until a larger, multicenter trial is undertaken.[59]

Peripheral nerve stimulation (PNS) has seen a dramatic increase in use over the last few years. Small, percutaneously implanted systems that provide electrical impulses to peripheral nerves have supplanted the need for open surgical procedures. The authors' experience includes primarily axillary nerve stimulation for shoulder pain with SPRINT from SPR Therapeutics. A relative benefit of this device is that it is placed percutaneously without surgical incision and is removed after 60 days, not requiring long-term implantation or surgical placement. This device was used primarily to treat nociceptive pain from weakness in tetraplegia. The use of PNS has been described in several pain syndromes, including poststroke shoulder pain, phantom limb pain, low back pain, and so forth.[60,61] There is 1 case report describing the use of PNS in shoulder pain following SCI.[62] This intervention may be well poised to play a significant role in pain management of the SCI patients in the future. Both authors have used this technique with meaningful results in their spinal cord–injured patients. Dr Saulino has experience with Bioness implanted over both the femoral and the sciatic nerves to treat lower-extremity neuropathic pain in complete and incomplete SCI patients. The Bioness device requires permanent surgical implantation. Although risks are relatively low with PNS, possible nerve injury, vascular injury, and device malfunction are all possible complications of PNS therapy. Good ultrasound skills are required in order to safely implant these devices near most peripheral nerves. The authors would like to stress that the data on this technique and treatment are extremely preliminary and require much more rigorous study and exploration.

SUMMARY

SCI-associated neuropathic pain is clearly a challenging pain syndrome. This review has demonstrated a wide array of potential interventions. Further investigation by both the SCI and the pain communities is warranted in an effort to further delineate the nature of this problem and create more effective treatment strategies. Physiatrists are uniquely positioned to participate in this process and should engage this process vigorously.

DISCLOSURE

E. Shaw disclosures: Boston Scientific (speakers bureau), Ter Sera (consultant, speakers bureau), BDSI (speakers bureau), SPR Therapeutics (speakers bureau); M. Saulino disclosures: Medtronic Inc (speakers bureau, clinical investigator), Ipsen (speaker bureau), Bioness (clinical investigator), SPR Therapeutics (speakers bureau).

REFERENCES

1. Gajraj NM. Pregabalin: its pharmacology and use in pain management. Anesth Analg 2007;105(6):1805–15.
2. Goodman CW, Brett AS. A clinical overview of off-label use of gabapentinoid drugs. JAMA Intern Med 2019;179(5):695–701.
3. Yu X, Liu T, Zhao D, et al. Efficacy and safety of pregabalin in neuropathic pain followed spinal cord injury: a review and meta-analysis of randomized controlled trials. Clin J Pain 2019;35(3):272–8.
4. Freynhagen R, Serpell M, Emir B, et al. A comprehensive drug safety evaluation of pregabalin in peripheral neuropathic pain. Pain Pract 2015;15(1):47–57.
5. Calandre EP, Rico-Villademoros F, Slim M. Alpha2delta ligands, gabapentin, pregabalin and mirogabalin: a review of their clinical pharmacology and therapeutic use. Expert Rev Neurother 2016;16(11):1263–77.
6. Levendoglu F, Ogun CO, Ozerbil O, et al. Gabapentin is a first line drug for the treatment of neuropathic pain in spinal cord injury. Spine (Phila Pa 1976) 2004; 29(7):743–51.
7. Tai Q, Kirshblum S, Chen B, et al. Gabapentin in the treatment of neuropathic pain after spinal cord injury: a prospective, randomized, double-blind, crossover trial. J Spinal Cord Med 2002;25(2):100–5.
8. To TP, Lim TC, Hill ST, et al. Gabapentin for neuropathic pain following spinal cord injury. Spinal Cord 2002;40(6):282–5.
9. Putzke JD, Richards JS, Kezar L, et al. Long-term use of gabapentin for treatment of pain after traumatic spinal cord injury. Clin J Pain 2002;18(2):116–21.
10. Shem K, Barncord S, Flavin K, et al. Adverse cognitive effect of gabapentin in individuals with spinal cord injury: preliminary findings. Spinal Cord Ser Cases 2018;4:9, 018-0038-y. [eCollection 2018].
11. Warner FM, Cragg JJ, Jutzeler CR, et al. Early administration of gabapentinoids improves motor recovery after human spinal cord injury. Cell Rep 2017;18(7): 1614–8.
12. Cragg JJ, Haefeli J, Jutzeler CR, et al. Effects of pain and pain management on motor recovery of spinal cord-injured patients: a longitudinal study. Neurorehabil Neural Repair 2016;30(8):753–61.
13. Rauck R, Coffey RJ, Schultz DM, et al. Intrathecal gabapentin to treat chronic intractable noncancer pain. Anesthesiology 2013;119(3):675–86.
14. Sindrup SH, Jensen TS. Efficacy of pharmacological treatments of neuropathic pain: an update and effect related to mechanism of drug action. Pain 1999; 83(3):389–400.
15. Rintala DH, Holmes SA, Courtade D, et al. Comparison of the effectiveness of amitriptyline and gabapentin on chronic neuropathic pain in persons with spinal cord injury. Arch Phys Med Rehabil 2007;88(12):1547–60.
16. Cardenas DD, Warms CA, Turner JA, et al. Efficacy of amitriptyline for relief of pain in spinal cord injury: results of a randomized controlled trial. Pain 2002; 96(3):365–73.
17. Mico JA, Ardid D, Berrocoso E, et al. Antidepressants and pain. Trends Pharmacol Sci 2006;27(7):348–54.
18. McKinley EC, Richardson EJ, McGwin G, et al. Evaluating the effectiveness of antidepressant therapy adjuvant to gabapentin and pregabalin for treatment of SCI-related neuropathic pain. J Spinal Cord Med 2018;41(6):637–44.

19. Vranken JH, Hollmann MW, van der Vegt MH, et al. Duloxetine in patients with central neuropathic pain caused by spinal cord injury or stroke: a randomized, double-blind, placebo-controlled trial. Pain 2011;152(2):267–73.

20. Fann JR, Bombardier CH, Richards JS, et al. Venlafaxine extended-release for depression following spinal cord injury: a randomized clinical trial. JAMA Psychiatry 2015;72(3):247–58.

21. Stahl SM, Grady MM, Moret C, et al. SNRIs: their pharmacology, clinical efficacy, and tolerability in comparison with other classes of antidepressants. CNS Spectr 2005;10(9):732–47.

22. Hallinan R, Osborn M, Cohen M, et al. Increasing the benefits and reducing the harms of prescription opioid analgesics. Drug Alcohol Rev 2011;30(3):315–23.

23. Hand BN, Krause JS, Simpson KN. Dose and duration of opioid use in propensity score-matched, privately insured opioid users with and without spinal cord injury. Arch Phys Med Rehabil 2018;99(5):855–61.

24. Walters JB, Montagnini M. Current concepts in the management of opioid-induced constipation. J Opioid Manag 2010;6(6):435–44.

25. Woller SA, Hook MA. Opioid administration following spinal cord injury: implications for pain and locomotor recovery. Exp Neurol 2013;247:328–41.

26. Eisenberg E, McNicol E, Carr DB. Opioids for neuropathic pain. Cochrane Database Syst Rev 2006;(3):CD006146.

27. Hatch MN, Raad J, Suda K, et al. Evaluating the use of Medicare Part D in the veteran population with spinal cord injury/disorder. Arch Phys Med Rehabil 2018;99(6):1099–107.

28. Duehmke RM, Derry S, Wiffen PJ, et al. Tramadol for neuropathic pain in adults. Cochrane Database Syst Rev 2017;6:CD003726.

29. Norrbrink C, Lundeberg T. Tramadol in neuropathic pain after spinal cord injury: a randomized, double-blind, placebo-controlled trial. Clin J Pain 2009;25(3):177–84.

30. Leppert W. Tramadol as an analgesic for mild to moderate cancer pain. Pharmacol Rep 2009;61(6):978–92.

31. Chaves RHF, Souza CC, Furlaneto IP, et al. Influence of tramadol on functional recovery of acute spinal cord injury in rats. Acta Cir Bras 2018;33(12):1087–94.

32. Ward AB, Kadies M. The management of pain in spasticity. Disabil Rehabil 2002;24(8):443–53.

33. Kamen L, Henney HR 3rd, Runyan JD. A practical overview of tizanidine use for spasticity secondary to multiple sclerosis, stroke, and spinal cord injury. Curr Med Res Opin 2008;24(2):425–39.

34. Duffell LD, Brown GL, Mirbagheri MM. Facilitatory effects of anti-spastic medication on robotic locomotor training in people with chronic incomplete spinal cord injury. J Neuroeng Rehabil 2015;12:29, 015-0018-4.

35. Yan X, Lan J, Liu Y, et al. Efficacy and safety of botulinum toxin type A in spasticity caused by spinal cord injury: a randomized, controlled trial. Med Sci Monit 2018;24:8160–71.

36. Wheeler A, Smith HS. Botulinum toxins: mechanisms of action, antinociception and clinical applications. Toxicology 2013;306:124–46.

37. Park J, Park HJ. Botulinum toxin for the treatment of neuropathic pain. Toxins (Basel) 2017;9(9). https://doi.org/10.3390/toxins9090260.

38. Han ZA, Song DH, Oh HM, et al. Botulinum toxin type A for neuropathic pain in patients with spinal cord injury. Ann Neurol 2016;79(4):569–78.

39. Yang ML, Li JJ, So KF, et al. Efficacy and safety of lithium carbonate treatment of chronic spinal cord injuries: a double-blind, randomized, placebo-controlled clinical trial. Spinal Cord 2012;50(2):141–6.

40. Shimizu T, Shibata M, Wakisaka S, et al. Intrathecal lithium reduces neuropathic pain responses in a rat model of peripheral neuropathy. Pain 2000;85(1–2):59–64.

41. Rozak MR, Shaw E. Chronic Central Neuropathic Pain Significantly Reduced With Lithium Carbonate: A Case Series. American Journal of Physical Medicine and Rehabilitation 2019;98(3 Suppl 1):a1–158.

42. Rintala DH, Fiess RN, Tan G, et al. Effect of dronabinol on central neuropathic pain after spinal cord injury: a pilot study. Am J Phys Med Rehabil 2010; 89(10):840–8.

43. Notcutt W, Langford R, Davies P, et al. A placebo-controlled, parallel-group, randomized withdrawal study of subjects with symptoms of spasticity due to multiple sclerosis who are receiving long-term Sativex(R) (nabiximols). Mult Scler 2012; 18(2):219–28.

44. Langford RM, Mares J, Novotna A, et al. A double-blind, randomized, placebo-controlled, parallel-group study of THC/CBD oromucosal spray in combination with the existing treatment regimen, in the relief of central neuropathic pain in patients with multiple sclerosis. J Neurol 2013;260(4):984–97.

45. Richardson EJ, Richards JS, Stewart CC, et al. Effects of nicotine on spinal cord injury pain: a randomized, double-blind, placebo controlled crossover trial. Top Spinal Cord Inj Rehabil 2012;18(2):101–5.

46. Coffey JR, Cahill D, Steers W, et al. Intrathecal baclofen for intractable spasticity of spinal origin: results of a long-term multicenter study. J Neurosurg 1993;78(2): 226–32.

47. Ordia JI, Fischer E, Adamski E, et al. Continuous intrathecal baclofen infusion by a programmable pump in 131 consecutive patients with severe spasticity of spinal origin. Neuromudulation 2002;5(1):16–24.

48. Saulino M. The use of intrathecal baclofen in pain management. Pain Manag 2012;2(6):603–8.

49. Deer TR, Pope JE, Hayek SM, et al. The Polyanalgesic Consensus Conference (PACC): recommendations on intrathecal drug infusion systems best practices and guidelines. Neuromodulation 2017;20(4):405–6.

50. Konrad PE, Huffman JM, Stearns LM, et al. Intrathecal drug delivery systems (IDDS): the Implantable Systems Performance Registry (ISPR). Neuromodulation 2016;19(8):848–56.

51. Wallace MS, Charapata SG, Fisher R, et al. Intrathecal ziconotide in the treatment of chronic nonmalignant pain: a randomized, double-blind, placebo-controlled clinical trial. Neuromodulation 2006;9(2):75–86.

52. Saulino M. Successful reduction of neuropathic pain associated with spinal cord injury via of a combination of intrathecal hydromorphone and ziconotide: a case report. Spinal Cord 2007;45(11):749–52.

53. Brinzeu A, Berthiller J, Caillet JB, et al. Ziconotide for spinal cord injury-related pain. Eur J Pain 2019;23(9):1688–700.

54. Shaw E. Ziconitide for Managing Central Neuropathic Pain Associated With Multiple Sclerosis: A Case Series. Presented at the AAPM 2011 Annual Meeting. National Harbor, March 24-27, 2011.

55. Sjolund BH. Pain and rehabilitation after spinal cord injury: the case of sensory spasticity? Brain Res Brain Res Rev 2002;40(1–3):250–6.

56. Barolat G, Singh-Sahni K, Staas WE Jr, et al. Epidural spinal cord stimulation in the management of spasms in spinal cord injury: a prospective study. Stereotact Funct Neurosurg 1995;64(3):153–64.

57. Shaw E. Clinical outcomes of spinal cord stimulation (SCS) in patients with chronic spinal cord injury in Abstracts from the 10th World Congress of the International Neuromodulation Society: Spine. Neuromodulation 2011;14(5):444–84.

58. Lagauche D, Facione J, Albert T, et al. The chronic neuropathic pain of spinal cord injury: which efficiency of neuropathic stimulation? Ann Phys Rehabil Med 2009;52(2):180–7.

59. Walters BC. Oscillating field stimulation in the treatment of spinal cord injury. PM R 2010;2(12 Suppl 2):S286–91.

60. Chakravarthy K, Nava A, Christo PJ, et al. Review of recent advances in peripheral nerve stimulation (PNS). Curr Pain Headache Rep 2016;20(11):60, 016-0590-8.

61. Pope JE, Carlson JD, Rosenberg WS, et al. Peripheral nerve stimulation for pain in extremities: an update. Prog Neurol Surg 2015;29:139–57.

62. Mehech D, Mejia M, Nemunaitis GA, et al. Percutaneous peripheral nerve stimulation for treatment of shoulder pain after spinal cord injury: a case report. J Spinal Cord Med 2018;41(1):119–24.

Conventional Respiratory Management of Spinal Cord Injury

John R. Bach, MD[a],*, Lindsay Burke, BA, MD[b], Michael Chiou, MD[c]

KEYWORDS

- Ventilatory support • Respiratory management • Spinal cord injury
- Respiratory support

KEY POINTS

- Long-term respiratory management outcomes for patients with high-level spinal cord injury have not significantly improved over the past 40 years.
- Patients who develop ventilatory failure are conventionally intubated for ventilatory support and airway suctioning, and if ventilator unweanable, undergo tracheotomy.
- Respiratory muscle training appears to increase respiratory muscle strength and endurance for the time that the patients perform the exercises.

Acute and long-term respiratory complications of spinal cord injury (SCI) are the main causes of death, and the incidence of the latter has not significantly decreased over the past 40 years.[1,2] Injury to both the anterior horn cells at C3 to C5 cervical levels and the adjacent lateral tracts of the spinal cord impair respiratory muscle function. With conventional management, that is, without access to noninvasive ventilatory support (NVS) or means to normalize cough flows by using mechanical insufflation-exsufflation (MIE), in the year following injury for complete tetraplegia, mortality is 93 (25%) of 382 from pneumonia and 132 (33%) of 382 from respiratory failure.[1,3] Long-term, the most frequent cause of death is respiratory complications, accounting for approximately 25% of mortality, as it has over the past 40 years.[1,2]

PATHOPHYSIOLOGY

There are 3 respiratory muscle groups: the inspiratory muscles, the expiratory muscles for coughing (predominantly abdominal), and the bulbar-innervated muscles (BIM) that

[a] Department of Physical Medicine and Rehabilitation, Rutgers University New Jersey Medical School, Behavioral Health Sciences Building, 183 South Orange Avenue, Newark, NJ 07103, USA; [b] Department of Medicine, Morristown Medical Center, 100 Madison Ave, Morristown, NJ 07960, USA; [c] Department of PM&R, Icahn School of Medicine at Mount Sinai, 3 East 101st Street, New York, NY 10029, USA
* Corresponding author.
E-mail address: bachjr@njms.rutgers.edu

Phys Med Rehabil Clin N Am 31 (2020) 379–395
https://doi.org/10.1016/j.pmr.2020.04.004
1047-9651/20/© 2020 Elsevier Inc. All rights reserved.

protect the airways. Inspiratory and expiratory muscle function can be entirely wiped out for lesions above the C3 level but BIM function is spared for any lesions that do not extend into the brain stem unless intubation and tracheotomy have caused irreparable damage to the strap muscles of the neck and the glottis. Patients managed with tracheostomy tubes have a 37% incidence of aspiration, and even after decannulation, the incidence remains 7% indefinitely.[4] Therefore, BIM are often affected in conventionally managed patients, that is, ventilator-dependent patients undergoing tracheotomies and not extubated to NVS.

The diaphragm is innervated by C3 to C5 levels. The parasternal and external intercostal muscles of the upper rib cage that stabilize the chest wall to prevent paradoxic breathing are innervated by T1 to T6 levels. The sternocleidomastoids are innervated by the spinal accessory nerve from C2 and C3 roots. They can lift the shoulders, extend the cervical spine, and expand the upper rib cage to stabilize and lift the chest wall as the diaphragm descends. The scalene muscles, innervated from C3 to C8 nerve roots, also lift the upper ribs to expand the chest. These accessory muscles can ventilate the lungs while the patient is upright even when the diaphragm is completely paralyzed. The same can be said for the tongue when it is used for glossopharyngeal ("frog") breathing.

The diaphragm is responsible for normal tidal breathing and for two-thirds of normal inspiratory capacity. Impairment of intercostal muscles and pelvic floor muscles that prevent protrusion of abdominal contents into the pelvis as the diaphragm descends, decrease the vital capacity (VC) even when the diaphragm and other accessory respiratory muscles are intact.

The VC is greater in the supine position for patients with SCI, as abdominal contents displace the diaphragm cephalad, lengthening it to a more favorable length-tension position. If the diaphragm is very weak or completely paralyzed, the accessory muscles can ventilate the lungs as noted, but this is fatiguing. With lumbar spine injuries, pelvic floor stabilization is lost.

With complete cervical lesions above the C2 level, the VC is often 0 mL. Patients with complete lesions at C5-6, on the other hand, are typically left with approximately 30% of normal VC in the sitting position and more when supine. The VC is usually less in the sitting position because abdominal contents sag and the diaphragm has less excursion to generate subatmospheric pressures for air to enter the lungs. On the other hand, patients with weak diaphragms but relatively intact accessory muscle function can increase tidal volumes and VC when sitting over what they have when supine.

The pulmonary morbidity and mortality for patients with SCI are often caused by chronic aspiration due to invasive airway tubes and inadequately prevented and treated upper respiratory infections (URIs) that cause airway mucous congestion, atelectasis, and pneumonia largely due to ineffective cough flows.[5,6] Cough peak flows (CPFs) more than 270 to 300 L/m are needed to expel airway debris to prevent pneumonia for adults.

The trachea divides approximately 27 times (**Fig. 1**). The first 6 divisions can be cleared only by creating adequate CPF. The next 21 divisions can be cleared only by the mucociliary elevator. Conventional airway mobilization methods are directed toward the latter rather than the former, none of which can effectively substitute for ineffective coughing, which may be the most important reason that respiratory prognoses have not improved.

EVALUATION

Outpatients are conventionally sent for pulmonary function testing, which is designed to evaluate for lung and airways disease for which there is an oxygenation

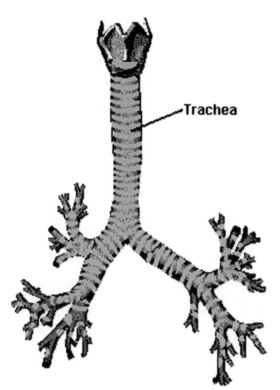

Fig. 1. The 27 divisions of the airways and the angle take off of the right main stem bronchus that the suction catheter enters 90% of the time.

requirement: forced VC (FVC), maximum inspiratory and expiratory pressures measured at the mouth, maximum expiratory flow rates, bronchodilator responses for reversible bronchospasm including exercise challenges, lung diffusion, plethysmography (chest and abdominal movements that can be falsely attributed to obstructive apneas and hypopneas rather than muscle weakness), gas exchange when arterial blood gas analyses are performed, none of which are needed for patients with ventilatory pump failure. Widely accepted guidelines suggest that FVC less than 50% of predicted normal justifies introduction of bilevel positive airway pressure (PAP) to treat the apneas and hypopneas of sleep-disordered breathing (SDB), a category that patients with ventilatory pump failure are conventionally lumped into. Specific evaluation for patients with pump failure is discussed in the John R. Bach and colleagues' article, "Noninvasive Respiratory Management of Spinal Cord Injury," elsewhere in this issue.

CONVENTIONAL INTERVENTIONS
Physical Therapeutic Interventions

Patients with SCI, who do not have tracheostomy tubes to impair their BIM and cause aspiration and mucociliary dysfunction, should, when medically stable, have essentially normal airways. Therefore, there is neither theoretic reason why, nor evidence that, routine chest oscillation, percussion, and vibration benefit them unless they have acute pulmonary disease or are overwhelmed with peripheral secretions. These techniques do not prevent intercurrent URIs or other complications. Although it is understood that an unopposed parasympathetic nervous system of high-level patients with SCI can stimulate copious volumes of submucosal gland mucus, as an acute (emergency) airway defense reflex mediated by vagal pathways in response to aspiration of foreign material, for stable high-level patients with SCI not experiencing acute challenges to the airways, gland secretion is under the control of local reflexes and appears to depend disproportionately on noncholinergic mechanisms. Most airway secretion is triggered by vasoactive intestinal polypeptides and tachykinins.[7] Thus, the stable high-level SCI patient without a tracheostomy tube to cause aspiration does not usually require manually or mechanically assisted coughing on a routine basis, whereas with a tube, frequent daily applications of physical therapeutic techniques and MIE may be needed to facilitate airway clearance.[7]

There are 9 postural drainage positions (**Fig. 2**) and the patient is placed in each for approximately 20 minutes to facilitate migration of secretions out of the lungs. The gravity drainage can be enhanced by percussion, vibration, and oscillation. However, although these techniques can facilitate secretion clearance from the peripheral 21 airway divisions, they do not substitute for effective coughing to clear the 6 central airway divisions.

Respiratory muscle training (RMT) has been used for more than 50 years for patients with SCI, chronic obstructive pulmonary disease (COPD), neuromuscular disease (NMD), and other conditions. For patients with COPD and NMD, it can improve endurance but not muscle strength.[8,9] The VC of patients with SCI can improve spontaneously even without routine administration of lung volume recruitment (LVR), perhaps for as long as 8 years,[10] so any effects of RMT can be more difficult to appreciate. It does appear, though, on the basis of metaanalyses and other studies, that RMT

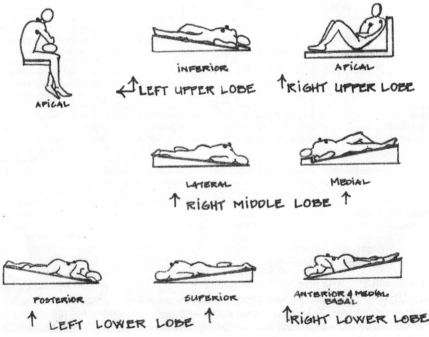

Fig. 2. The 9 positions of postural drainage. (*Courtesy of* L. Bach, Montreal, Canada.)

may indeed increase respiratory strength for patients with SCI.[11–13] Only 1 review of 5 of 11 studies suggested, however, that besides increasing maximum inspiratory and expiratory pressures and FVC, respiratory complications also decreased.[12] No increases in CPF were reported. It is very unlikely that RMT could ever prevent pneumonias and acute respiratory failure (ARF) as effectively as NVS and MIE. Further, any benefits of RMT are also quickly lost with cessation of training, so they would have to kept up for life.[11] Although long-term prognoses have not been reported to be improved for these patients, on the other hand, there does not appear to be any harm in the training itself.

Medications and Oxygen

Bronchospasm in SCI is typically due to loss of sympathetic lung innervation and responds to beta-2 agonists and ipratropium bromide. The latter also provides greater reduction in central airway resistance and less airway hyperresponsiveness to methacholine.[11] The use of bronchodilators appears to enhance MIE effectiveness for patients with SCI, especially during URIs. However, bronchodilators also can cause anxiety, tachycardia, and gastrointestinal distress.

Supplemental oxygen therapy (O2) can lead to ventilatory failure by suppressing ventilatory drive. It can exacerbate hypercapnia by more than 100 mm Hg and quickly result in obtundation and CO_2 narcosis.[14] Thus, O2 is not a substitute for ventilatory support or airway clearance. If NVS and MIE do not reverse the hypoxia and the patient is hypercapnic, O2 administration can be given only if the clinician is ready to intubate for the possibly sudden hypercapnic respiratory failure that the O2 can provoke.

Increasing Cough Flows

Manually assisted coughing

"Quad coughing" or manually assisted coughing can greatly increase cough flows and make the difference between developing pneumonia or not. Although a normal cough volume is 2.3 L of air,[15] and patients with less than 1.5 L of VC often have markedly diminished CPF even without expiratory muscle weakness,[16] air stacking to deep lung volumes is not conventionally administered (see the John R. Bach and colleagues' article, "Noninvasive Respiratory Management of Spinal Cord Injury," elsewhere in this issue). Nevertheless, abdominal thrusts with or without concomitant chest thrusts can increase CPF and often make them functional even without air stacking. Effective CPF exceed 300 L/m and there is little danger when cough flows are at least 270 L/m but as CPF decreases below 200 L/m with age, risk of pneumonia and ARF increase.[16–22] Indeed, 30% of otherwise healthy old people in nursing homes die of pneumonia in part because of ineffective cough flows.[23]

Mechanical insufflation-exsufflation

Although MIE is not yet a conventional intervention, especially in critical care, it is increasingly being used for outpatients, more as a technique of physical therapy, that is, on a twice-daily or thrice-daily schedule and at grossly inadequate settings, than for cough assistance. Twice-daily or thrice-daily MIE for patients with airway secretions is like having bronchitis and only coughing on schedule 2 or 3 times a day. Survival would be impossible. Amazingly, a patient with severe scoliosis operated on in a major New York City hospital had her MIE settings changed to 40 cm H2O pressures and 10 seconds of insufflation to 10 seconds of exsufflation. It did not occur to the clinicians that that would only permit her to take 3 breaths a minute. Obviously, she could not even get through the first 10-second insufflation. Any pressures less than 40 cm H2O are never the most effective. Although often described as a complication of "noninvasive ventilation," secretion encumbrance actually results from failure to use MIE effectively via both invasive and noninvasive interfaces. Correct MIE applications are discussed in the John R. Bach and colleagues' article, "Noninvasive Respiratory Management of Spinal Cord Injury," elsewhere in this issue.

Expiratory muscle electrical stimulation

Although this can hardly be considered conventional at this point, magnetic stimulation or surface electrical stimulation over the abdominal wall and over the dorsal epidural surface of the cord has been reported to increase expiratory flows to 6.4 to 7.4 L/s at airway pressures of 90 to 132 cm H2O for patients unable to generate more than 2 or 3 L/s of unassisted cough flows. Patients are also able to trigger the device independently.[24,25] These flows and pressures are comparable to those from optimally used MIE, so this may be an effective way to generate cough flows for patients with SCI whose lower motor neurons, peripheral nerves, and muscle physiology are normal. It remains to be seen if this intervention can translate into decreased pneumonia and ARF rates.

Although the patients can slowly develop symptomatic chronic alveolar hypoventilation for which they are likely to seek help and be placed on conventional bilevel PAP but not NVS, URIs and general anesthesia can cause sudden ARF mainly by causing VC and CPF to decrease and impairing mucus expulsion.[26,27] Unfortunately, while continuous NVS (CNVS) and MIE with oximetry feedback (see the John R. Bach and colleagues' article, "Noninvasive Respiratory Management of Spinal Cord Injury," elsewhere in this issue) are increasingly being used at optimal settings for patients with NMDs,[21] it is not for patients with SCI, and, thus, the lack of improvement in long-term prognoses.

Ventilatory Assistance

Conventional ventilatory assistance is invariably limited to continuous positive airway pressure (CPAP) and low-span bilevel PAP. The CPAP is a pneumatic splint to keep the airway open, but it does not assist breathing. The bilevel PAP, which is typically used at low spans (pressure support levels) of less than 15 cm H2O, provides minimal and often inadequate assistance to prevent ARF and result in intubation. Patients with inspiratory muscle paralysis need NVS settings that will be described in the John R. Bach and colleagues' article, "Noninvasive Respiratory Management of Spinal Cord Injury," elsewhere in this issue.

PHRENIC NERVE PACING

> "Pacing is a drastic and dangerous procedure. The risks are enormous. Batteries fail. The procedure frees you from the ventilator, but the outcome can be fatal."
> —Christopher Reeve in Still Me

Phrenic nerve pacing and diaphragm pacing, which also stimulates the phrenic nerves at the muscle's motor points, can provide up to all-day ventilatory support for some high-level patients with SCI. Ideally, it should be used by patients with SCI with less than 200 mL of VC who require 24-hour support with little if any ventilator-free breathing ability (VFBA). Because phrenic/diaphragm pacing causes severe obstructive sleep apneas because the subatmospheric pressures it creates in the upper airway causes it to collapse without the normal activation of airway dilator muscles by normal spontaneous inhalation, clinicians conventionally leave tracheostomy tubes in, or if the tubes are removed, CPAP may be used. Although there is a role for pacing for patients with C1-2 tetraplegia who cannot use mouthpiece NVS, there should be no role for it for patients with significant VFBA who can use noninvasive support, as is discussed in the John R. Bach and colleagues' article, "Noninvasive Respiratory Management of Spinal Cord Injury," elsewhere in this issue.

SLEEP-DISORDERED BREATHING

One-third to one-half of patients with SCI have sleep disrupted by pain, spasticity, medications, and SDB, that is, central and obstructive sleep apneas and hypopneas. Their number, per hour, is classified as the apnea-hypopnea index (AHI). The SDB results in episodic O2 desaturations, large intrathoracic pressure swings, increased sympathetic activity, sleep fragmentation, decreased quality of life, difficulty concentrating, depression, risk of cardiovascular events, and typical symptoms.[28,29]

Patients tend to be symptomatic when the sleep AHI exceeds 5 to 10. Among patients with SCI with incidence of SDB of 40% to 75% is much greater than normal.[30,31] This is possibly due to the effect of benzodiazepines, narcotics, antispasticity and antiarrhythmia medications, greater cervical and neck adiposity,[32] more time spent sleeping supine, dyscoordination between breathing and pharyngeal dilators, and muscles damaged by previous intubation and tracheostomy tubes.[33]

Polysomnographic titration of apneas and hypopneas by CPAP, which is useful for treating simple obstructive sleep events, or bilevel PAP, which assists lung ventilation but is not conventionally used at adequate settings for support or rest, are typically prescribed. There are numerous commercially available vented nasal interfaces (eg, CPAP "masks"), to deliver CPAP and bilevel PAP via passive ventilator circuits (circuits without exhalation valves). The expiratory (E)PAP is counterproductive for patients with weak muscles, however.[34] Oral appliances that bring the jaw forward to open the airway can also decrease the AHI.[35]

Besides obstructive and central events, hypoventilation can occur due to respiratory muscle weakness and Cheyne-Stokes respiration. Aging patients with SCI who already have diminished VCs have advancing respiratory muscle weakness as well. They have at least the normal annual rate of loss of VC of 1% for men and 1.2% for women. Symptomatic sleep hypoventilation can occur for which routine polysomnographic titrations of bilevel PAP settings may normalize AHI but not CO_2 levels. At this point, either the inspiratory (I)PAP of bilevel PAP needs to be increased to more than 20 cm H2O or the patient transitioned to an active ventilator circuit and use a non-vented interface for NVS during sleep, as is described in the John R. Bach and colleagues' article, "Noninvasive Respiratory Management of Spinal Cord Injury," elsewhere in this issue. Neither is typically done, because routine polysomnography does not monitor CO_2 levels. Typically the IPAP and EPAP are increased together to often intolerable levels, for example, IPAP 21, EPAP 17 cm H2O, without increasing the bilevel span (IPAP minus EPAP) to adequately assist breathing and decrease the CO_2. When hypercapnia and dyspnea extend into daytime hours and during URIs, low-span bilevel PAP becomes completely inadequate and intubation becomes likely for these patients.

Intercurrent Upper Respiratory Tract Infections

In one longitudinal study of 8775 acute care visits to a Department of Veterans Affairs Hospital, URI-pneumonias and ARF accounted for 49% of visits and the overall mortality was 7.9%.[36] Yet, for noninvasively managed patients with NMDs, respiratory mortality is greatly reduced.[21,37] Unfortunately, conventional respiratory management of SCI does not use the protocols used for patients with NMDs.

Conventional management usually entails obtaining a chest radiograph and prescribing antibiotics and perhaps chest physical therapy and quad coughing. Patients are hospitalized if they have pneumonia but may not be hospitalized if the radiograph is clear and they are not in acute distress. Bronchodilators and possibly bronchodilator/steroid inhalers are prescribed. Deep airway suctioning may be recommended. Most often, little is done to increase cough flows, the inadequacy of which may be a principal reason for pneumonia, as it is for patients with respiratory muscle weakness from NMDs.[22]

ACUTE PATIENT ASSESSMENT AND MANAGEMENT
Initial

The vast majority of high-level patients with SCI who are apneic at the time of injury die before making it to a hospital. Otherwise, ventilatory support is often needed 12 hours to 6 days postinjury with spinal shock and ascending cord edema transiently extending the level of neurologic impairment.

Signs of ventilatory insufficiency include orthopnea, tachypnea, paradoxical breathing, hypophonia, nasal flaring, use of accessory respiratory muscles, cyanosis, flushing or pallor, elevated CO_2 levels, O2 desaturation, airway congestion, and respiratory distress. O2 saturation is typically monitored and imaging performed to assess diaphragm function, but, most importantly, VC and CPF are not conventionally followed. Accessory muscle use may be present[38] but it is tiring and the patient's dyspnea is treated with supplemental O2 rather than NVS. O2 is conventionally administered whether or not the patient is hypoxic.

During this period, VC and CPF often decrease, and atelectasis, pneumonia, and ventilatory failure often develop because only low-span bilevel PAP is administered. Concomitant chest, head, skeletal, thoracic, and abdominal trauma, as well as injuries to soft tissue organs can necessitate surgical procedures under general anesthesia and contribute to morbidity and mortality.[38,39] Many patients require spine stabilization procedures. Although intubation is necessary for these procedures, the current treatment paradigm is to follow intubation with a tracheotomy to facilitate further surgical interventions, as well as to provide up to continuous tracheostomy mechanical ventilatory support (CTMV). This can be unnecessary.[40]

The supplemental O2 diminishes ventilatory drive, even more so when combined with narcotics and other sedating medications. Without primary cardiac disease, any O2 desaturation below 95% in ambient air that is not artifact MUST be due to hypoventilation (hypercapnia), airway secretions, and/or lung disease (atelectasis, lung collapse, pneumonia). These are caused by ineffective ventilatory support and ineffective airway clearance because supplemental O2 is administered instead of NVS and MIE.[37,41] The O2 can cause the CO_2 of a patient with hypercapnic SCI to increase by more than 120 mm Hg and result in CO_2 narcosis and ARF.[14]

Intubation and Extubation

Although intubation is not needed for uncomplicated high-level patients with SCI (see the John R. Bach and colleagues' article, "Noninvasive Respiratory Management of Spinal Cord Injury," elsewhere in this issue), SCI is most often complicated by traumatic brain injury and coma, chest trauma, severe anxiety at least in part due to inadequate ventilatory assistance, orthopedic complications, multiorgan insufficiency, adult respiratory distress syndrome for approximately 17% of high-level patients with SCI,[41] and need for high-dose narcotics, all of which can render noninvasive management ineffective. More than 50% of patients with cervical spine injuries are intubated.[42,43]

Intubation is done to provide ventilatory support and for secretion management by suctioning. Ironically, although grossly inadequate bilevel PAP settings, for example, IPAP 12, EPAP 6 cm H2O, are used before ventilatory failure results in intubation, ventilatory support settings of approximately 20 cm H2O are administered while patients are intubated.[44] Often, even while patients are intubated, permissive hypercapnia secondary to tidal volume settings of 6 to 8 mL/kg are used for fear of barotrauma, which is rare for patients with healthy lungs, such as uncomplicated patients with SCI.[45] With these minimal ventilator-delivered volumes and the fact that LVR is not conventionally administered, the lungs stiffen, shrink, and lose compliance.[46] This also results in tachypnea, fatigue, inadequate respiratory muscle rest, and loss of pulmonary compliance, all of which hamper ventilator weaning.[46] More than 20 years ago, high-volume ventilation was recommended to facilitate weaning,[47] often with increased dead space to avoid hyperventilation, but the reports had significant limitations and constant high volumes can deplete surfactant. Nevertheless there was no significant barotrauma.

The second reason for intubation is to facilitate secretion clearance, much of which is caused by the invasive airway tube itself. Instead of using ambient air oximetry feedback with O2 saturations less than 95% signaling airway congestion and the need for MIE and suctioning to reverse the O2 desaturations, typically supplemental O2 is simply increased as the patient spirals downward into ARF. The O2 is paramount to putting a Band-Aid on a cancer of hypoventilation and secretions. Suctioning via any invasive interface misses the left main stem bronchus approximately 90% of the time, resulting in more than 80% of pneumonias occurring in the left lungs.[48] Suctioning also increases airway resistance, probably from bronchoconstriction triggered by constriction of the bronchial muscles in response to irritation and triggering of the bronchial stretch receptors.[49] The greater than -200 cm H2O pressures crossing the catheter portals tear out cilia and disrupt the function of the mucociliary elevator itself. For more than 80 ventilator unweanable patients who refused tracheotomies and were transferred to our center for extubation to CNVS and MIE, after first normalizing the CO_2, then placing the patients on Fio_2 21%, O2 saturation baseline levels were less than 95% for 84% of patients,[25] because O2 was used to keep the baseline normal rather than MIE via the tubes. For patients in spinal shock, though, both airway suctioning and MIE can cause severe bradycardias. Anticholinergic medications can prevent this.

Typically, once intubated and surgical interventions are completed, ventilator weaning is attempted. Many protocols have been described. The most common is the use of synchronized intermittent mandatory ventilation, which allows the patient to trigger pressure-supported breaths above the set back-up rate of intermittent positive pressure breaths. The back-up rate and pressure support levels are typically decreased as tolerated, that is, unless excessive tachypnea, hypercapnia, O2 desaturation, and distress occur. This approach neither provides optimal muscle rest nor exercise. A key principle of physical medicine and rehabilitation is to strengthen muscles by rest and exercise, not by stressing them by continuously applying suboptimal assistance.

Ventilator disconnection and breathing while receiving a continuous flow of O2 or, better, compressed humidified air via an open tracheostomy tube collar exercises weak respiratory muscles of patients with diminished VC. These autonomous breathing "sprints" are interspersed with periods of ventilatory support to rest the muscles. This approach is considered the most effective way to wean patients from ventilatory support.[50,51] It also satisfies the principle of rest and exercise provided that the rest is delivered at full ventilatory support settings and only for periods of 30 to 60 minutes, so not so long as to cause further deconditioning or disuse atrophy of respiratory muscles.

For extubation attempts without undergoing tracheotomy, typically, conventional ventilator weaning parameters and spontaneous breathing trials need to be passed. These parameters assess the ability of the patient to breathe autonomously and the patient must have minimal airway secretions and have the ability to expel them. If patients wean expeditiously, do not develop pneumonia or other respiratory complications, and need no further surgeries, then they may be successfully extubated despite receiving the supplemental O2, CPAP, and low-span bilevel PAP. However, any apparent delay in weaning, even if caused by a build-up of secretions and atelectasis that would have been signaled by dips in ambient air O2 saturation below 95% and that could have been reversed by using MIE via the tube, results in the conventional thinking that tracheotomy is indicated. Because of the severe long-term morbidity and mortality due to tracheostomy tubes, however, tracheotomy may not be the better option if unweanable patients can meet extubation criteria to CNVS and MIE in a month or so while surgical interventions are completed (see the John R. Bach and colleagues' article, "Noninvasive Respiratory Management of Spinal Cord Injury," elsewhere in this issue), but this is unconventional thinking to put it mildly.[26,52] Further, because upper airway complications are greatest in patients undergoing tracheotomy following intubation rather than undergoing intubation only or elective tracheotomy,[48] and it is far easier to extubate ventilator unweanable patients to CNVS and MIE than to decannulate them to CNVS and MIE, greater efforts should be made to extubate to CNVS and MIE rather than to tracheostomy mechanical ventilatory support (TMV). The clinicians placing the tubes are not the ones who will manage the subsequent complications caused by them. Tracheotomies are so routine that we have had perfectly stable, BIM intact, mid-cervical patients with SCI with more than 2 L of VC and absolutely no dysphagia consent to tracheotomies and gastrostomy tubes only to withdraw their consents when, as consultants, we told them that they were unnecessary.

TRACHEOSTOMY

Many patients who have undergone tracheotomies must retain the tubes because of inability to cooperate, severe BIM dysfunction, tracheal stenosis, or severe trachiectasis, tracheomalacia, or other severe complications caused by the tube. These patients can benefit from full ventilatory support, that is, up to full CTMV, with cuffs inflated, deflated, or via cuffless tubes (**Fig. 3**).[53,54]

Cuff deflation or removal is not routine, conventional management. Yet, because most patients who can speak and swallow can be decannulated whether ventilator-dependent or not as considered in the John R. Bach and colleagues' article, "Noninvasive Respiratory Management of Spinal Cord Injury," elsewhere in this issue, cuff deflation or removal should always be considered, because most life-threatening complications of tracheostomy tubes are due to the cuff.

When the cuff is deflated, or removed, settings, generally 10 to 15 mL/kg before deflation, need to be markedly increased to compensate for leak around the tube and to optimize speech production. A wider-diameter tube can be placed if leak is excessive or a smaller one placed to increase leak if leak is inadequate for speech and effective clearance of airway debris above the cuff. Fenestrated cuffless tubes can be used for patients who practice NVS for eventual decannulation, but this is not conventionally done. Ambient air O2 saturation and occasionally end-tidal CO_2 can be monitored to ensure normal ventilation.

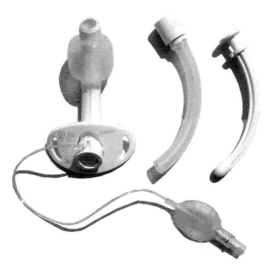

Fig. 3. A typical tracheostomy tube with an obturator, inner cannula, and inflated cuff that can cause trachiectasis, tracheomalacia, and tracheal rupture.

The most common mistakes are to provide supplemental O2 instead of MIE via the tube for airway secretion clearance (see the John R. Bach and colleagues' article, "Noninvasive Respiratory Management of Spinal Cord Injury," elsewhere in this issue), use settings inadequate to normalize CO_2 levels, and to not prescribe passive LVR via the tube. These patients, who conventionally receive approximately a constant 7 to 10 mg/kg of ventilator-delivered volume via TMV for normal alveolar ventilation (CO_2) almost invariably ask for more air with time and become grossly overventilated,[55] often with Pa_{CO_2} levels to less than 20 mm Hg. The hyperventilation is thought to be due to some combination of lack of tidal volume variability, tube-induced airway secretion congestion diminishing respiratory exchange, bypassing upper airway afferents, and lack of glottis closure to hold thoracolumbar pressures needed to cough.[55] The chronic hyperventilation increases ventilator dependence and impedes ventilator weaning.

Rapid disuse atrophy of diaphragm fibers are observed after only 18 hours of invasive mechanical ventilation and it continues indefinitely.[54] VC also decreases because of airway mucus functionally blocking respiratory exchange, because mucociliary clearance is impaired by inflammation caused by the tube. Thus, many SCI CTMV users we have extubated or decannulated to CNVS and MIE weaned to part-time NVS despite having as little as 250 mL of VC.[21,26,27,52,55,56] Indeed, in 1954, it was reported that tracheotomy can cause permanent ventilator dependence and prevent ventilator weaning.[57] The chronic hypocapnia and compensatory metabolic acidosis renders TMV users more dependent on ventilatory support.[55,58–61]

Wright suggested that loss of Hering Breuer triggering during constant volume invasive mechanical ventilation plays a central role in the production of breathlessness and demands to ever increase minute ventilation.[61] Thus, decreased control of inspiratory effort and tidal volumes may increase inspiratory cell activity to produce dyspnea at hypocapnic levels. Chemosensation and thoracic stretch reflexes continuously drive respiration. Varying tidal volumes, pressures, timing, and sequences may be needed for air satiety. Any mechanical ventilation system, such as TMV or iron lung use, that does not permit control and variable respiration, results in demands for "more air" and, ultimately hyperventilation.[62–64]

DECANNULATION

Decannulation is not conventionally done unless the patient is entirely ventilator weaned and it is typically done by steps, that is, converting to cuffless tubes and changing the tubes to progressively smaller diameters. In reality, either a patient needs a tracheostomy tube because of severe upper motor neuron impairment or does not need one. No patients with MIE-expiratory flows of more than 200 L/m need tracheostomy tubes irrespective of extent of dependence on mechanical ventilation.[65] Unfortunately, there has as yet been no paradigm shift to this principle.

TRACHEOSTOMY MANAGEMENT OUTCOMES

There has been no improvement in long-term mortality since the 1980s, including in the age-adjusted mortality rate for respiratory complications. The gap in life expectancy between the able-bodied and persons with SCI has been increasing in large part due to respiratory causes.[66] Using model SCI system data with a 2019 updated life expectancy calculator, we find that a 21-year-old male SCI survivor with complete C1-4 tetraplegia injured 1 year ago and not using a ventilator can expect to live to age 53.1 and a woman to 56.2, but using TMV both men and women can expect to survive only 16 years, to age 37.3. For SCI survivors whose cause of death is known, respiratory causes account for more than 65% of the deaths.[2,67]

Presumably much of the excess mortality is due to the same tracheostomy tube–related complications that cause it for patients with neuromuscular diseases.[37] Respiratory issues cause the deaths of up to 90% of conventionally managed patients with many NMDs,[21,68] with approximately 80% of the TMV users dying because of tube-related complications.[22,68]

Whiteneck and colleagues[69] reported that 55% of 76 CTMV-dependent patients with SCI had annual pulmonary complications and averaged 22 hospitalization days yearly. The URI incidence has been reported to be 18% to 25% per year for patients with SCI, and pneumonia and atelectasis 10% per year.[70,71] Survival percentages at 1, 3, 5, and 7 years postinjury were 86%, 70%, 63%, and 59%, with deaths mostly from respiratory causes.[72] Deaths by accidental tube disconnection are common.[73] Carter and colleagues[73] reported 17 deaths in 35 SCI CTMV-dependent patients with or without pacemakers in an average of 1.5 years postinjury. They felt that more than 50% of the deaths were sudden and directly due to the tube itself, including from accidental disconnection, mucus plugging, tracheomalacia, tracheal stenosis, hemorrhage, and so forth. Thus, as for CTMV-dependent patients with NMDs, the incidence of tube-related deaths in SCI is also very high.

Whereas most adult patients with as little as 250 to 300 mL of VC may use NVS around-the-clock but have significant VFBA, this is never the case for SCI CTMV users with these VCs who have none at all, are typically hyperventilated, and who become immediately dyspneic on any disconnection. We have had SCI CTMV users with 900 mL of VC and normal BIMs. This would never be the case for patients managed by CNVS without tubes.

Despite our challenge to rehabilitation, spinal cord services in 2006 to essentially create tracheostomy tube–free centers[74] and the fact that CNVS including via mouthpiece was first described for high-level patients with SCI in 1969,[75] only 11 other ventilator "unweanable" patients with SCI have been reported to have been decannulated to CNVS and MIE in one center in Portugal since 2006.[59]

QUALITY OF LIFE

Happiness is reality divided by expectation. While on the morning of the SCI, life expectations were normal but with SCI reality suddenly became terrible. With time, expectations decrease to match reality and patients again develop positive life satisfaction. While for the first 2 years postinjury, 40% of tetraplegics consider suicide, after this, Krause[76] reported positive life satisfaction and little suicidal ideation. Age also negatively impacts subjective well-being.[77]

In a study by Hall and colleagues[78] who evaluated individuals with chronic C1-C4 SCI tetraplegia 14 and 24 years postinjury, the quality of life was rated as high in both ventilator-dependent and autonomously breathing individuals. Moreover, Bach and Tilton[79] found that long-term life satisfaction and well-being were considered to be positive by most individuals with tetraplegia, ventilator-dependent or not. Whiteneck and colleagues[69] reported that 15 of 20 patients with SCI more than 20 years postinjury rated their quality of life as good or excellent on a 5-point scale. There were no significant differences by level of injury but satisfaction correlated inversely with age. Interestingly, in studies from the 2 centers, ventilator-dependent high-level individuals with tetraplegia were significantly more satisfied with their lives than were ventilator-free individuals with tetraplegia.[72,79] Bach and Tilton[79] reported that it was correlated to their greater satisfaction with family life. It seems that the constant struggle of lower-level ventilator-free cervical patients with SCI to attain more function creates frustrations that the higher-level ventilator-dependent patients do not have. The latter's lives are more fragile, and this may give cause for greater appreciation to be alive on a day-to-day basis. On the other hand, all studies comparing quality of life and life satisfaction for invasive versus noninvasive ventilator-supported individuals have noted that both are superior in the latter.[79–81]

DISCLOSURE

The authors have nothing to disclose.

REFERENCES

1. Devivo MJ. Epidemiology of traumatic spinal cord injury: trends and future implications. Spinal Cord 2012;50(5):365–72.

2. Center NSCIS. Annual statistical report for the spinal cord injury model systems public version. Birmingham (AL): University of Alabama at Birmingham; 2018.

3. Hagen EM, Lie SA, Rekand T, et al. Mortality after traumatic spinal cord injury: 50 years of follow-up. J Neurol Neurosurg Psychiatry 2010;81(4):368–73.

4. Kirshblum S, Johnston MV, Brown J, et al. Predictors of dysphagia after spinal cord injury. Arch Phys Med Rehabil 1999;80(9):1101–5.

5. Jackson AB, Groomes TE. Incidence of respiratory complications following spinal cord injury. Arch Phys Med Rehabil 1994;75(3):270–5.

6. Bach JR. Noninvasive respiratory management of high level spinal cord injury. J Spinal Cord Med 2012;35(2):72–80.

7. Postma K, Haisma JA, Hopman MT, et al. Resistive inspiratory muscle training in people with spinal cord injury during inpatient rehabilitation: a randomized controlled trial. Phys Ther 2014;94(12):1709–19.

8. Martin AJ, Stern L, Yeates J, et al. Respiratory muscle training in Duchenne muscular dystrophy. Dev Med Child Neurol 1986;28(3):314–8.

9. DiMarco AF, Kelling JS, DiMarco MS, et al. The effects of inspiratory resistive training on respiratory muscle function in patients with muscular dystrophy. Muscle Nerve 1985;8(4):284–90.

10. Bach JR. Inappropriate weaning and late onset ventilatory failure of individuals with traumatic spinal cord injury. Paraplegia 1993;31(7):430–8.

11. Rutchik A, Weissman AR, Almenoff PL, et al. Resistive inspiratory muscle training in subjects with chronic cervical spinal cord injury. Arch Phys Med Rehabil 1998; 79(3):293–7.

12. Tamplin J, Berlowitz DJ. A systematic review and meta-analysis of the effects of respiratory muscle training on pulmonary function in tetraplegia. Spinal Cord 2014;52(3):175.

13. Gross D, Ladd HW, Riley EJ, et al. The effect of training on strength and endurance of the diaphragm in quadriplegia. Am J Med 1980;68(1):27–35.

14. Chiou M, Bach JR, Saporito LR, et al. Quantitation of Oxygen induced hypercapnia in respiratory pump failure. Rev Port Pneumol (2006) 2016;22(5):262–5.

15. Leith D. Lung biology in health and disease: respiratory defense mechanisms, vol. 2. New York: Marcel Dekker; 1977.

16. Bach JR. Mechanical insufflation-exsufflation. Comparison of peak expiratory flows with manually assisted and unassisted coughing techniques. Chest 1993; 104(5):1553–62.

17. Kirby NA, Barnerias MJ, Siebens AA. An evaluation of assisted cough in quadriparetic patients. Arch Phys Med Rehabil 1966;47(11):705–10.

18. Bach JR, Smith WH, Michaels J, et al. Airway secretion clearance by mechanical exsufflation for post-poliomyelitis ventilator-assisted individuals. Arch Phys Med Rehabil 1993;74(2):170–7.

19. Sortor S, McKenzie M. Toward independence: assisted cough (video). Dallas (TX): BioScience Communications of Dallas; 1986.

20. Bach JR, Martinez D. Duchenne muscular dystrophy: continuous noninvasive ventilatory support prolongs survival. Respir Care 2011;56(6):744–50.

21. Bach JR. New approaches in the rehabilitation of the traumatic high level quadriplegic. Am J Phys Med Rehabil 1991;70(1):13–9.

22. Bach JR. Update and perspectives on noninvasive respiratory muscle aids: part 2–the expiratory muscle aids. Chest 1994;105(5):1538–44.

23. Wang T-G, Bach JR. Pulmonary dysfunction in residents of chronic care facilities. Taiwan Journal of Rehabilitation 1993;(21):67–73.

24. DiMarco AF, Kowalski KE, Geertman RT, et al. Lower thoracic spinal cord stimulation to restore cough in patients with spinal cord injury: results of a National Institutes of Health-sponsored clinical trial. Part I: methodology and effectiveness of expiratory muscle activation. Arch Phys Med Rehabil 2009;90:717–25.

25. DiMarco AF, Kowalski KE, Geertman RT, et al. Lower thoracic spinal cord stimulation to restore cough in patients with spinal cord injury: results of a National Institutes of Health-sponsored clinical trial. Part II: clinical outcomes. Arch Phys Med Rehabil 2009;90:726–32.

26. Bach JR, Goncalves MR, Hamdani I, et al. Extubation of patients with neuromuscular weakness: a new management paradigm. Chest 2010;137(5):1033–9.

27. Bach JR, Sinquee DM, Saporito LR, et al. Efficacy of mechanical insufflation-exsufflation in extubating unweanable subjects with restrictive pulmonary disorders. Respir Care 2015;60(4):477–83.

28. Kryger MHRT, Roth T, Dement WC, editors. Principles and practice of sleep medicine. 6th edition. Cambridge (MA): Elsevier; 2016.

29. BaHammam AS. Factors that may influence apnea-hypopnea index in patients with acute myocardial infarction. Chest 2009;136(5):1444–5.
30. Garvey JF, Pengo MF, Drakatos P, et al. Epidemiological aspects of obstructive sleep apnea. J Thorac Dis 2015;7(5):920.
31. Young T, Palta M, Dempsey J, et al. The occurrence of sleep-disordered breathing among middle-aged adults. N Engl J Med 1993;328(17):1230–5.
32. Spungen AM, Adkins RH, Stewart CA, et al. Factors influencing body composition in persons with spinal cord injury: a cross-sectional study. J Appl Physiol (1985) 2003;95(6):2398–407.
33. Cahan C, Gothe B, Decker M, et al. Arterial oxygen saturation over time and sleep studies in quadriplegic patients. Spinal Cord 1993;31(3):172.
34. Crescimanno G, Greco F, Arrisicato S, et al. Effects of positive end expiratory pressure administration during non-invasive ventilation in patients affected by amyotrophic lateral sclerosis: A randomized crossover study. Respirology 2016;21(7):1307–13.
35. Ferguson KA, Cartwright R, Rogers R, et al. Oral appliances for snoring and obstructive sleep apnea: a review. Sleep 2006;29(2):244–62.
36. Weaver FM, Smith B, Evans CT, et al. Outcomes of outpatient visits for acute respiratory illness in veterans with spinal cord injuries and disorders. Am J Phys Med Rehabil 2006;85(9):718–26.
37. Bach JR. Noninvasive respiratory management of patients with neuromuscular disease. Ann Rehabil Med 2017;41(4):519–38.
38. Silver JR. Chest injuries and complications in the early stages of spinal cord injury. Paraplegia 1968;5(4):226–45.
39. McSweeney T. The early management of associated injuries in the presence of co-incident damage to the spinal cord. Paraplegia 1968;5(4):189–96.
40. Bach JR, Hunt D, Horton JA 3rd. Traumatic tetraplegia: noninvasive respiratory management in the acute setting. Am J Phys Med Rehabil 2002;81(10):792–7.
41. Veeravagu A, Jiang B, Rincon F, et al. Acute respiratory distress syndrome and acute lung injury in patients with vertebral column fracture(s) and spinal cord injury: a nationwide inpatient sample study. Spinal Cord 2013;51(6):461–5.
42. Seidl RO, Wolf D, Nusser-Muller-Busch R, et al. Airway management in acute tetraplegics: a retrospective study. Eur Spine J 2010;19(7):1073–8.
43. Royster R, Barboi C, Peruzzi W. Critical care in the acute cervical spinal cord injury. Top Spinal Cord Inj Rehabil 2004;9(3):11–32.
44. Bach JR. Continuous noninvasive ventilation for patients with neuromuscular disease and spinal cord injury. Semin Respir Crit Care Med 2002;23(3):283–92.
45. Suri P, Burns SP, Bach JR. Pneumothorax associated with mechanical insufflation-exsufflation and related factors. Am J Phys Med Rehabil 2008;87(11):951–5.
46. Bach JR, Kang SW. Disorders of ventilation : weakness, stiffness, and mobilization. Chest 2000;117(2):301–3.
47. Peterson P, Brooks C, Mellick D, et al. Protocol for ventilator management in high tetraplegia. Top Spinal Cord Inj Rehabil 1997;2(3):101–6.
48. Fishburn MJ, Marino RJ, Ditunno JF Jr. Atelectasis and pneumonia in acute spinal cord injury. Arch Phys Med Rehabil 1990;71(3):197–200.
49. Woodburne CR, Powaser MM. Mechanisms responsible for the sustained fall in arterial oxygen tension after endotracheal suctioning in dogs. Nurs Res 1980;29(5):312–6.
50. Brochard L, Rauss A, Benito S, et al. Comparison of three methods of gradual withdrawal from ventilatory support during weaning from mechanical ventilation. Am J Respir Crit Care Med 1994;150(4):896–903.

51. Jubran A, Grant BJ, Duffner LA, et al. Effect of pressure support vs unassisted breathing through a tracheostomy collar on weaning duration in patients requiring prolonged mechanical ventilation: a randomized trial. JAMA 2013;309(7):671–7.
52. Bach JR, Alba AS. Noninvasive options for ventilatory support of the traumatic high level quadriplegic patient. Chest 1990;98(3):613–9.
53. Respiratory management following spinal cord injury: a clinical practice guideline for health-care professionals. J Spinal Cord Med 2005;28(3):259–93.
54. Bach JR, Alba AS. Tracheostomy ventilation: a study of efficacy with deflated cuffs and cuffless tubes. Chest 1990;97(3):679–83.
55. Haber II, Bach JR. Absence of chronic hypocapnia with long-term noninvasive intermittent positive pressure ventilation. Arch Phys Med Rehabil 1992;73:970.
56. Schepens T, Verbrugghe W, Dams K, et al. The course of diaphragm atrophy in ventilated patients assessed with ultrasound: a longitudinal cohort study. Crit Care 2015;19:422.
57. Hodes HL, et al. Treatment of respiratory difficulty in poliomyelitis. In: Poliomyelitis: papers and discussions presented at the third international poliomyelitis conference. Philadelphia: Lippincott; 1955. p. 91–113.
58. Esquinas Rodriguez AM, Pravinkumar E. Mechanical insufflation-exsufflation in prevention of post-extubation acute respiratory failure: most welcome but must be used cautiously in critically ill patients. Crit Care 2012;16(3):431.
59. Bach JR, Saporito LR, Shah HR, et al. Decanulation of patients with severe respiratory muscle insufficiency: efficacy of mechanical insufflation-exsufflation. J Rehabil Med 2014;46(10):1037–41.
60. Haber II, Bach JR. Normalization of blood carbon dioxide levels by transition from conventional ventilatory support to noninvasive inspiratory aids. Arch Phys Med Rehabil 1994;75(10):1145–50.
61. Wright GW, Branscomb BV. The origin of the sensations of dyspnea. Trans Am Clin Climatol Assoc 1954;66:116–25.
62. Bach JR, Haber II, Wang TG, et al. Alveolar ventilation as a function of ventilatory support method. Eur J Phys Rehabil Med 1995;5(3):80–4.
63. Watt JW, Silva P. Respiratory alkalosis and associated electrolytes in long-term ventilator dependent persons with tetraplegia. Spinal Cord 2001;39(11):557–63.
64. Iscoe S, Fisher JA. Hyperoxia-induced hypocapnia: an underappreciated risk. Chest 2005;128(1):430–3.
65. Bach JR, Giménez GC, Chiou M. Mechanical In-exsufflation-Expiratory Flows as Indication for Tracheostomy Tube Decannulation: Case Studies. Am J Phys Med Rehabil 2019;98(3):e18–20.
66. Shavelle RM, DeVivo MJ, Brooks JC, et al. Improvements in long-term survival after spinal cord injury? Arch Phys Med Rehabil 2015;96(4):645–51.
67. Garshick E, Kelley A, Cohen SA, et al. A prospective assessment of mortality in chronic spinal cord injury. Spinal Cord 2005;43(7):408–16.
68. Bach JR. Amyotrophic lateral sclerosis. Communication status and survival with ventilatory support. Am J Phys Med Rehabil 1993;72(6):343–9.
69. Whiteneck GG, Charlifue SW, Frankel HL, et al. Mortality, morbidity, and psychosocial outcomes of persons spinal cord injured more than 20 years ago. Paraplegia 1992;30(9):617–30.
70. McKinley WO, Jackson AB, Cardenas DD, et al. Long-term medical complications after traumatic spinal cord injury: a regional model systems analysis. Arch Phys Med Rehabil 1999;80(11):1402–10.

71. Meyers AR, Bisbee A, Winter M. The "Boston model" of managed care and spinal cord injury: a cross-sectional study of the outcomes of risk-based, prepaid, managed care. Arch Phys Med Rehabil 1999;80(11):1450–6.

72. Splaingard ML, Frates RC Jr, Harrison GM, et al. Home positive-pressure ventilation. Twenty years' experience. Chest 1983;84(4):376–82.

73. Carter RE, Donovan WH, Halstead L, et al. Comparative study of electrophrenic nerve stimulation and mechanical ventilatory support in traumatic spinal cord injury. Paraplegia 1987;25:86–91.

74. Bach JR. Prevention of respiratory complications of spinal cord injury: a challenge to "model" spinal cord units. J Spinal Cord Med 2006;29(1):3–4.

75. Alba A, Solomon M, Trainor F. Management of respiratory insufficiency in spinal cord lesions. Paper presented at: Proceedings of the 17th Veteran's Administration Spinal Cord Injury Conference 1969.

76. Krause JS. Longitudinal changes in adjustment after spinal cord injury: a 15-year study. Arch Phys Med Rehabil 1992;73(6):564–8.

77. Hall KM, Knudsen ST, Wright J, et al. Follow-up study of individuals with high tetraplegia (C1-C4) 14 to 24 years postinjury. Arch Phys Med Rehabil 1999;80(11):1507–13.

78. Bach JR, Tilton MC. Life satisfaction and well-being measures in ventilator assisted individuals with traumatic tetraplegia. Arch Phys Med Rehabil 1994;75(6):626–32.

79. Bach JR, Campagnolo DI, Hoeman S. Life satisfaction of individuals with Duchenne muscular dystrophy using long-term mechanical ventilatory support. Am J Phys Med Rehabil 1991;70(3):129–35.

80. Bach JR. A comparison of long-term ventilatory support alternatives from the perspective of the patient and care giver. Chest 1993;104(6):1702–6.

81. Campagnolo DIBJ, Bach JR. Assessment of life satisfaction for ventilator-supported polio patients. Arch Phys Med Rehabil 1991;72:801.

Noninvasive Respiratory Management of Spinal Cord Injury

John R. Bach, MD[a],*, Lindsay Burke, BA, MD[a], Michael Chiou, MD[b]

KEYWORDS

- Noninvasive ventilatory support • Spinal cord injury • Respiratory support
- Mechanical insufflation-exsufflation • Mouthpiece ventilation

KEY POINTS

- Ventilator-dependent patients with high-level spinal cord injury can be managed without tracheostomy tubes.
- Ventilator unweanable patients can be extubated and/or decannulated of invasive airway tubes to noninvasive ventilatory support.
- Noninvasive ventilation is being used as continuous positive airway pressure (CPAP) and bilevel PAP but not for ventilatory support.
- Mechanical insufflation-exsufflation is crucial for long-term noninvasive ventilatory support as well as for extubation and decannulation of ventilator-dependent patients.

Because respiratory complications remain the number one cause of death after spinal cord injury (SCI), both in the acute stage and long term, and morbidity and mortality have not significantly decreased over the last 40 years,[1,2] this article offers a rational noninvasive alternative, well documented for patients with neuromuscular disorders. Physical medicine inspiratory and expiratory muscle aids involve the application of pressures to the body and/or airways to assist or fully support inspiratory and expiratory muscles rather than resort to invasive airway tubes. The 4 goals of noninvasive management are to maintain or improve pulmonary compliance and lung volumes by lung volume recruitment (LVR), to maintain normal alveolar ventilation around-the-clock using noninvasive interfaces, to provide effective cough flows to prevent pneumonia and episodes of acute respiratory failure (ARF), and to train patients who have little to no vital capacity (VC) and who would

[a] Department of Physical Medicine and Rehabilitation, Rutgers University New Jersey Medical School, Behavioral Health Sciences Building, 183 South Orange Avenue, Newark, NJ 07103, USA; [b] Department of PM&R, Icahn School of Medicine at Mount Sinai, 3 East 101th Street, New York, NY 10029, USA
* Corresponding author.
E-mail address: bachjr@njms.rutgers.edu

Phys Med Rehabil Clin N Am 31 (2020) 397–413
https://doi.org/10.1016/j.pmr.2020.03.006
1047-9651/20/© 2020 Elsevier Inc. All rights reserved.

otherwise be apneic in the event of disconnection from continuous tracheostomy mechanical ventilation (CTMV), the ability to breathe without a ventilator by using bulbar innervated muscles (BIM).

NONINVASIVE INTERVENTIONS
Lung Volume Recruitment and Manually Assisted Coughing

Over time, the tendons, ligaments, and joints of the rib cage stiffen, which along with chest wall spasticity decreases lung capacity and pulmonary compliance.[3–5] Whether in acute care or long-term, LVR is important to maintain lung health, compliance, and lung volumes, and it increases cough flows, VC, and vocalization. It can be active or passive.

Active LVR is achieved by the air stacking of consecutive volumes of air delivered by volume preset ventilation or a manual resuscitator. The maximum air volume that the glottis can hold by air stacking is termed the maximum insufflation capacity (MIC). As it increases with routine 3 times daily practice, VC and cough peak flows (CPF) increase and atelectasis decreases.[6,7] Patients can speak louder and longer. The MIC-VC difference is a direct function of glottis and BIM integrity. If a patient can air stack when stable, transitioning from extubation to continuous noninvasive ventilatory support (CNVS) is easier if ever intubation becomes necessary. The LVR can be provided via mouthpiece, lip cover, or nasal/oronasal interfaces, as can NVS.

For patients who cannot air stack because of impaired glottis closure, passive LVR is performed by using a manual resuscitator with blocked exhalation valve to prevent exhalation until maximum lung volumes are attained or the air can also be delivered as an insufflation to 60 to 70 cm H2O via mechanical insufflation-exsufflation (MIE). Adequate delivery can be noted by feeling the resistance of lung recoil while squeezing the manual resuscitator to inflate the lungs. Patients using TMV also require passive LVR by routinely delivering sighs to approach predicted inspiratory capacities but this is rarely done so lungs of TMV users stiffen and shrink.

The greater the cough flow, the more effective the cough. Patients with CPF less than 300 L/m have increased risk of pneumonia and ARF. Bronchodilators, chest percussion and vibration, and supplemental O2 do not address the problem, which is a reason that conventional management outcomes have not improved. Manually assisted coughing is the application of an abdominal thrust after active LVR, or "air stacking," to a deep lung volume. It typically increases cough flows to effective levels, because patients with SCI usually have intact glottis function to hold the thoracoabdominal pressures, as manual thrusts to the abdomen provide effective cough flows after air stacking. When these patients have adequate help at home to apply manually assisted cough flows greater than 300 L/m, essentially around-the-clock as needed during upper respiratory tract infections (URIs), they may not need MIE.

Glossopharyngeal Breathing

Glossopharyngeal breathing (GPB) or "frog breathing" can be used instead of ventilators for mechanical ventilatory support, as a backup for ventilator failure, and for autonomous air stacking. The tongue pistons boluses of air past the glottis and into the lungs. It is learned by imitating the therapist or any available frog. Frog breathing supplements autonomous tidal volumes for active LVR and can be used when awake all day instead of a ventilator for patients with as little as no measurable VC. Patients who master GPB awaken from sleep using GPB to ventilate their lungs to discover that their ventilators are off. This is not possible for patients using CTMV, and it is a major reason to decannulate patients with tracheostomy tubes and switch them to

NVS/CNVS. Because they generally have good BIM function, up to 70% of SCI CNVS users can master GPB to breathe free of ventilatory support.[3,8–12]

Mechanical Insufflation-Exsufflation

MIE is forced passive inflation followed by forced passive deflation of the lungs using an MIE device at positive, immediately followed by negative, 40 to 70 cm H_2O pressures via invasive or noninvasive interfaces. Forty to sixty centimeters H_2O is insufflated and exsufflated via noninvasive interfaces and 60 to 70 cm H_2O via invasive interfaces (airway tubes). Insufflation and exsufflation times for automatic, rather than manual, MIE should not be set until determined by observing the time it takes for full clinical chest expansion than full clinical chest deflation for powerful exsufflation flows (MIE-EF). The insufflations and exsufflations should not take so much time that users do not get enough minute ventilation and become short of breath. Hyperventilation is avoided by brief pauses after every 3 to 5 cycles for the patient to return to normal ventilation. One treatment consists of multiple 3 to 5 cycle periods of MIE via oronasal interfaces and/or simple mouthpieces until no more secretions are expelled. Unlike suctioning, MIE clears both left and right airways without discomfort or trauma and patients prefer it.[13] Effective clearance of airway secretions with MIE improves VC, pulmonary flow rates,[14] and oxyhemoglobin saturation (O_2 saturation [sat])[15,16] and facilitates ventilator weaning by clearing both left and right airways.[17,18]

NONINVASIVE VENTILATORY SUPPORT
Intermittent Noninvasive Positive Pressure Ventilation for Noninvasive Ventilory Support

Although symptomatic hypoventilation begins during sleep, many patients who have less VC when sitting first use NVS during the daytime to facilitate eating, speech, coughing, and for air stacking for LVR. With weakness, tachypnea can exceed 40 per minute, leaving only a second for swallowing food. NVS eases tachypnea, dyspnea, and can make swallowing safer. It is prescribed at volumes of 700 mL to 1800 mL with a physiologic backup rate, usually 10 to 12/min. Specifically trained respiratory therapists introduce mouthpiece (**Fig. 1**) and nasal NVS and determine the patient-preferred settings in the outpatient clinic or in the patients' homes. Most of the adults settle on inspiratory volumes of 1200 to 1300 mL, which they can receive via angled mouthpieces, straw-type conduits, or nasal prongs during the day. Besides facilitating air stacking, the relatively large volumes permit patients to physiologically vary tidal volumes.

Some neck movement and lip function are needed for effective mouthpiece NVS. To master mouthpiece NVS the patient must move the soft palate posteriocranially to seal off the nasopharynx from leak out of the nose. The glottis must also open to permit air entry. These normally reflex movements are lost for patients being transitioned from CTMV and must be relearned after decannulation because during TMV with an inflated cuff the glottis remains closed.[19,20] The mouthpiece is fixed adjacent to the mouth by a metal clamp or microphone holder attached to a wheelchair. The mouthpiece can also be fixed onto sip and puff, chin, or tongue controls of motorized wheelchairs.

Most patients use nasal NVS for sleep. Unlike CPAP and low-span (low pressure support) bilevel PAP that often does not adequately relieve tachypnea, NVS settings relieve the patient from struggling to breathe. Patients using NVS no longer trigger the ventilator at rates much greater than physiologic breathing or the ventilator back-up rates that are set. Volume preset ventilation facilitates air stacking for LVR,

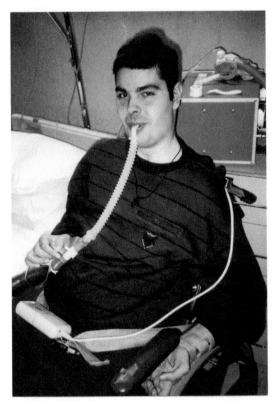

Fig. 1. A 22-year-old C1-C2 AIS A traumatic tetraplegic on continuous tracheostomy ventilation for 1 year when an ATROTECH Atrostin Phrenic Nerve Stimulator was placed but only used for 5 hours per day due to shoulder and chest pain. However, 3 years later, with a VC of 650 mL, a fenestrated, cuffless tube was placed; he practiced noninvasive ventilatory support (NVS), was able to air stack to 1300 mL, satisfied all **Table 1** criteria, and was decannulated to volume-preset NVS at 1400 mL rate 15/min via 15 mm angled mouthpiece (see here) during the day and a Lipseal (see **Fig. 3**) during sleep. The stoma closed and after 3 days of continuous NVS his vital capacity increased to 1100 mL and he required fewer and fewer mouthpiece-assisted breaths and weaned to nocturnal-only NSV. He mastered frog breathing and was discharged home 5 days postdecannulation. He stopped pacing permanently and used NVS for sleep, maintaining a mean O2 saturation of 96%, via a Lipseal interface.

raising voice volume, and coughing overnight. If it causes persistent abdominal distension during sleep, patients are switched to pressure assist/control ventilation at less than 25 cm H2O, the normal maximum pressure for gastroesophageal sphincter integrity. Most patients use the same daytime volume preset settings for sleep as well. About 3% of sleep nasal NVS users require oronasal interfaces to prevent excessive leak.[21] Maintaining normal daytime CO2 also helps sustain ventilatory drive. Excessive air leakage is prevented by the alert though sleeping brain's ventilatory drive being undiminished by avoiding sedatives and O2. Brief arousals, of which the patient is mostly unaware, cut off the leak and reverse O2 desaturations. Mouthpiece/lip cover and nasal NVS are open systems that necessitate central nervous system reflexes to prevent excessive leakage during sleep.[22] Excessive leakage is only that which results in

O2 desaturations severe enough to cause arousals of which the patient becomes aware or results in a return of symptoms.

The Trilogy ventilator (Respironics Inc., Murrysville, PA, USA) has a Kiss Trigger that permits air delivery by simply touching (grabbing) the mouthpiece with the lips so that backup rates can be set to zero and nuisance alarms turned off. Although CTMV users require alarms and on accidental disconnection the low pressure alarm may not sound due to back pressure from air leak against the skin or dressing covering the tube, sleeping CNVS users can rely on an alert central nervous system to arouse them for GPB. The only alarm needed for CNVS users is an O2 sat alarm so the many other alarms, including the exhaled volume alarm, sound unnecessarily, as the patients generally exhale into the atmosphere rather than into the tubing. With age and further muscle weakness, complicating conditions, and especially during URIs patients can become CNVS dependent without any hospitalization.[23]

Nasal NVS is typically used for daytime as well as sleep support by patients who do not want to or cannot grab a mouthpiece because of oral and neck muscle weakness and/or inadequate jaw opening. As such, daytime nasal CNVS is a viable and desirable alternative to tracheotomy. When using nasal NVS around-the-clock the nasal interfaces must be alternated to avoid excessive skin pressures and breakdowns. Nasal prongs and nostril covering systems are typically used during daytime hours and "mask" designs for sleep.

With age and further weakness and debility, sleep NVS users can gradually become dyspneic when attempting to discontinue nasal NVS in the morning and extend its use. These patients also typically become CNVS dependent during intercurrent URIs. When long-term daytime aid is needed, transition to the use of an intermittent abdominal pressure ventilator (IAPV) is encouraged (**Fig. 2**).

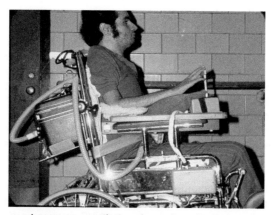

Fig. 2. Continuous tracheostomy ventilation-dependent (CTMV) 17-year-old C2 complete tetraplegic developed severe trachiectasis, chronic bronchitis, and 2 respiratory arrests from airway mucous plugging that caused partial cortical blindness, then had an implanted phrenic pacemaker that never functioned adequately. After 2 years of CTMV and practicing noninvasive ventilatory support (NVS) he was decannulated, transitioned to sleep lipseal NVS and daytime intermittent abdominal pressure ventilator (see here), and his pacemaker was removed. Although his supine vital capacity (VC) remained unmeasurable, following decannulation he used accessory muscles while sitting for 420 mL along with frog breathing most of the day for 32 years.

The Intermittent Abdominal Pressure Ventilator

The pneumatic IAPV (PIAPV) operates by about 2.5 L of air being delivered from a portable ventilator into an elastic air sac in a corset (see **Fig. 2**). The sac is cyclically inflated, moving the diaphragm upwards. Subsequently the sac empties and the diaphragm descends causing air to enter the upper airways. A trunk angle of 30° or more from the horizontal is necessary for effectiveness. The patient can add autonomous breathing and GPB to the PIAPV-derived volumes of 300 mL to as much as 1200 mL.[24] Patients with little ventilator-free breathing ability (VFBA) often prefer it to NVS for daytime support. A new mechanical IAPV is in development.[25] The IAPVs do not interfere with eating or gastrostomy tubes and are useful to treat constipation as well and during labor for CNVS-dependent women in labor as well.[26]

Managing Sleep-Disordered Breathing or Hypoventilation

Aging patients with SCI often develop symptomatic sleep-disordered breathing (SDB) before hypoventilation but eventually both sleep and daytime hypercapnia and hypoxia can occur.[27] Polysomnograms are only useful when pulmonary function is essentially normal, and there is no daytime O2 desaturation or CO2 retention, to treat the simple central and obstructive apneas of SDB. They are not warranted to evaluate patients with reduced VC because routine polysomnograms do not distinguish between apneas and hypopneas from SDB from those caused by respiratory muscle weakness. This leads to inappropriate administration of O2, CPAP, and/or bilevel PAP instead of NVS. Whether for treating SDB or hypoventilation, NVS normalizes the apnea-hypopnea index (AHI), better rests respiratory muscles, and can provide up to CNVS when patients need it during URIs.

Although the AHI can be normalized and symptoms often relieved early on by titrating the AHI to less than 5 using low-span bilevel PAP, when hypoventilation predominates the bilevel PAP often does not normalize sleep CO2 levels or daytime blood gases. It is debatable whether low-span bilevel PAP should ever be used instead of NVS settings that better rest and support the muscles and can normalize blood gases day and night.

Although bilevel PAP is delivered via vented nasal interfaces and passive ventilator circuits, sleep NVS is delivered via lip cover, nasal, or oronasal interfaces via active ventilator circuits, that is, ventilator circuits with exhalation valves, and nonvented interfaces are used.[23,28] When used with an active circuit the portals of vented interfaces must be sealed by tape. Several interfaces should be tried and the patient should alternate their use.

Suboptimal humidification dries out and irritates nasal mucous membranes, causes sore throat, and results in vasodilatation and nasal congestion. Heated humidification may be indicated.[29] Decongestants can help relieve sinus irritation and nasal congestion. Switching to a lip cover–only interface can relieve sinus pressure, nasal congestion, and the nasal bridge discomfort associated with bilevel PAP or NVS.

Although often described as a complication of "noninvasive ventilation," secretion encumbrance actually results from failure to use NVS settings and/or MIE effectively via both invasive and noninvasive interfaces. Patients with severe intrinsic lung disease requiring O2 should use oronasal interfaces for NVS. Uncontrolled seizures and substance abuse are relative contraindications for daytime NVS.[12]

Phrenic Nerve Pacing

Phrenic nerve pacing and diaphragm pacing (which also paces the phrenic nerve) are not noninvasive but can provide all-day ventilatory support for some patients with high-level SCI. In the author's opinion, however, they should be used in conjunction with decannulation and NVS particularly for patients whose VCs are less than 200 mL. These patients usually have no ability to rotate the neck to grab mouthpieces for daytime NVS (**Table 1**). Nasal NVS can be used for sleep along with daytime pacing to avoid the severe sleep obstructive apneas caused by pacing. Because pacers can fail suddenly, they cause sleep apneas, and the patients may have no ventilator free breathing ability, they leave the tracheostomy tubes in. Rather than resort to CPAP to treat pacer-associated obstructive events, NVS, which is essentially only the inspiratory phase of CPAP, can be safely used during sleep even for patients with no measurable VC. Likewise, IAPVs and NVS can be used instead of pacing during the day as well. Once introduced to IAPVs and NVS, patients with some VFBA with VCs greater than 250 mL often prefer to use IAPVs or mouthpiece NVS and stop using pacers permanently (see **Fig. 1**), especially when they cause shoulder, chest, and abdominal pain, and their use, along with the tracheostomy tube, prevents mastery of GPB for security and VFBA.[12] The pacing also does not permit the deep breaths needed for coughing, speaking loudly, and LVR, and they can cause infections and other complications. In the author's opinion there is no role for pacers for patients who can use mouthpiece NVS, IAPVs, and who have significant VFBA. Unfortunately, unlike for tracheotomies and pacing, there is no financial incentive for noninvasive management.

The Oximetry Continuous Noninvasive Ventilatory Support/Mechanical Insufflation-Exsufflation Protocol

Because patients with SCI have ventilatory pump failure rather than intrinsic lung disease, oxygen supplementation should never be administered as an alternative to NVS and MIE to keep O2 sat ($\geq$95%) and CO2 normal during daytime hours or, for that matter, during sleep. O2 supplementation during sleep can cause NVS to be ineffective.[22] Once artifact is ruled out, O2 sat less than 95% is due to hypoventilation (hypercapnia), airway encumberment (secretions), and if the latter is not adequately managed, eventually gross atelectasis and/or pneumonia. A protocol using oximetry feedback to maintain normal O2 sat using NVS/CNVS and MIE as needed can prevent pneumonia and ARF and can greatly facilitate successful extubation and decannulation of patients with SCI even when they are not weanable from ventilatory support.[17,18] Without using this protocol, which has been very effective for patients with neuromuscular disorders,[23,30] respiratory complications continue to be one of the 3 main causes for hospitalizations after the first-year postinjury,[31,32] and mortality rates of 8.5% have been reported.[33] Patients often require CNVS during URIs, which they also use for air stacking to increase cough flows. If, when using NVS, the O2 sat does not renormalize greater than 94%, the desaturation is not due to hypoventilation but probably due to airway mucus. This indicates need for manually assisted coughing and/or effective

Table 1			
Respiratory management indications for patients with spinal cord injury			
Level of Lesion	**VC (in mL)**	**Function (Bulbar/Neck)**	**Ventilation (Daytime/Nocturnal)**
Above C1	0	-/-	CTMV/CTMV
C1-C2	< 200	+/-	EPP/DP/EPP/DP/NVS
C3 or lower	> 200	+/+	NVS/IAPV/NVS

Abbreviations: DP, diaphragm pacing; EPP, electrophrenic pacing.

MIE. If hospitalized, the patient's primary care providers must continue to use the oximetry CNVS/MIE protocol provided that supplemental O2 is not needed to maintain O2 sat greater than 90% and the patient is not in acute distress, in which case, intubation is probably required.

Management Goals

The management goals are to increase cough flows, maximize pulmonary compliance and lung volumes, and maintain normal blood gases around-the-clock. All are accomplished by NVS/CNVS and MIE for cognitively intact patients with SCI. As noted, mouthpiece NVS is not always possible for C1 and C2 tetraplegic patients with no neck excursion. Although the IAPV, nasal NVS, and GPB can be used for daytime support, because mouthpiece NVS is the most important method for daytime support, an alternative approach for the C1-C2 patient is phrenic nerve or diaphragm pacing during the day and decannulation and nasal NVS for sleep (see **Table 1**).

ACUTE PATIENT ASSESSMENT AND MANAGEMENT
Initial

Symptoms and signs of ventilatory insufficiency were noted in the John R. Bach and colleagues'article, "Conventional Respiratory Management of Spinal Cord Injury," in this issue. Although O2 sat is commonly monitored in the acute care setting, VC, CPF, and CO2 should also be monitored. The patient's CO2 can be measured by end-tidal or transcutaneous monitoring as well as by arterial blood gas sampling but the latter is usually unnecessary provided that supplemental O2 is avoided. A CO2 increase by 8 to 10 mm Hg will normally cause dyspnea. Venous bicarbonate levels can also provide useful information.

The VC is measured every 8 hours (nursing shift) until it is stable or increasing. If the VC becomes less than 1000 mL and accessory muscle use occurs,[34] the patient often becomes tired and dyspneic and should be set up and trained to use mouthpiece and nasal NVS (**Fig. 3**) when awake and possibly for sleep as well.[23] Initial NVS use can gradually increase to CNVS dependence with spinal shock and ascending cord edema.[23] If immediate surgery is needed or there are severe complicating injuries, noninvasive management is not initially possible.

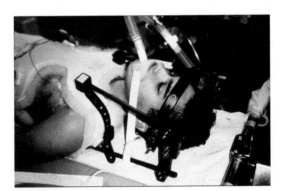

Fig. 3. A 15-year-old traumatic tetraplegic developed dyspnea with VC becoming less than 750 mL and eventually to 200 mL, treated by mouthpiece (daytime) and nasal (sleep) CNVS despite no VFBA. He remained CNVS dependent until postinjury day 15 when his vital capacity increased to 940 mL; daytime NVS was discontinued; and on day 16 with 1070 mL he discontinued NVS and never developed any airway secretions requiring clearance.[29]

NVS settings are high, 700 to 1500 mL, or pressure support about 20 cm H2O. Nevertheless, patients tend not to be overventilated because with intact ventilatory drive they take as much of the air as they need and let the rest leak. O2 therapy and/or sedative and narcotic medications can greatly exacerbate hypercapnia[35] and by causing excessive leakage, can render nasal NVS ineffective.[22] However, the interface can be switched to a tight-fitting oronasal interface for a closed system of support for sleep to maintain effective ventilation despite O2 therapy. As long as the patient is alert and cooperative, mouthpiece and nasal NVS are effective and intubation may be avoided. If the soft palate is incompetent to seal off the nasopharynx from excessive leak of mouthpiece NVS, then only nasal and oronasal NVS can be used.[22]

For patients in spinal shock, both airway suctioning and MIE can cause symptomatic bradycardias. Anticholinergic medications can alleviate this and permit effective MIE and suctioning for secretion clearance. Patients who become NVS/CNVS dependent who do not have lung damage usually do not develop any airway secretions to expel because they do not have invasive airway tubes to cause them and their BIM should be intact to swallow them (see **Fig. 3**).

It is a common mistake to use CPAP or low span bilevel PAP in the critical care setting. Neither of these fully rests or supports respiratory muscles, and supplemental O2 does not treat the airway secretions or hypoventilation that is causing the O2 desaturation. It is tantamount to placing a Band-Aid on a cancer of hypercapnia and airway secretions and worse. The O2 can increase CO2 of a hypercapnic patient with SCI by more than 120 mm Hg and CO2 narcosis.[35] Although low-span (<15 mm Hg) bilevel PAP can at times be adequate to avert intubation and even permit successful extubation, this is not the case for more severe inspiratory muscle paralysis that causes ventilator dependence and necessitates NVS settings, especially when airways are not cleared by normalizing O2 sat by using MIE.

When volume-targeted bilevel PAP is administered, tidal volumes are minimal, LVR impossible, and lungs can stiffen, shrink, and lose compliance.[3] It can not be overemphasized that for patients without primary cardiac disease, O2 desaturations in ambient air indicate NVS and MIE, not low-span bilevel PAP and O2 administration.[23,35]

Intubation

Intubation is done to provide ventilatory support and for secretion management. For some uncomplicated patients intubation can be avoided by up to CNVS and MIE (see **Figs. 1** and **3**) but conditions of most patients with high-level SCI are complicated and they require surgery under general anesthesia. More than 50% of patients with cervical spine injuries are intubated[36,37] but very few need tracheotomies.

Patients who were not NVS dependent before being intubated may wean from support by being placed on CPAP mode with minimal, if any, pressure support to see if they can pass spontaneous breathing trials and ventilator weaning parameters. If they wean quickly, they can be extubated without NVS although CPF are usually ineffective so manually assisted coughing and MIE are likely to be necessary. However, ventilator weaning parameters and spontaneous breathing trials are unnecessary for patients who satisfy CNVS-specific extubation criteria, many of whom who are not weanable from ventilatory support.[17,18]

Weaning an intubated patient with low VC should not even be attempted before the O2 sat baseline remains normal in ambient air by using MIE because if the intrinsic lung disease and airway secretions that are causing a decrease in O2 sat are not cleared before extubation, they will be more difficult to manage after it and tracheotomy will be thought to be needed. Although O2 supplementation is not hazardous for intubated patients being treated for intrinsic lung diseases such as pneumonia, it should be discontinued, as the use of MIE at 60 to 70 cm H2O used via the tube every 1 to 2 hours clears the secretions. The O2 sat baseline usually normalizes in 1 to 3 days and the patient satisfies extubation criteria to CNVS and MIE (**Box 1**) whether ventilator weanable or not.[17,18] Thus, intubated patients are prepared for extubation by normalizing the CO2 using NVS settings at physiologic backup rates, then normalizing O2 sat and clearing any pneumonia in large part by using MIE via the tube along with antibiotics and other conventional care.

More than 83% of unweanable patients who fail one or more extubation attempts to bilevel PAP, CPAP, and O2; who refuse tracheotomies; and who are transferred to our units for extubation to CNVS and MIE have O2 sat baselines less than 95% after their CO2 is normalized and the supplemental O2 is eliminated that they are invariably receiving on arrival.[17,18] Had the referring units used MIE via the tubes and followed published protocols and extubation criteria (see **Box 1**) they would also have been able to successfully extubate these unweanable patients without resort to tracheotomies. The primary reason for extubation failure is failure of the clinicians to use MIE both via the translaryngeal tube at 60 to 70 cm H2O to prepare the patient for extubation and subsequently use it postextubation as well as failure to extubate to CNVS.[17,18] Indeed, most of the patients with high-level SCI who may have failed to ventilator wean and even those who do wean but undergo tracheotomy anyway can be decannulated and learn GPB for VFBA. Even if it takes a month or so to permit surgical interventions, in the author's opinion, patients should be extubated to CNVS and MIE rather than undergo tracheotomy to avoid its life-threatening complications over time.[17,19]

Postextubation

Postextubation to CNVS and MIE patients wean themselves as possible by taking fewer and fewer mouthpiece-delivered breaths or by shorter and shorter periods of nasal NVS as tolerated. If O2 sat drops less than 95%, the care providers are taught to consider reasons such as oral air leakage, interface leakage, tube condensation and pooling, decreased peak airway pressures from leakage or inadequate settings, CO2 retention, and need for more aggressive airway secretion management. Care

---

Box 1
Extubation/decannulation criteria for unweanable patients

1. Fully alert and cooperative, minimal to no sedative medications

2. Afebrile and normal white blood cell count

3. No oxygen requirement for oxyhemoglobin saturation $\geq 95\%$

4. $Paco_2$ 40 mm Hg or less at peak inspiratory pressures less than 30 cm H2O (except if morbidly obese) using up to full ventilatory support as needed

5. Oxyhemoglobin saturation $\geq 95\%$ for 12 hours or more in ambient air

6. All oxyhemoglobin desaturations less than 95% reversed by MIE and suctioning via the airway tube with inflated cuff

7. For intubated patient—a positive leak test with the cuff deflated

8. For patient with tracheostomy—cough peak flows unassisted or assisted or mechanical insufflation-exsufflation flows exceeding 160 L/m with the tube removed, ostomy covered, and patient receiving NVS as needed.

providers use the oximetry CNVS/MIE protocol in the intensive care unit to keep the airways clear and ambient air O2 sat normal.[17,18] Overnight, provided that sedatives, narcotics, and O2 are avoided, heavy mucous accumulation will arouse the patient to request MIE to renormalize O2 sat so oximetry alarms can be set in the low 80s. The family or primary care providers quickly learn that, because they are doing most of the work anyway, the patients can most often be best and most safely cared for at home as long as baseline ambient air O_2 sat remains normal. Even if patients do not wean at all, they return home using CNVS and MIE.

The success rate using this protocol for first attempts at extubation in individuals with high cervical SCI who are unable to pass spontaneous weaning trials before or after extubation has been 100% (32 of 32).[17,18] Overall, 254 of 257 ventilator unweanable patients with ventilatory pump failure have been reported to have been extubated to CNVS and MIE by this protocol including the 32 with SCI.[17,18] Their families provided most of the postextubation care for 24 hours after which the secretions die down. Thus, MIE is most important for preparing patients for extubation or decannulation and is crucial for successful extubation and decannulation of unweanable patients.[17,18] Because many of our patients have had to wait intubated for 1 to 6 months before their insurance approved the transfers and all were successfully extubated to CNVS and MIE including 32 patients with SCI in 1 to 11 days, no harm was caused by the prolonged intubations.[17,18]

Because it is easier to extubate unweanable patients than to decannulate them, and because most respiratory morbidity and mortality is from the cuffed tubes, it may certainly be time for a paradigm shift to more humane noninvasive management. Invasive management has never been shown to be superior to CNVS and MIE; rather it has been the contrary.[16,23,30,38]

Long-Term Outpatient Assessment and Management

VC can increase for up to 8 years in patients after high cervical level SCI; patients may wean entirely several years after injury. More commonly, as the VC decreases with age the patient becomes symptomatic for symptoms of SDB and/or hypoventilation and requires NVS later in life.[27] Patients with SCI with 1000 mL of VC at age 20 years are typically normocapnic and asymptomatic but by age 50 years they are more likely to be symptomatic for hypoventilation and have frequent sleep O2 desaturations and hypercapnia with the same VC.[35,39]

Their evaluations need to be specific for patients with ventilatory pump failure and not include traditional pulmonary function testing that evaluates for lung and airways diseases rather than for muscle dysfunction. Specific outpatient evaluation to assess for and prevent respiratory complications includes monitoring of CPF, age, basal metabolic index (BMI), O2 sat, and CO2 levels; spirometric assessment of active and passive LVR, GPB, and VC in various positions including supine and with orthotics such as thoracolumbar braces on and off when present; and BIM assessment. For patients with weak lips, active LVR (air stacking) is performed via nasal, lip cover, or oronasal interfaces. The BIM function is assessed by the determination of the MIC, VC difference, a direct function of glottis, and BIM integrity.

An abdominal binder can support the abdominal contents by limiting expansion of the abdominal wall to prevent diaphragm sagging when seated. This tends to expand the lower rib cage more with the descent of the diaphragm to increase total lung capacity and rib-cage dimensions in tetraplegics.[40] Any lower lobe atelectasis caused by the binder is countered by LVR.

Absolute VC can be more useful than percentage of predicted normal VC. The authors first described SCI late-onset SDB with hypoventilation and diminished VCs in

1991.[27,41–43] In general, symptomatic adults with less than 1000 mL of VC sitting or supine or a VC 20% greater when sitting than when supine, because of accessory muscle rather than diaphragm sparing, should be offered sleep nasal NVS rather than sleep sitting up or being confined to side lying. As noted previously, excessive use of accessory musculature can be alleviated by using an IAPV or daytime mouthpiece and/or nasal NVS.

Arterial blood gases are typically unnecessary for patients with SCI because oximetry and capnography/transcutaneous CO_2 along with venous bicarb levels can provide the needed information unless there is an oxygenation requirement, which should be corrected with effective management.

As in acute care, patients with decreased VC are trained in air stacking, GPB, manually assisted coughing, and MIE. CO_2, O_2 sat, CPF, and spirometry are assessed annually. If CPF, whether unassisted or assisted, do not exceed 300 L/m, patients are trained in MIE and provided with immediate access to it if only needed during intercurrent URIs.

If symptoms are unclear, CO_2 and O_2 sat levels are monitored during sleep. When sleep EtCO2 exceeds 50 mm Hg and there are many O_2 desaturations or baseline less than 95%, even if symptoms are equivocal, a trial of sleep nasal NVS should be urged. Many patients only realize that they are symptomatic after feeling better using nasal NVS.

With time and further decreases in VC, daytime CO_2, after being corrected by sleep NVS, can very gradually increase again and with age lesser levels of hypercapnia are needed for symptomatic daytime O_2 desaturation to occur and result in sleep NVS being extended into daytime hours.[23] Obesity and scoliosis further exacerbate problem. For intercurrent URIs the above-described oximetry CNVS/ MIE protocol must be used. It can prevent ARF more than 90% of the time.[44] Despite hyperpyrexia and elevated white blood cell counts, baseline O_2 sat can return to normal and hospitalization be avoided by the protocol despite continuous ventilator dependence.[23,45] As the O_2 baseline returns to normal, most patients gradually wean back to the usual pre-URI ventilatory assistance regimen until the next URI.

Decannulation

Although decreasing synchronized intermittent mandatory ventilation rates and pressure support levels are a most frequent invasive ventilation weaning strategy, this approach permits neither optimal respiratory muscle rest nor exercise. An arguably better strategy is to place weaning patients on trach collar with compressed humidified air in Fio_2 21% until they become dyspneic and O2 sat baseline becomes less than 95%, then placing them back on support settings for 30 minutes before taking them off again for the next sprint. Typically the ventilator free sprints become longer between 30 min support sessions until they wean.[46–48]

Whether they wean or not, they are still candidates for decannulation and transition to NVS/CNVS. Because NVS is preferred by all over TMV for safety, security, appearance, swallowing, speech, comfort, appearance, and overall,[49] decannulation can be offered to those who wish it, are cognitively intact, can rotate the neck sufficiently to grab a mouthpiece fixed near the mouth, and when the upper airway is patent as seen by having MIE-EF exceed at least 150 L/m(Gonçalves MR, Bach JR, Ishikawa Y, et al. Mechanical insufflation-exsufflation expiratory flow generation for patients with respiratory muscle weakness/paralysis.[50] Even patients who cannot rotate their necks to safely use mouthpiece NVS and who cannot use GPB can use phrenic pacemakers during the day and nasal or oronasal NVS for sleep. Dependence on CNVS is unsafe for patients with seizure disorders or who are severely cognitively impaired. Decannulation criteria are very similar to those for extubation (see **Box 1**).

Decannulation approaches have been described in detail. Initially we decannulated CTMV-dependent patients in critical care units but more recently, of the last 61, 51 were decannulated in the outpatient clinic after weeks to months of practice using mouthpiece and/or nasal CNVS with fenestrated cuffless tube or Olympic trach buttons in place. With criteria satisfied (see **Box 1**) and the patient experienced in NVS and MIE, the tubes were removed. Pressure dressings were applied until the ostomies closed so that the CNVS did not blow out of the stoma.[51] Duoderm (3M Inc., St. Paul, MN) covered the ostomy with a cane tip over that with the tips walls cut short. Over that is placed adhesive tape and a figure of 8 ace bandage for counter pressure to the NVS. The stomas close entirely or to a pinhole in 3 days. If not closed in 2 months, they are sutured closed. Former CTMV users continue to use CNVS as outpatients, indefinitely.[51]

In one study in which 25 SCI CTMV users were decannulated, switched to CNVS, and had their ostomies closed despite VCs of 50 mL to 740 mL, 7 of the 25 injured at 25.1 ± 12.1 years of age were CNVS dependent for a mean of 12.4 ± 6.3 (1–22) years after decannulation and the others weaned to less than CNVS. Five of the seven mastered GPB for VFBA. All 25 were CNVS dependent at extubation and became CNVS dependent and required MIE during intercurrent URIs. Two patients were CNVS dependent for 18 and 30.1 years. Twenty of the twenty-five were discharged to private residencies. Two patients died due to decubiti and seizures, respectively. From the same study, 28 patients continued CTMV from age 30.2 ± 20 years for 7.1 ± 5.2 years. Five were lost to follow-up; 13 died in 3.8 ± 2.8 years (6 from pneumonia, 2 from cancer, 2 accidental disconnection, 2 tracheal hemorrhage, 1 vent dysfunction, and 1 unknown). Thus, at least 11 of 28 TMV users died from tube complications.[19]

In another study 24 of 34 CTMV-dependent patients with high-level SCI since age 29.8 ± 18.4 years were switched to CNVS and decannulated despite mean VC of 606 ± 458 (0-1150) mL. The patients had less than 3 hours of VFBA, 11 had none, and 4 had 0 mL of VC. The IAPV was the predominant method of daytime support for 7 patients. There were 2 hospital admissions for respiratory complications over the next 45 patient-years of noninvasive management. Five of six patients with no VFBA and mean VC 402 mL mastered GPB to volumes of 2205 mL and used it for VFBA.[20]

In another early study, 67 CTMV-dependent patients including 24 with high-level SCI with mean VC 671 mL were decannulated to CNVS.[21] All weaned to sleep NVS but 7 needed it day and night for a mean 8.8 (3 weeks to 32) years. In yet another, 4 high-level patients were decannulated to CNVS and MIE, but one was recannulated within 12 hours due to severe abdominal distension despite gastrostomy tube placement and cardiovascular instability associated with digital stimulation for bowel evacuation and turns in bed.[51]

Acute respiratory failure typically due to intercurrent pneumonias is a frequently cited cause of death in conventionally managed patients with SCI as it was for patients with neuromuscular diseases before their management by up to CNVS and MIE.[52] Besides the 120 patients who used both TMV and NVS for at least 1 month preferring the latter,[49] noninvasive management also facilitates discharge of these patients into the community, whereas tracheostomy can proscribe many activities and is a great cost saving measure as well as facilitates better quality of life.[44,53]

Although tracheostomy tubes are unnecessary for ventilatory support for mentally competent patients, they are needed for patients with severe tracheal stenosis or other fixed upper airway obstruction.

Noninvasive Management Outcomes

Although respiratory prognoses for invasively managed patients are very poor, comparing invasive and noninvasive survival outcomes for SCI is problematic because these patients die for so many reasons. Although respiratory causes are the most frequent causes, they are still only responsible for about 25% of mortality.[1,2] Another problem in comparing the approaches is that the tube makes patients more dependent on TMV, whereas its removal results in increases in VC, in large part due to less airway secretion congestion, and facilitates weaning to less than CNVS.[23] Although most adult patients with as little as 250 to 300 mL of VC may use NVS around-the-clock but have significant VFBA, this is never the case for SCI CTMV users who have no VFBA at all with these VCs, are typically hyperventilated, and who become immediately dyspneic on disconnection. The authors have had SCI CTMV users with 900 mL of VC and normal BMIs. This would never be the case for patients managed by NVS/CNVS.

Knowing the short duration of survival using CTMV, it would be interesting to note how long CNVS users can survive even though many wean to NVS and can no longer be considered CNVS dependent. From 2 studies alone patients with high-level SCI following decannulation were CNVS dependent for 132 patient-years with at least 2 patients CNVS dependent for 27 and 32 years, respectively. The latter patient mastered GPB for up to all-day VFBA.[19,20]

Despite our challenge to rehabilitation spinal cord services to essentially create tracheostomy tube-free centers in 2006 and the fact that CNVS including via mouthpiece was first described for high-level SCI patients in 1969,[54] only 11 other ventilator "unweanable" patients with SCI have been reported to have been decannulated to CNVS and MIE in one center in Portugal at this time.[51,55]

Quality of Life

As noted in John R. Bach and colleagues'article, "Conventional Respiratory Management of Spinal Cord Injury," in this issue, although it seems that constant struggle of lower level ventilator-free patients with cervical SCI to attain more function creates frustrations that the higher level ventilator-dependent patients do not have; quality of life and life satisfaction are also significantly greater when managed noninvasively.[36,49,56] This, combined with the fact that long-term survival of SCI TMV users is extremely poor with no significant improvement in long-term respiratory morbidity and mortality rates over the last 4 years and the fact that noninvasively managed patients with neuromuscular disorders are now surviving far longer than those managed by tracheostomies, for example, 10 years longer for Duchenne muscular dystrophy,[57] 25 years for severe spinal muscular atrophy type 1,[58] and others surviving using CNVS for more than 65 years,[23] it seems reasonable to suggest that a noninvasive approach might provide similar benefits for the high-level SCI population as well.

DISCLOSURE

The authors have nothing to disclose.

REFERENCES

1. Center NSCIS. Annual statistical report for the spinal cord injury model systems public version. Birmingham (AL): University of Alabama at Birmingham; 2018.
2. Devivo MJ. Epidemiology of traumatic spinal cord injury: trends and future implications. Spinal Cord 2012;50(5):365–72.

3. Bach JR, Kang SW. Disorders of ventilation: weakness, stiffness, and mobilization. Chest 2000;117(2):301–3.
4. Axen K, Pineda H, Shunfenthal I, et al. Diaphragmatic function following cervical cord injury: neutrally mediated improvement in vital capacity measurements. Arch Phys Med Rehabil 1985;66:219–22.
5. Estenne M, DeTroyer A. The effects of tetraplegia. Am Rev Respir Dis 1986;134: 121–4.
6. Chiou M, Bach JR, Jethani L, et al. Active lung volume recruitment to preserve vital capacity in Duchenne muscular dystrophy. J Rehabil Med 2017;49:49–53.
7. Kang SW, Bach JR. Maximum insufflation capacity. Chest 2000;118:61–5.
8. Dail C, Rodgers M, Guess V, et al. Glossopharyngeal breathing. Downey (CA): Rancho Los Amigos Hospital, Department of Physical Therapy; 1979.
9. Dail CW, Affeldt JE. Glossopharyngeal breathing [Video]. Los Angeles (CA): College of Medical Evangelists, Department of Visual Education; 1954.
10. Webber B, Higgens J. Glossopharyngeal breathing what, when and how?[Video]. West Sussex (England): Aslan Studios Ltd.; 1999.
11. Bach JR, Bianchi C. Prevention of pectus excavatum for children with spinal muscular atrophy type 1. Am J Phys Med Rehabil 2003;82:815–9.
12. Bach JR. Noninvasive respiratory management of high level spinal cord injury. J SpinalCord Med 2012;35(2):72–80.
13. Garstang SV, Kirshblum SC, Wood KE. Patient preference for in exsufflation for secretion management with spinal cord injury. J SpinalCord Med 2000;23:80–5.
14. Welch JR, DeCesare R, Hess D. Pulse oximetry: instrumentation and clinical applications. Respir Care 1990;35:584–94.
15. Bach JR. Respiratory muscle aids: patient evaluation and the oximetry, respiratory aid protocol. In: Bach JR, editor. Noninvasive mechanical ventilation. Philadelphia: Hanley & Belfus; 2002. p. 165–88.
16. Bach JR, Rajaraman R, Ballanger F, et al. Neuromuscular ventilatory insufficiency: the effect of home mechanical ventilator use vs. oxygen therapy on pneumonia and hospitalization rates. Am J Phys Med Rehabil 1998;77(1):8–19.
17. Bach JR, Gonçalves MR, Hamdani I, et al. Extubation of unweanable patients with neuromuscular weakness: a new management paradigm. Chest 2010;137(5): 1033–9.
18. Bach JR, Sinquee D, Saporito LR, et al. Efficacy of mechanical insufflation-exsufflation in extubating unweanable subjects with restrictive pulmonary disorders. Respir Care 2015;60(4):477–83.
19. Bach JR, Alba AS. Noninvasive options for ventilatory support of the traumatic high level quadriplegic patient. Chest 1990;98:613–9.
20. Bach JR. New approaches in the rehabilitation of the traumatic high level quadriplegic. Am J Phys Med Rehabil 1991;70(1):13–20.
21. Bach JR, Alba AS, Saporito LR. Intermittent positive pressure ventilation via the mouth as an alternative to tracheostomy for 257 ventilator users. Chest 1993; 103:174–82.
22. Bach JR, Robert D, Leger P, et al. Sleep fragmentation in kyphoscoliotic individuals with alveolar hypoventilation treated by NIPPV. Chest 1995;107:1552–8.
23. Bach JR. Noninvasive respiratory management of patients with neuromuscular disease. Ann Rehabil Med 2017;41(4):1–20.
24. Bach JR, Alba AS. Intermittent abdominal pressure ventilator in a regimen of noninvasive ventilatory support. Chest 1991;99:630–6.
25. Bach JR, Radbourne M. A mechanical intermittent abdominal pressure ventilator. Am J Phys Med Rehabil 2019;98(12):e144–6.

26. Bach JR. Successful pregnancies for ventilator users. Am J Phys Med Rehabil 2003;82(3):226–9.
27. Bach JR. Inappropriate weaning and late onset ventilatory failure of individuals with traumatic quadriplegia. Paraplegia 1993;31(7):430–8.
28. Allen J. Pulmonary complications of neuromuscular disease: a respiratory mechanics perspective. Paediatr Respir Rev 2010;11:18–23.
29. Richards GN, Cistulli PA, Ungar RG, et al. Mouth leak with nasal continuous positive airway pressure increases nasal airway resistance. Am J Respir Crit Care Med 1996;154:182–6.
30. Bach JR, Martinez D. Duchenne muscular dystrophy: prolongation of survival by noninvasive interventions. Respir Care 2011;56(6):744–50 [Arch Phys Med Rehabil 1971;52:333-336].
31. Cardenas DD, Huffman JM, Kirshblum S, et al. Etiology and incidence of rehospitalization after traumatic spinal cord injury: a multicenter analysis. Arch Phys Med Rehabil 2004;85:1757–63.
32. Chang HT, Evans CT, Weaver FM, et al. Etiology and outcomes of veterans with spinal cord injury and disorders hospitalized with community-acquired pneumonia. Arch Phys Med Rehabil 2005;86(2):262–7.
33. Meyers AB, Bisbee A, Winter M. The "Boston Model" of managed care spinal cord injury: a cross-sectional study of the outcomes of risk-based, pre-paid, managed care. Arch Phys Med Rehabil 1999;80:1450–6.
34. Bach JR, Hunt D, Horton JA III. Traumatic tetraplegia: noninvasive respiratory management in the acute setting. Am J Phys Med Rehabil 2002;81(10):792–7.
35. Chiou M, Bach JR, Saporito LR, et al. Quantitation of Oxygen induced hypercapnia in respiratory pump failure. Rev Portug Pneumol (2006) 2016;22(5):262–5.
36. Seidl RO, Wolf D, Nusser-Muller-Busch R, et al. Airway management in acute tetraplegics: a retrospective study. Eur Spine J 2010;19(7):1073–8.
37. Royster RA, Barboi C, Peruzzi WT. Critical care in the acute cervical spinal cord injury. Top Spinal Cord Inj Rehabil 2004;9:11–32.
38. Bach JR. Amyotrophic lateral sclerosis: communication status and survival with ventilatory support. Am J Phys Med Rehabil 1993;72(6):343–9.
39. Bach JR, Alba AS. Management of chronic alveolar hypoventilation by nasal ventilation. Chest 1990;97(1):52–7.
40. McCool FD, Pichurko BM, Slutsky AS, et al. Changes in lung volume and rib cage configuration with abdominal binding in quadriplegia. J Appl Physiol 1985;60: 1198–202.
41. 14th Annual Scientific Meeting of the American Spinal Injury Association, San Diego, May 2, 1988.
42. Bach JR, Sortor S, Sipski M. Sleep blood gas monitoring of high cervical quadriplegic patients with respiratory insufficiency by non-invasive techniques. Proc 1988;102–3.
43. Bach JR, Wang TG. Pulmonary function and sleep disordered breathing in traumatic tetraplegics: a longitudinal study. Arch Phys Med Rehabil 1994;75(3): 279–84.
44. Bach JR, Martinez D. Duchenne muscular dystrophy: continuous noninvasive ventilatory support prolongs survival. Respir Care 2011;56(6):744–50.
45. Bach JR, Ishikawa Y, Kim H. Prevention of pulmonary morbidity for patients with Duchenne muscular dystrophy. Chest 1997;112:1024–8.
46. Esteban A, Frutos F, Tobin MJ, et al. A comparison of four methods of weaning patients from mechanical ventilation.Spanish Lung Failure Collaborative Group. N Engl J Med 1995;332(6):345–50.

47. Brochard L, Rauss A, Benito S, et al. Comparison of three methods of gradual withdrawal from ventilatory support during weaning from mechanical ventilation. Am J Respir Crit Care 1994;150(4):896–903.

48. Jubran A, Grant BJ, Duffner LA, et al. Effect of pressure support vs. unassisted breathing through a treacheostomy collar on weaning duration in patients requiring prolonged mechanical ventilation: a randomized trial. JAMA 2013; 309:671–7.

49. Bach JR. A comparison of long-term ventilatory support alternatives from the perspective of the patient and care giver. Chest 1993;104(6):1702–6.

50. Bach JR, Giménez GC, Chiou M. Mechanical in-exsufflation-expiratory flows as indication for tracheostomy tube decannulation: case studies. Am J Phys Med Rehabil 2019;98:e18–20.

51. Bach JR, Saporito LR, Shah HR, et al. Decanulation of patients with severe respiratory muscle insufficiency: efficacy of mechanical insufflation-exsufflation. J Rehabil Med 2014;46:1037–41.

52. Ryu JS, Park SR, Choi KH. Prediction of laryngeal aspiration using voice analysis. Am J Phys Med Rehabil 2004;83:753–7.

53. Bach JR, Intintola P, Alba AS, et al. The ventilator-assisted individual: cost analysis of institutionalization versus rehabilitation and in-home management. Chest 1992;101(1):26–30.

54. Alba A, Solomon M, Trainor FS. Management of respiratory insufficiency in spinal cord lesions, In: Proceedings of the 17th Veteran's Administration Spinal Cord Injury Conference, U.S. Government Printing Office 0-436-398. Las Vegas, October 20, 1969.

55. Bach JR. Prevention of respiratory complications of spinal cord injury: a challenge to "model" spinal cord injury units. J SpinalCord Med 2006;29(1):3–4.

56. Bach JR, Tilton MC. Life satisfaction and well-being measures in ventilator assisted individuals with traumatic tetraplegia. Arch Phys Med Rehabil 1994;75: 626–32.

57. Ishikawa Y, Miura T, Ishikawa Y, et al. Duchenne muscular dystrophy: survival by cardio-respiratory interventions. Neuromuscul Disord 2011;21:47–51.

58. Bach JR. Point: Is Non-invasive ventilation always the most appropriate manner of long-term ventilation for infants with Spinal Muscular Atrophy Type 1? Yes, almost always? Chest 2016;151(5):962–5.

Cardiometabolic Disease and Dysfunction Following Spinal Cord Injury

Origins and Guideline-Based Countermeasures

Mark S. Nash, PhD[a,b,c,d],*, David R. Gater Jr, MD, PhD[a,b,c,e]

KEYWORDS

- Spinal cord injuries • Cardiometabolic disease • Cardiovascular disease • Exercise
- Nutrition • Pharmacotherapy

KEY POINTS

- The health risks and guideline diagnosis of the cardiometabolic syndrome (CMS) are commonly observable after spinal cord injuries (SCIs) and disorders.
- Intense exercise and nutritional modification after SCI represent first-line countermeasures to the CMS and its risk determinants.
- Early surveillance of cardiometabolic risks should be undertaken to identify and treat the risks of overweight/obesity and insulin resistance.
- Pharmacotherapy and bariatric surgery represent alternatives to exercise and nutrition, although at higher risks and untested effectiveness.

CARDIOENDOCRINE DISEASE
The Cardiometabolic Syndrome After Spinal Cord Injury

The cardiometabolic syndrome (CMS) is a coalescing of cardiovascular (CV), renal, metabolic, prothrombotic, and inflammatory health risks.[1] **Fig. 1** shows the general health indicators and component risks for the CMS, where co-occurrence of 3 (or more) of the following health risks typically defines the syndrome: abdominal (central) obesity, hypertension, insulin resistance, and dyslipidemia (dyslipidemia being either hypertriglyceridemia or low high-density lipoproteinemia). When coexpressed, these risks become a distinct disease entity defined by many authoritative bodies, including

[a] Departments of Neurological Surgery and Physical Medicine & Rehabilitation; [b] The Miami Project to Cure Paralysis; [c] The NIDILRR Model SCI System, University of Miami Leonard M. Miller School; [d] 1095 Northwest 14th Terrace, R-48, Miami, FL 33136, USA; [e] 1120 Northwest 14th Street, CRC 958, Miami, FL 33136, USA
* Corresponding author. University of Miami Miller School of Medicine, Lois Pope Life Center, 1095 Northwest 14th Terrace, R-48, Miami, FL 33136.
E-mail address: mnash@med.miami.edu

Phys Med Rehabil Clin N Am 31 (2020) 415–436
https://doi.org/10.1016/j.pmr.2020.04.005
1047-9651/20/© 2020 Elsevier Inc. All rights reserved.

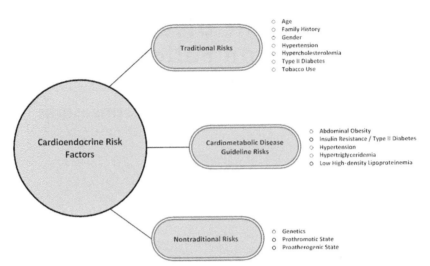

Fig. 1. Interrelated component risks of the cardiometabolic disease. (*Adapted from* Després JP, Lemieux I. Abdominal obesity and metabolic syndrome. Nature. 2006;444(7121):881–887; with permission.)

the World Health Organization (WHO).[2] Although the definitions for CMS shown in **Table 1** are not yet harmonized,[3] any coalescing of risk factors worsens a CV disease (CVD) prognosis. In particular, a CMS diagnosis poses a health risk equivalent to that of either type 2 diabetes or existing coronary disease. The syndrome is currently reported in 22.9% of the US adult population,[4] is increased by 50% after spinal cord injury (SCI), and is expanding at a rate that resembles a pandemic of infectious diseases.[5]

CMS is known to develop from a mismatch between daily energy intake and energy expenditure,[6] making persons with SCI a high-risk target for the disorder. The primary metabolic abnormality of the syndrome is insulin resistance, whereas the unified cause is excessive body fat mass associated with visceral and ectopic fat depots. Combined overweight and obesity in persons with chronic SCI describes 60% to 80% of the population,[7,8] with the most common period for body mass gain occurring 2 to 7 months after discharge from postinjury rehabilitation.[9,10] Even though the CMS diagnosis is based on a sum-of-risks strategy, the 5 component risks are not equally weighted, with sarcopenic obesity[11] (a highly prevalent finding after SCI[12–16]) being the most powerful contributor, followed by insulin resistance.

All-cause disorders of the cardioendocrine system have been reported in persons with SCI since the early 1980s[17,18] and are thought to hasten CV-related morbidity and mortality.[19–21] The genesis of these disorders is primarily attributed to CMS risk factors observed in the nondisabled population, although reported at a significantly increased prevalence after SCI.[7] These risks include atherogenic dyslipidemia with low levels of the cardioprotective high-density lipoprotein cholesterol (HDL-C).[22–28]

Nonguideline Cardiometabolic Syndrome Risks of Sedentary Lifestyle and Imprudent Nutrition After Spinal Cord Injury

Although the 5 component risks of the cardiometabolic disease (CMD) do not include physical deconditioning, it is still considered a significant cause of obesity, insulin resistance, hypertension, and dyslipidemia.[22,29] The same is known for hypercaloric

Table 1
Guideline definition of cardiometabolic disease in the general population

Authority		Diagnosis
AHA/NHLBI[122,123]	Three or more of:	Waist circumference[a]: • Men: >102 cm (40 inches) • Women: >88 cm (35 inches) Plasma triglycerides: ≥150 mg/dL (1.7 mmol/L) Reduced HDL ("good") cholesterol: Men: <40 mg/dL (1.03 mmol/L) Women: <50 mg/dL (1.29 mmol/L) Increased BP: ≥130/85 mm Hg or use of medication for hypertension Fasting glucose ≥100 mg/dL (5.6 mmol/L) or use of medication for hyperglycemia

Abbreviations: AHA, American Heart Association; BP, blood pressure; HDL, high-density lipoprotein; NHLBI, National Heart, Lung, and Blood Institute.

[a] NOTE: Use of waist circumference is not validated in persons with SCI. For adults with SCI substitute definitions of obesity using: a: greater than 22% BF body fat when using 3- or 4- compartment modeling, or (b) BMI ≥22 kg/m².

Data from Refs.[68,122,123]

nutrition relative to daily need.[9,30] Several factors point to physical deconditioning after SCI as a significant contributor to a CMS diagnosis. The SCI population was long ago identified at the lowest end of the human fitness continuum, making physical deconditioning suspect as a cause for CMS-related risks.[24,31–33] Further, the most common dyslipidemia reported after SCI is low HDL-C,[23,25,34] which is often comorbid with poor cardiorespiratory fitness in persons without disability.[35–37]

In addition to physical inactivity, dietary habits and nutritional status strongly influence the CMS condition.[38] Changes in the post-SCI metabolic milieu (eg, loss of metabolically active tissue and altered fuel homeostasis), physical barriers (eg, access to food shopping and grocery store shelving), environment (eg, institutional food), functional challenges (eg, difficulties encountered in preparing food), and social factors (eg, food provided as comfort by family/friends),[39] favor a so-called obesogenic environment,[39] and make lifelong healthy nutrition habits a lifelong challenge.

Guidelines for Addressing Cardiometabolic Syndrome Risks After Spinal Cord Injury

Given the well-documented CMS risks after SCI and the lack of a unified treatment strategy for its composite and individualized risks, The Consortium for Spinal Cord Medicine recently convened an expert panel to develop guidelines for identification and management of cardiometabolic risk after SCI.[40] These guidelines (from now on the Paralyzed Veterans of America [PVA] guidelines) and others form the basis for the remaining information presented in this article.

DEFINITION AND SURVEILLANCE OF CARDIOMETABOLIC SYNDROME

The recently published PVA guidelines[40] recommend the use of the American Heart Association (AHA) definition for determining CMS in persons with SCI (**Table 2**). Because waist circumference is not a validated proxy for obesity in SCI, the PVA guidelines assumed definitions of obesity as (1) greater than 22% body fat when using 3-compartment or 4-compartment modeling, or (2) body mass index (BMI) greater than or equal to 22 kg/m². **Table 3** identifies timing for postinjury surveillance and periodic follow-up for the CMS diagnosis and component risks.

LIFESTYLE INTERVENTION

Although physical activity is a recognized countermeasure to excessive energy intake, some persons with SCI cannot effectively balance energy intake and expenditure with physical activity alone. A high level of injury,[41] overuse injuries,[42,43] and documented barriers to exercise may further diminish exercise benefits.[44–47] Appreciating that energy expenditure from upper-body physical activity rarely compensates for excessive caloric intake, nutritional modification may represent a needed collateral target for obesity management and CMD prevention in individuals with SCI. Because the use of, and guidelines for, exercise after SCI have recently been reviewed,[48–52] the balance of this article addresses nutrition within the lifestyle plan, and other nonexercise intervention strategies (**Table 4**).

Nutritional Intervention and Energetics as Countermeasure to Cardiometabolic Syndrome After Spinal Cord Injury

Obesity in persons with SCI is ultimately the result of a positive energy balance in which markedly diminished energy expenditure is exceeded by caloric intake. An individual's total daily energy expenditure (TDEE) comprises their resting metabolic rate (RMR), the thermic effect of physical activity (TEA), and the thermic effect of food digestion (TEF). RMR reflects the calories needed by the body to maintain essential life functions at rest and incorporates metabolic activity from muscles, bones, and organs (ie, fat-free mass [FFM]) to sustain life. For most populations, there exists a tight correlation between FFM and RMR, which is independent of age, race, or gender.[53] Several factors make this relationship less predictable after SCI. Spastic paralysis resulting from the SCI results in obligatory sarcopenia in all myotomes below the level of the injury,[11] with profound loss of metabolically active skeletal muscle, including the diaphragm, intercostal muscles, and myocardium at high cervical levels of SCI.[54] Mechanical unloading, diminished neurogenic activation, and intermittent pathologic bursts of sympathetic activity further contribute to bone loss, particularly in the lower extremities where bone mineral content plateaus at roughly two-thirds of normal within 2 years after SCI (ie, virtually at fracture threshold).[55] Higher levels of SCI diminish autonomic control of the sympathetic nervous system, which arises from the thoracolumbar regions of the cord. Because the sympathetic nervous system activates adrenergic fight-or-flight responses, higher levels of SCI interrupt these energy-consuming sympathetic nervous system responses, further reducing metabolic energy expenditure. Parasympathetic dominance of the autonomic nervous system ultimately results in diminished heart rate and contractility, neurogenic hypotension, and neurogenic obstructive lung disease.[56–58]

In daily activity, upper extremity exercise burns fewer calories than lower extremity exercise because of reduced muscle mass and workload, even at similar heart rates. As with RMR, SCI results in marked reductions of TEA because of reduced total FFM but is also limited by blunted sympathetic responses that diminish cardiopulmonary exercise responses. Relatively unopposed parasympathetic dominance at baseline and during exercise results in diminished vascular tone on both arterial and venous systems, effectively reducing both afterload and preload exposure of myocardium with a resulting adaptive myocardial atrophy. Chronotropic responses are also blunted because of diminished adrenergic stimulation of the sinoatrial node, such that /min even during maximal exertion. Upper extremity exercise under these physiologic conditions results in venous pooling at lower extremities and inferior vena cava that is further exacerbated by the absence of lower extremity muscle contractions caused by paralysis. Although nondisabled individuals see both increased heart rate and

Table 2
Recommended schedule for surveillance and follow-up of cardiometabolic risk after spinal cord injury

Risk	Test	Patients	Initial	Follow-up
CMD	3+ risk components (discussed later)	All	See individual risk components	
CMD Risk Components				
Impaired fasting glucose, prediabetes, and diabetes	FPG, OGTT, or HbA1c	Asymptomatic adults with SCI	Screen adults with SCI for diabetes and prediabetes, and repeat testing at least every 3 y if tests are normal	
		Individuals having confirmed prediabetes, diabetes, or CMD		Annual testing and ongoing management. Institute lifestyle management and, if necessary, drug therapy (see **Table 4**)
Obesity	Multicompartment modeling or BMI	All	At discharge from rehabilitation	Annual testing, or when evidence of increased risk is identified
Dyslipidemia	Fasting lipid panel preferred; but at minimum HDL-C and TG			
Hypertension	BP			Measured at every routine visit (and at least annually). Increased BP readings should be confirmed on a separate visit to diagnose hypertension. Repeat BP measurements over time and measure BP in both the supine and seated positions to account for postural influences and BP variability caused by autonomic instability
Lifestyle Risk Factors				

(continued on next page)

Table 2
(continued)

Risk	Test	Patients	Initial	Follow-up
Suboptimal nutrition	Maintenance of stable body fat mass or whole-body mass throughout the lifespan	All	Medically supervised nutrition plan beginning in rehabilitation, or as soon as possible	Continuous throughout the lifespan
Physical deconditioning	Exercise testing if practical	All, insofar as feasible and practical	Recommendations for therapeutic or recreational exercise initiated by the time of rehabilitation discharge	Annual assessment with continuous follow-up throughout the lifespan

Abbreviations: BMI, body mass index; CMD, cardiometabolic disease; FPG, fasting plasma glucose; HbA1c, glycated hemoglobin; OGTT, oral glucose tolerance test (2 hours, 75 g of glucose); TG, triglycerides.

Data from Nash MS, Groah SL, Gater DR, et al. Identification and Management of Cardiometabolic Risk after Spinal Cord Injury Clinical Practice Guideline for Health Care Providers. J Spinal Cord Med. 2019;42(5):643-77.

Table 3
Criteria for the diagnosis of prediabetes and diabetes

Criterion	Prediabetes	Diabetes
HbA1c (%)	5.7–6.4	≥6.5
FPG	100–125 mg/dL (95.6–6.9 mmol/L)	≥126 mg/dL (7.0 mmol/L)
OGTT	140–199 mg/dL (7.8–11.0 mmol/L)	≥200 mg/dL (11/.1 mmol/L)[a]
RPG	—	≥200 mg/dL (11/.1 mmol/L)[b]

Abbreviation: RPG, random plasma glucose.
[a] In the absence of unequivocal hyperglycemia, results should be confirmed by repeat testing.
[b] Only diagnostic in patients with classic symptoms of hyperglycemia or hyperglycemic crisis.
Data from Nash MS, Groah SL, Gater DR, et al. Identification and Management of Cardiometabolic Risk after Spinal Cord Injury Clinical Practice Guideline for Health Care Providers. J Spinal Cord Med. 2019;42(5):643-77.

stroke volume during progressively increased upper extremity work, CV responses are blunted for persons with SCI, and blood pressure (BP) decreases with progressively increased loads, potentially leading to presyncopal/syncopal events caused by diminished cerebral perfusion. TEA is further limited by neurogenic restrictive (abdominal and intercostal muscle paralysis) and obstructive (parasympathetic dominant bronchoconstriction with mucus secretion) lung disease, both of which restrict respiration for persons with high SCI. A compendium of physical activity for persons with SCI has been developed that estimates the increased energy expenditure associated with everyday activities and exercise; notably, RMR was calculated at 2.7 mL O_2/kg/min for SCI compared with the usual 3.5 mL O_2/kg/min RMR value in nondisabled individuals.[59]

Lower extremity functional electrical stimulation (FES) has been used to improve TEA for persons with upper motor neuron injuries but activates motor units in direct contrast to the Henneman size principle because electricity flows through the path of least resistance.[60,61] Although physiologic recruitment of motor units occurs in a sequence of smaller, slower, fatigue-resistant fiber types with progressive activation of larger, faster, and fatigable fiber types, FES activates the fastest, most fatigable motor units first. Ultimately, FES is limited in its ability to sustain energy-expending physical activity but also limited in its ability to cause muscle hypertrophy because of blunted anabolic hormonal responses after SCI. Relative to nondisabled individuals, those with SCI are less likely to hypertrophy muscle or significantly improve TEA energy expenditure through physical activity or exercise.[62–64]

Even the TEF is diminished following SCI, likely because of a combination of sympathetic blunting, increased adiposity, and reduced size and composition of foods ingested.[65] Although TEF only represents 8% to 10% of TDEE, even this minimal reduction in energy expenditure can result in significant accumulation of adipose tissue over time. Since the Harris-Benedict equation was introduced more than 100 years ago, estimates for human basal metabolism have attempted to predict TDEE.[66,67] However, the predictive equations have not taken into account body composition differences other than height and weight, such that metabolically active tissues (FFM) were not distinguished from adipose tissue that is metabolically inert.[62] Because SCI profoundly changes body composition, such equations are of minimal value, and recent guidelines recommend indirect calorimetry as an essential measurement to determine RMR in this unique population.[68] A recent systematic analysis of SCI-specific predictive equations corroborated significant error introduced in studies comparing estimated versus measured resting energy expenditure (REE).[69] Once

Table 4
Recommended lifestyle management and pharmacotherapy for persons with spinal cord injury

Cardiometabolic Risk	Goal	Primary Management: Lifestyle Intervention	
		Nutrition	Exercise
CMD diagnosis	Reduce number of risk components to <3	Institute the following nutritional adjustments beginning as soon as possible after the SCI: (1) for all individuals, adopt a heart-healthy nutrition plan focusing on fruits, vegetables, whole grains, low-fat dairy, poultry, fish, legumes, nontropical vegetable oils, and nuts while (2) limiting sweets and sugar-sweetened beverages, fried foods, and red meats; (3) limit saturated fat to 5%–6% of total caloric intake; and (4) limit daily sodium intake to ≤2400 mg for individuals with hypertension	Encourage participation at least 150 min/wk of moderate-intensity physical exercise according to ability, beginning as soon as possible following acute SCI. The 150-min/wk guideline can be satisfied by sessions of 30–60 min performed 3–5 d/wk, or by exercising for at least 3, 10-min sessions per day. When individuals with SCI are not able to meet these guidelines, they should engage in regular physical activity according to their abilities and should avoid inactivity
Overweight or obese	Reduce body fat mass to achieve <22%, or a BMI <22 kg/m^2		
Insulin resistance, type 2 prediabetes, or type 2 diabetes	Reduce FBG to ≤100 mg/dL and HbA1c <7%		
Dyslipidemia	Reduce TG to ≤150 mg/dL and increase HDL-C to ≥40 mg/dL (men) and ≥50 mg/dL (women)		
Hypertension	Reduce BP$_{SYSTOLIC}$ to <140 mm Hg and BP$_{DIASTOLIC}$ to <90 mm Hg		

Risk	Goal	Secondary Management: Pharmacotherapy
CMD diagnosis	As above	Treat specific CMD risk component
Overweight or obese		None recommended
Insulin resistance, type 2 prediabetes, or type 2 diabetes		Metformin (Glucophage) as the first-line agent for treatment of HbA1c >7%, unless contraindicated or poorly tolerated. If the maximum tolerated dose of metformin fails to achieve goals, add a second (and possibly a third) agent according to ADA Standards of Medical Care
Dyslipidemia		Patient selection for pharmacotherapy should be guided by other factors commonly seen in SCI, such as low levels of HDL-C and high levels of C-reactive protein. Statin monotherapy should be initiated using at least a moderate-intensity statin (eg, rosuvastatin 10–20 mg/d)
Hypertension		JNC-8 guidelines[111] recommend initial antihypertensive treatment with a thiazide-type diuretic, CCB, ACEI, or ARB in the nonblack population, and either a thiazide-type diuretic or CCB in the black population. Consider SCI-related factors when selecting an antihypertensive agent, such as the effect of thiazide diuretics on bladder management

Abbreviations: ACEI, angiotensin-converting enzyme inhibitor; ADA, American Diabetes Association; ARB, angiotensin receptor blocker; BMI, body mass index (kg/m²); CCB, calcium channel blocker; FBG, fasting blood glucose; JNC-8, Eighth Joint National Committee, evidence-based guideline for the management of high BP in adults.

Data from Nash MS, Groah SL, Gater DR, et al. Identification and Management of Cardiometabolic Risk after Spinal Cord Injury Clinical Practice Guideline for Health Care Providers. J Spinal Cord Med 2019;42(5):643-77; and James PA, Oparil S, Carter BL, et al. 2014 evidence-based guideline for the management of high blood pressure in adults: report from the panel members appointed to the Eighth Joint National Committee (JNC 8). J Am Med Assoc 2014;311(5):507-20.

REE has been determined, a conversion factor of 1.2 is typically used to estimate TDEE,[70,71] but the authors recently suggested a conversion factor of 1.15 as being more accurate for SCI TDEE, because of the profound body composition, metabolic, and adrenergic differences associated with SCI.[72]

On the other side of the energy balance equation is energy intake, which considers the quantity and caloric density of all ingested macronutrients. Carbohydrates and proteins have similar caloric densities of 4 kcal/g of tissue, whereas fats and alcohol have caloric densities of 9 kcal/g and 7 kcal/g, respectively. Multiple nutrition tables and software programs have been developed to allow accurate assessment of dietary macronutrients and micronutrients, but these processes depend on the accuracy of reporting through dietary recall. Food frequency questionnaires of 1-day, 3-day, and 7-day dietary recall have been validated in the nondisabled literature against known quantities of food prepared in a metabolic kitchen, but such rigor has yet to be reported in the SCI population. Macronutrients digested and absorbed in the gut are processed by the body and either immediately used for reparative and metabolic functions or stored as future fuel sources. Carbohydrates are stored in limited amounts as glycogen in liver and muscle to fuel glycolytic energy pathways, but are also used indirectly to facilitate oxidation of fat; excess dietary carbohydrates are stored as fat. Amino acids from dietary proteins are essential for synthesizing enzymes, structural proteins, and hormones; excess protein is stored as fat with excess nitrogen excreted in feces or urine. Dietary fats are readily digested and packaged into water-soluble chylomicrons that can be transported to the liver and adipose tissue for processing and storage. Regardless of diet composition, once energy needs are met, excess calories are stored as adipose tissue. Of note, structural storage of both glycogen and proteins requires concomitant water storage. In contrast, adipose tissue is 90% triglycerides, with small amounts of diglycerides, monoglycerides, cholesterol, phospholipids, free fatty acids, protein, and water. Adipose tissue has a low molecular density of 0.901 g/mL such that energy storage in the form of fat is more efficient because it weighs less than higher-density tissues such as muscle (1.340 g/mL) or bone (3.038 g/mL),[73] but the efficiency of storage also challenges the oxidation of fats at times when caloric need exceeds intake.

Nutritional guidelines for SCI were provided by the Academy of Nutrition and Dietetics in 2009, but were nonspecific and reflected guidelines for the nondisabled population except for protein recommendations because of paralysis-induced sarcopenia and reduced protein reserves.[74] Since that time, several studies have reported nutritional practices for persons with SCI, including both macronutrients and micronutrients, but energy balance was not always included as an essential entity.[9,75–79] A recent meta-analysis comparing persons with SCI with the 2015 to 2020 Dietary Guidelines of America showed positive energy balance for those with SCI despite reduced caloric intake, with excess protein and carbohydrate, lower fiber intake, and several vitamin deficiencies, including vitamins A, B_5, B_7, C, D, and E.[80] Calcium, magnesium, and potassium intakes were also noted to be less than recommended daily allowances compared with guidelines of nondisabled populations. Although previous studies for persons with SCI showed excess dietary fat ingestion, including saturated fat,[9,79,81] the meta-analysis indicated fat intake within recommended guidelines.[80]

To achieve sustainable fat loss, a negative energy balance targeting 100 to 200 kcal/d ought to reduce body mass by 450 to 900 g/wk (1–2 pounds/wk).[14] Weight loss in excess of these recommendations is likely to result in the undesirable loss of muscle and water, further reducing RMR, which would necessitate concomitant reductions in energy intake. Ideally, persons with SCI should target a body composition of less than

22% body fat for men (<35% body fat for women), or a BMI less than or equal to 22 kg/m^2.[68] The 2015 to 2020 Dietary Guidelines for America recommended low-energy, high-nutrient-density foods, including a variety of foods in recommended amounts across and within all food groups.[82] Recent guidelines to reduce cardiometabolic risk for persons with SCI recommend limiting sweets, sugar-sweetened beverages, and red meats, while adopting a heart-healthy nutrition plan focusing on fruits, vegetables, whole grains, low-fat dairy, poultry, fish, legumes, nontropical vegetable oils, and nuts.[68] Saturated fats should be limited to less than 6% of total caloric intake, sodium intake should be limited to less than or equal to 2400 mg for persons with hypertension, and the DASH (Dietary Approaches to Stop Hypertension) nutritional plan or Mediterranean dietary plan should be adopted if hypertension or other cardiometabolic risk factors are present.[68]

ALTERNATIVE INTERVENTIONS FOR CARDIOMETABOLIC SYNDROME RISKS
Secondary Management: Pharmacotherapy for Overweight/Obesity After Spinal Cord Injury

Although comprehensive lifestyle intervention incorporating exercise and nutrition is the preferred approach for CMS intervention,[83] a failure to satisfy targets using this strategy then defaults to pharmacotherapy as secondary management. In most cases, the selection of a therapeutic agent for the PVA guidelines was made by guideline approaches and good medical practices adopted for the nondisabled population. Various pharmacologic agents,[84] nutraceuticals,[85,86] and herbal medicines[87] are currently available for use in obesity management.

All US Food and Drug Administration (FDA)–approved medications for chronic weight management in obese adults are recommended as an aide to a reduced-calorie diet and increased physical activity, or for overweight adults having at least 1 weight-related condition such as hypertension, type-2 diabetes, or dyslipidemia.[88] Discussed next are FDA-approved drugs for treating obese and overweight adults without a disability and their potential hazards for use by persons with SCI.

Orlistat (Xenical and Alli) is a gastrointestinal lipase inhibitor that reduces the absorption of dietary fat by approximately 30%.[89] Orlistat has not undergone testing for safety, tolerance, or effectiveness in persons with SCI. The efficacy of orlistat for long-term weight loss was established in several clinical trials,[90,91] although a meta-analysis incorporating 5 studies of 11,000 participants reported common gastrointestinal side effects including diarrhea, fecal incontinence, oily spotting, flatulence, bloating, and dyspepsia.[92,93] Stringent dietary management focusing on restriction of fat intake must are needed to lessen, but not necessarily eliminate, these risks. The use of this drug in persons with a neurogenic bowel, autonomic dysreflexia, and insensate skin may be life disrupting, socially distressing, and potentially hazardous.

Phentermine/topiramate (Qsymia) is a multitherapy pharmaceutical containing a low dose of the centrally acting appetite suppressant phentermine and the antiepileptic agent topiramate. This combination is useful for the long-term treatment of obesity,[94,95] although the efficacy, tolerance, and safety of this combination have not undergone testing in persons with SCI. Sympathomimetic properties of phentermine pose risks for insomnia, xerostomia, dizziness, palpitation, hand tremor, and increase of BP and pulse rate.[96,97] Topiramate is an antiseizure agent that may have additive effects for other analeptics, such as used for neuropathic pain. Tricyclic antidepressants and serotonin reuptake inhibitors potentiate the effects of phentermine and have significant adverse interactions with the phentermine/topiramate combination. The use of this agent in persons with SCI who have altered autonomic function and may be taking other medications that interact with phentermine/topiramate should be considered potentially hazardous.

Bupropion/naltrexone (Contrave) is a multitherapy agent containing naltrexone, a synthetic opioid antagonist, and bupropion, a norepinephrine-dopamine reuptake inhibitor and nicotinic acetylcholine receptor antagonist. The combination has not undergone testing for safety, tolerance, or effectiveness in persons with SCI. In 2 published clinical trials,[98,99] nausea was reported in 27% to 34% of trial participants, and a headache was reported more often in treatment groups (24% of participants) than in placebo subjects. Bupropion/naltrexone has the potential for adverse interactions with benzodiazepines, analeptics, and antidepressants, and may pose hazards when administered to patients with neurogenic bowel.

In summary, drugs prescribed for treating obesity have not undergone essential clinical testing for safety, tolerance, and effectiveness in the SCI population. All have adverse effects that may substantially affect the health, daily function, safety, and comfort of people with SCI. The described agents have extensive drug-drug interactions with agents contained within the pharmacopeia that are typically used to treat SCI. The medical and social risks of drug use in persons with SCI may outweigh reported benefits on body mass reduction or CVD risk abatement.

Pharmacotherapy for Dysglycemia

The disproportionate prevalence of diabetes and the CMD after SCI emphasizes a need for broadened surveillance and treatment of dysglycemia starting from the time of injury. Pharmacotherapy should be used where comprehensive lifestyle intervention has failed to meet clinical targets. Reducing hemoglobin A1c (HbA1c) level to less than 7% in adults without disabilities slows the microvascular progression of diabetes, and, if implemented soon after the diabetes diagnosis and sustained through the lifespan, results in a modest reduction of macrovascular disease. Guidelines prefer the more conservative HbA1c goal of less than 6.5% for individuals without significant hypoglycemia or other treatment adverse effects.[100] These patients may include those with short duration of diabetes, suitable treatment results accompanying lifestyle or metformin monotherapy, long life expectancy, or absence of significant CVD.

In general, the "Pharmacologic Therapy for Type 2 Diabetes: Synopsis of the 2017 American Diabetes Association Standards of Medical Care in Diabetes"[101] made several recommendations, which are discussed next.

Metformin should be the preferred initial pharmacologic agent for the treatment of HbA1c level greater than 7% unless contraindicated or poorly tolerated. If the maximum tolerated dosage of metformin fails to achieve treatment goals, the addition of a second and possibly a third agent should conform to the most recent treatment guidelines. General warnings for gastrointestinal complications and volume depletion accompany metformin monotherapy, which may be more impactful on persons with SCI and include risks of resting and orthostatic hypotension. A greater risk of hypoglycemia should be anticipated with multitherapy approaches, especially when incorporating sulfonylureas and basal insulin as second-line agents. Risks for genitourinary infection, volume depletion, and resting and orthostatic hypotension may be more pronounced in persons with SCI in the general population and should be judiciously monitored.

Caution should also be exercised when using multitherapy approaches that are more likely to precipitate hypoglycemia and patient-specific characteristics where drug selection may invoke resting and postural hypotension, lymphedema, heart failure, and urinary tract infections. Long-term use of metformin may be associated with biochemical vitamin B_{12} deficiency, which may require checks for appropriate levels.

Treatment plans should consider initiating insulin therapy (with or without additional agents) in patients with newly diagnosed type 2 diabetes who are symptomatic, have HbA1c level greater than or equal to 10% (86 mmol/mol), or blood glucose levels greater than or equal to 300 mg/dL (16.7 mmol/L). If noninsulin monotherapy at the maximum tolerated dose does not achieve or maintain the HbA1c target after 3 months, add a second oral agent, a glucagonlike peptide-1 receptor agonist, or basal insulin. In patients with long-standing, suboptimally controlled type 2 diabetes and an established atherosclerotic CVD, empagliflozin or liraglutide should be considered because they reduce CV and all-cause mortality when added to standard care.

Pharmacotherapy for Dyslipidemia

Selection of patients for treatment of dyslipidemia is often based on the use of CV risk equations developed for use by nondisabled populations, and therefore with uncertain ability to generalize and calibrate to assess risks in those with SCI.[7,102] Moreover, most risk equations, except the Reynolds Risk Score, do not account for the inflammation and lipid interactions and neglect to incorporate the risks associated with remnant particles or postprandial lipemia.[103,104] Given these limitations, typical thresholds for the initiation of pharmacologic treatment of dyslipidemia developed in nondisabled populations may not apply to SCI.

Limited evidence has tested rates of treatment and control of dyslipidemia in SCI, with available evidence suggesting that a therapeutic gap is present,[105,106] consistent with data from the National Health and Nutrition Examination Survey in nondisabled persons. The use of traditional therapeutic agents potentially effective in SCI-associated dyslipidemia includes statins, fibric acid derivatives, and niacin. Statin drugs are effective for dyslipidemia and reduce the risk of CV events. Limited outcomes data in patients with SCI suggest that statins may reduce all-cause mortality.[107] Once initiated, statin therapy should be monitored in accordance with the product information per the FDA. A notable exception may be for heightened surveillance of myopathy using creatine kinase monitoring because of the limitations for assessing pain and weakness in the SCI population. There are no outcomes data in the treatment of dyslipidemia in SCI using nonstatin therapies, such as niacin or fibric acid derivatives. Niacin tolerably improves the dyslipidemic risk profile in SCI.[108] Recent evidence suggests that fenofibrate is both well tolerated and effective for promoting favorable changes in serum lipoprotein profiles and ratios in persons with early SCI.[109,110] The PVA guidelines encouraged patient selection for pharmacotherapy using factors commonly seen in SCI, such as low levels of HDL-C and high levels of C-reactive protein. If using a statin, initiate monotherapy using at least a moderate-intensity statin (eg, rosuvastatin 10–20 mg/d).

Pharmacotherapy for Hypertension

Abundant evidence from randomized controlled trials (RCTs) in the general population has shown the benefit of antihypertensive drug treatment in improving important health outcomes in people with hypertension. Baseline BP is often lower in people with tetraplegia and high paraplegia than in the general population, but evidence to support a different threshold for treating high BP in individuals with SCI is lacking. The PVA guidelines recommend applying evidence-based guidelines for treating hypertension in the general population to those with SCI. Current guidelines for initiating pharmacologic treatment of hypertension by most major organizations recommend 140/90 mm Hg as the threshold for pharmacologic treatment and a target goal for most adults with hypertension. However, there are differences and areas of controversy regarding treatment thresholds and targets for certain subpopulations between the different guidelines. For example, in age cutoff for a higher systolic BP target and treatment threshold, a lower BP threshold is recommended by some organizations for certain populations, including those with diabetes or chronic kidney disease.[111–114]

Consistent with the guidelines discussed earlier, the PVA guidelines recommend initiating pharmacologic treatment to decrease BP at systolic BP of 140 mm Hg or higher or diastolic BP of 90 mm Hg or higher in most adults with SCI. Although the panel recognized differences in treatment goals and targets for certain subpopulations between various guidelines, it did not endorse a specific guideline more than the others given the current lack of high-quality evidence to make that determination. For individual patients, clinicians should use a combination of factors to set BP goals, including scientific evidence, clinical judgment, and patient tolerance. In some patients, including those with albuminuria, chronic kidney disease, or additional CV risk factors, clinicians could consider a lower BP standard (eg, 130/80 mm Hg) if lower targets can be achieved without undue treatment burden, while recognizing that the benefit of pursuing these target levels using antihypertensive drugs is currently not established through RCTs.

The Eighth Joint National Committee (JNC-8) guidelines recommend initial antihypertensive treatment with a thiazide-type diuretic, calcium channel blocker (CCB), angiotensin-converting enzyme inhibitor (ACEI), or angiotensin receptor blocker (ARB) in the nonblack population, and either a thiazide-type diuretic or CCB in the black population.[111] In adults with chronic kidney disease, initial or add-on antihypertensive treatment should include an ACEI or ARB to improve kidney outcomes. Additional coexisting conditions may influence drug selection. For example, in patients with a history of myocardial infarction, a β-blocker and ARB or ACEI are indicated regardless of BP.[113]

Studies that have systematically tested antihypertensive agents in people with SCI are lacking. In the absence of such evidence, it is reasonable to apply guidelines for choosing antihypertensive agents in the general population to people with SCI. However, SCI-related factors may affect the choice of an antihypertensive agent in some circumstances. For example, a thiazide-type diuretic may not be the antihypertensive agent of choice in individuals who perform intermittent bladder catheterizations, because of its effect on increased urine volumes between catheterizations. Hyponatremia, hypokalemia, or decline in renal function sometimes occur during the first 9 months of thiazide use, and older patients may be especially vulnerable to renal-electrolyte disturbances, gout, hyperglycemia, and hypotension.

The main objective of hypertension treatment is to attain and maintain goal BP. JNC-8 guidelines recommend increasing the dose of the initial drug or adding a second drug if goal BP is not reached within a month of initiating treatment.[111] An ACEI and an ARB should not be used together in the same patient. If goal BP cannot be achieved with 2 drugs, a third drug should be added and titrated. Barry and colleagues[115] found that veterans with traumatic SCI were less likely to be prescribed more than 1 antihypertensive medication compared with matched controls. The investigators postulated that these findings could relate to concern over the propensity of these patients to develop hypotension. Although some patients with SCI who have coexisting orthostatic hypotension and supine hypertension require careful titration and trial of medications, clinicians should continue to assess BP and adjust the treatment regimen until goal BP is reached.

In cases of treatment-resistant hypertension, compliance and adherence to treatment regimen should be confirmed. Drug interactions (eg, nonsteroidal antiinflammatory drugs, illicit drugs, sympathomimetic agents, over-the-counter agents, and herbal supplements) may hamper BP control. Secondary causes of hypertension should be investigated. Referral to a hypertension specialist may be appropriate for patients whose BP cannot be controlled with the strategies discussed earlier.[113]

BARIATRIC SURGERY FOR CARDIOMETABOLIC DISEASE RISK

Current evidence fails to support the use of bariatric surgery for obesity management after SCI, except in cases of last resort where lifestyle intervention and pharmacotherapy have failed and where medical judgment compels intervention. Several case reports address population-specific perioperative or postoperative risks of the procedures,[116–118] but no level I, II, or III studies have investigated bariatric surgery to manage obesity after SCI. Current guidelines for determining bariatric surgery candidates and their perioperative/postoperative care use BMI and screening practices that are developed for the non-SCI population,[119,120] but do not address the complex care needs and unique risks associated with SCI. These hazards include deficits in mobility and activities of daily living, neurogenic bradycardia, neurogenic hypotension, adapted myocardial atrophy, circulatory hypokinesis, risks for autonomic dysreflexia, neurogenic restrictive and obstructive lung disease, neurogenic bladder, neurogenic bowel, neurogenic skin, sarcopenia, osteopenia/osteoporosis, and spasticity. The reported odds ratio for venous thromboembolism after bariatric surgery is 5.7 times that of the nondisabled population[121] and does not anticipate other surgical complications of abdominal pain/cramping, dumping syndrome, beriberi, postoperative adhesions, and loose stools. As such, practitioners should consider bariatric surgery as a last resort for persons with morbid obesity because of significant perioperative and postoperative risks. If bariatric surgery is considered, an SCI specialist should provide preoperative, perioperative, and postoperative consultative services to the surgical and anesthesia teams to alert them of unique population risks.

SUMMARY

An alarming number of individuals with SCI develop component risks for CMS at some point in their lives, the 2 most serious of which are sarcopenic obesity and insulin resistance. For many individuals with SCI, exercise offers an effective strategy for attenuation of these risks, with a benefit favored by the adoption of more intensive activity. Exercise in CMD management may be less useful for individuals with higher levels of injury, and in the background of adrenergic dysfunction. In these individuals, and when combined with balanced, calorie-regulated nutrition, the 2 interventions constitute a lifestyle intervention that favors a best practice appropriate to cardioendocrine disease management. When lifestyle intervention is ineffective for risk reduction, both pharmacotherapy and bariatric surgery become options for CMD risk reduction, but may also pose unique risks and as-yet unknown benefits for the SCI population.

DISCLOSURE

The authors have no conflicts to declare. The work is supported by grants from the Paralyzed Veterans of America (MSN); the U.S. Department of Defense CDMRP (MSN); Field-Initiated, DRRP, and SCIMS grants from the National Institute for Disability, Independent Living, and Rehabilitation Research (MSN and DRG; the Craig H. Nielsen Foundation (MSN), and the Miami Project to Cure Paralysis (MSN).

REFERENCES

1. Despres JP, Lemieux I, Bergeron J, et al. Abdominal obesity and the metabolic syndrome: contribution to global cardiometabolic risk. Arterioscler Thromb Vasc Biol 2008;28(6):1039–49.

2. Castro JP, El-Atat FA, McFarlane SI, et al. Cardiometabolic syndrome: pathophysiology and treatment. Curr Hypertens Rep 2003;5(5):393–401.

3. Mancia G, Bombelli M, Facchetti R, et al. Impact of different definitions of the metabolic syndrome on the prevalence of organ damage, cardiometabolic risk and cardiovascular events. J Hypertens 2010;28(5):999–1006.

4. Beltrán-Sánchez H, Harhay MO, Harhay MM, et al. Prevalence and trends of metabolic syndrome in the adult US population, 1999–2010. J Am Coll Cardiol 2013;62(8):697–703.

5. Dyson-Hudson T, Nash M. Guideline-driven assessment of cardiovascular disease and related risks after spinal cord injury. Top Spinal Cord Inj Rehabil 2009;14(3):32–45.

6. Bremer AA, Mietus-Snyder M, Lustig RH. Toward a unifying hypothesis of metabolic syndrome. Pediatrics 2012;129(3):557–70.

7. Nash MS, Tractenberg RE, Mendez AJ, et al. Cardiometabolic syndrome in people with spinal cord injury/disease: guideline-derived and nonguideline risk components in a pooled sample. Arch Phys Med Rehabil 2016;97(10): 1696–705.

8. Weaver FM, Collins EG, Kurichi J, et al. Prevalence of obesity and high blood pressure in veterans with spinal cord injuries and disorders: a retrospective review. Am J Phys Med Rehabil 2007;86(1):22–9.

9. Groah SL, Nash MS, Ljungberg IH, et al. Nutrient intake and body habitus after spinal cord injury: an analysis by sex and level of injury. J Spinal Cord Med 2009;32(1):25–33.

10. Groah SL, Nash MS, Ward EA, et al. Cardiometabolic risk in community-dwelling persons with chronic spinal cord injury. J Cardiopulm Rehabil Prev 2011;31(2): 73–80.

11. Pelletier CA, Miyatani M, Giangregorio L, et al. Sarcopenic obesity in adults with spinal cord injury: a cross-sectional study. Arch Phys Med Rehabil 2016;97(11): 1931–7.

12. Gorgey A, Gater D. Prevalence of obesity after spinal cord injury. Top Spinal Cord Inj Rehabil 2007;12(4):1–7.

13. Buchholz AC, Bugaresti JM. A review of body mass index and waist circumference as markers of obesity and coronary heart disease risk in persons with chronic spinal cord injury. Spinal Cord 2005;43(9):513–8.

14. Gater DR Jr. Obesity after spinal cord injury. Phys Med Rehabil Clin N Am 2007; 18(2):333–51, vii.

15. Nash MS, Gater DR. Exercise to reduce obesity in SCI. Top Spinal Cord Inj Rehabil 2007;12(4):76–93.

16. Kressler J, Cowan RE, Bigford GE, et al. Reducing cardiometabolic disease in spinal cord injury. Phys Med Rehabil Clin N Am 2014;25(3):573–604, viii.

17. Bauman WA, Spungen AM, Raza M, et al. Coronary artery disease: metabolic risk factors and latent disease in individuals with paraplegia. Mt Sinai J Med 1992;59(2):163–8.

18. Cowan RE, Nash MS. Cardiovascular disease, SCI and exercise: unique risks and focused countermeasures. Disabil Rehabil 2010;32(26):2228–36.

19. Bauman WA, Spungen AM. Coronary heart disease in individuals with spinal cord injury: assessment of risk factors. Spinal Cord 2008;46(7):466–76.

20. Banerjea R, Sambamoorthi U, Weaver F, et al. Risk of stroke, heart attack, and diabetes complications among veterans with spinal cord injury. Arch Phys Med Rehabil 2008;89(8):1448–53.

21. Nash MS, Horton JA, Cowan RE, et al. Recreational and Therapeutic Exercise after SCI. In: Kirshbaum S, Campagnolo DI, Healy R, et al, editors. Spinal Cord Medicine. Philadelphia: Lippincott, Williams, and Wilkins; 2011. p. 427–47.

22. Libin A, Tinsley E, Nash M, et al. Cardiometabolic risk clustering in spinal cord injury: results of exploratory factor analysis. Top Spinal Cord Inj Rehabil 2013; 19(3):183–94.

23. Bauman WA, Spungen AM, Zhong YG, et al. Depressed serum high density lipoprotein cholesterol levels in veterans with spinal cord injury. Paraplegia 1992; 30(10):697–703.

24. Brenes G, Dearwater S, Shapera R, et al. High density lipoprotein cholesterol concentrations in physically active and sedentary spinal cord injured patients. Arch Phys Med Rehabil 1986;67(7):445–50.

25. Nash MS, Mendez AJ. A guideline-driven assessment of need for cardiovascular disease risk intervention in persons with chronic paraplegia. Arch Phys Med Rehabil 2007;88(6):751–7.

26. Bauman WA, Adkins RH, Spungen AM, et al. Is immobilization associated with an abnormal lipoprotein profile? Observations from a diverse cohort. Spinal Cord 1999;37(7):485–93.

27. Bauman WA, Adkins RH, Spungen AM, et al. The effect of residual neurological deficit on serum lipoproteins in individuals with chronic spinal cord injury. Spinal Cord 1998;36(1):13–7.

28. Bauman WA, Spungen AM. Disorders of carbohydrate and lipid metabolism in veterans with paraplegia or quadriplegia: a model of premature aging. Metabolism 1994;43(6):749–56.

29. Nash MS, Cowan RE, Kressler J. Evidence-based and heuristic approaches for customization of care in cardiometabolic syndrome after spinal cord injury. J Spinal Cord Med 2012;35(5):278–92.

30. Levine AM, Nash MS, Green BA, et al. An examination of dietary intakes and nutritional status of chronic healthy spinal cord injured individuals. Paraplegia 1992;30(12):880–9.

31. Dearwater SR, LaPorte RE, Robertson RJ, et al. Activity in the spinal cord-injured patient: an epidemiologic analysis of metabolic parameters. Med Sci Sports Exerc 1986;18(5):541–4.

32. LaPorte RE, Adams LL, Savage DD, et al. The spectrum of physical activity, cardiovascular disease and health: an epidemiologic perspective. Am J Epidemiol 1984;120(4):507–17.

33. LaPorte RE, Brenes G, Dearwater S, et al. HDL cholesterol across a spectrum of physical activity from quadriplegia to marathon running. Lancet 1983;1(8335): 1212–3.

34. Zlotolow SP, Levy E, Bauman WA. The serum lipoprotein profile in veterans with paraplegia: the relationship to nutritional factors and body mass index. J Am Paraplegia Soc 1992;15(3):158–62.

35. Halle M, Berg A, Baumstark M, et al. Association of physical fitness with LDL and HDL subfractions in young healthy men. Int J Sports Med 1999;20(7):464–9.

36. Franks PW, Ekelund U, Brage S, et al. Does the association of habitual physical activity with the metabolic syndrome differ by level of cardiorespiratory fitness? Diabetes Care 2004;27(5):1187–93.

37. Carnethon MR, Gulati M, Greenland P. Prevalence and cardiovascular disease correlates of low cardiorespiratory fitness in adolescents and adults. J Am Med Assoc 2005;294(23):2981–8.

38. Liu L, Nunez AE. Cardiometabolic syndrome and its association with education, smoking, diet, physical activity, and social support: findings from the Pennsylvania 2007 BRFSS Survey. J Clin Hypertens 2010;12(7):556–64.

39. Feasel SGS. The impact of diet on cardiovascular disease risk in individuals with spinal cord injury. Top Spinal Cord Inj Rehabil 2009;14(3):56–68.

40. Nash MS, Groah SL, Gater DR Jr, et al. Identification and management of cardiometabolic risk after spinal cord injury: clinical practice guideline for health care providers. Top Spinal Cord Inj Rehabil 2018;24(4):379–423.

41. Noreau L, Shephard RJ, Simard C, et al. Relationship of impairment and functional ability to habitual activity and fitness following spinal cord injury. Int J Rehabil Res 1993;16(4):265–75.

42. Boninger ML, Dicianno BE, Cooper RA, et al. Shoulder magnetic resonance imaging abnormalities, wheelchair propulsion, and gender. Arch Phys Med Rehabil 2003;84(11):1615–20.

43. Ballinger DA, Rintala DH, Hart KA. The relation of shoulder pain and range-of-motion problems to functional limitations, disability, and perceived health of men with spinal cord injury: a multifaceted longitudinal study. Arch Phys Med Rehabil 2000;81(12):1575–81.

44. Scelza WM, Kalpakjian CZ, Zemper ED, et al. Perceived barriers to exercise in people with spinal cord injury. Am J Phys Med Rehabil 2005;84(8):576–83.

45. Cowan RE, Nash MS, Anderson KD. Exercise participation barrier prevalence and association with exercise participation status in individuals with spinal cord injury. Spinal Cord 2013;51(1):27–32.

46. Cowan RE, Nash MS, Anderson-Erisman K. Perceived exercise barriers and odds of exercise participation among persons with SCI living in high-income households. Top Spinal Cord Inj Rehabil 2012;18(2):126–7.

47. Kroll T, Kratz A, Kehn M, et al. Perceived exercise self-efficacy as a predictor of exercise behavior in individuals aging with spinal cord injury. Am J Phys Med Rehabil 2012;91(8):640–51.

48. Nash MS, Bilzon JLJ. Guideline approaches for cardioendocrine disease surveillance and treatment following spinal cord injury. Curr Phys Med Rehabil Rep 2018;6(4):264–76.

49. Gaspar R, Padula N, Freitas TB, et al. Physical exercise for individuals with spinal cord injury: systematic review based on the international classification of functioning, disability, and health. J Sport Rehabil 2019;28(5):505–16.

50. Nash MS, Bilzon JL. Therapeutic exercise after spinal cord injury. In: Kirshbaum S, Lin V, editors. Spinal cord medicine. 3rd edition. Philadelphia: Lippincott, Williams, and Wilkins; 2018. p. 831–48.

51. Ginis KAM, van der Scheer JW, Latimer-Cheung AE, et al. Evidence-based scientific exercise guidelines for adults with spinal cord injury: an update and a new guideline. Spinal cord 2018;56(4):308.

52. Rezende LS, Lima MB, Salvador EP. Interventions for promoting physical activity among individuals with spinal cord injury: a systematic review. J Phys Act Health 2018;15(12):954–9.

53. Wang ZM, Ying ZL, Westphal AB, et al. Specific metabolic rates of major organs and tissues across adulthood evaluation by mechanistic model of resting energy expenditure. Am J Clin Nutr 2010;92(6):1369–77.
54. Nash MS, Bilsker S, Marcillo AE, et al. Reversal of adaptive left-ventricular atrophy following electrically-stimulated exercise training in human tetraplegics. Paraplegia 1991;29(9):590–9.
55. Bauman WA, Nash MS. Endocrinology and metabolism of persons with spinal cord injury. In: Kirshbaum S, Lin V, editors. Spinal cord medicine. 3rd edition. Philadelphia: Lippincott, Williams, and Wilkins; 2018. p. 279–317.
56. Krassioukov AV, Karlsson AK, Wecht JM, et al. Assessment of autonomic dysfunction following spinal cord injury: rationale for additions to International Standards for Neurological Assessment. J Rehabil Res Dev 2007;44(1):103–12.
57. Schilero GJ, Bauman WA, Radulovic M. Traumatic spinal cord injury: pulmonary physiologic principles and management. Clin Chest Med 2018;39(2):411–25.
58. Reid WD, Brown JA, Konnyu KJ, et al. Physiotherapy secretion removal techniques in people with spinal cord injury: a systematic review. J Spinal Cord Med 2010;33(4):353–70.
59. Collins EG, Gater D, Kiratli J, et al. Energy cost of physical activities in persons with spinal cord injury. Med Sci Sports Exerc 2010;42(4):691–700.
60. Henneman E. The size-principle - a deterministic output emerges from a set of probabilistic connections. J Exp Biol 1985;115(MAR):105–12.
61. Gater DR, Dolbow D, Tsui B, et al. Functional electrical stimulation therapies after spinal cord injury. NeuroRehabilitation 2011;28(3):231–48.
62. Gater DR, Farkas GJ. Alterations in body composition after SCI and the mitigating role of exercise. In: Taylor JA, editor. The physiology of exercise in spinal cord injury. Boston: Springer; 2016. p. 175–98.
63. Gorgey AS, Dolbow DR, Dolbow JD, et al. Effects of spinal cord injury on body composition and metabolic profile - Part I. J Spinal Cord Med 2014;37(6): 693–702.
64. Gorgey AS, Dolbow DR, Dolbow JD, et al. The effects of electrical stimulation on body composition and metabolic profile after spinal cord injury - Part II. J Spinal Cord Med 2015;38(1):23–37.
65. Swaminathan R, King R, Holmfield J, et al. Thermic effect of feeding carbohydrate, fat, protein and mixed meal in lean and obese subjects. Am J Clin Nutr 1985;42(2):177–81.
66. Harris JA, Benedict FG. A biometric study of basal metabolism in man. Proc Nat Acad Sci USA 1918;12(4):370–3.
67. Mifflin MD, Stjeor ST, Hill LA, et al. A new predictive equation for resting energy-expenditure in healthy-individuals. Am J Clin Nutr 1990;51(2):241–7.
68. Nash MS, Groah SL, Gater DR, et al. Identification and management of cardiometabolic risk after spinal cord injury clinical practice guideline for health care providers. J Spinal Cord Med 2019;42(5):643–77.
69. Farkas GJ, Pitot MA, Gater DR. A systematic review of the accuracy of estimated and measured resting metabolic rate in chronic spinal cord injury. Int J Sport Nutr Exerc Metab 2019;29(5):548–58.
70. Cox SAR, Weiss SM, Posuniak EA, et al. Energy-expenditure after spinal-cord injury - an evaluation of stable rehabilitating patients. J Trauma 1985;25(5): 419–23.
71. Long CL, Schaffel N, Geiger JW, et al. Metabolic response to injury and illness: estimation of energy and protein needs from indirect calorimetry and nitrogen balance. J Parenter Eternal Nutr 1979;3(6):452–6.

72. Farkas GJ, Gorgey AS, Dolbow DR, et al. Caloric intake relative to total daily energy expenditure using a spinal cord injury–specific correction factor: an analysis by level of injury. Am J Phys Med Rehabil 2019;98(11):947–52.

73. Brozek J, Anderson JT, Keys A, et al. Densitometric analysis of body composition revision of some quantitative assumptions. Ann N Y Acad Sci 1963; 110(1):113.

74. Walters JL, Buchholz AC, Ginis KM. Evidence of dietary inadequacy in adults with chronic spinal cord injury. Spinal Cord 2009;47(4):318–22.

75. Gorgey AS, Caudill C, Sistrun S, et al. Frequency of dietary recalls, nutritional assessment, and body composition assessment in men with chronic spinal cord injury. Arch Phys Med Rehabil 2015;96(9):1646–53.

76. Gorgey AS, Mather KJ, Cupp HR, et al. Effects of resistance training on adiposity and metabolism after spinal cord injury. Med Sci Sports Exerc 2012; 44(1):165–74.

77. Lieberman J, David Goff J, Hammond F, et al. Dietary intake relative to cardiovascular disease risk factors in individuals with chronic spinal cord injury: a pilot study. Top Spinal Cord Inj Rehabil 2014;20(2):127–36.

78. Nightingale TE, Williams S, Thompson D, et al. Energy balance components in persons with paraplegia: daily variation and appropriate measurement duration. Int J Behav Nutr Phys Act 2017;14(1):132.

79. Sabour H, Soltani Z, Latifi S, et al. Dietary pattern as identified by factorial analysis and its association with lipid profile and fasting plasma glucose among Iranian individuals with spinal cord injury. J Spinal Cord Med 2016;39(4):433–42.

80. Farkas GJ, Pitot MA, Berg AS, et al. Nutritional status in chronic spinal cord injury: a systematic review and meta-analysis. Spinal Cord 2019;57(1):3–17.

81. Bigford G, Nash MS. Nutritional health considerations for persons with spinal cord injury. Top Spinal Cord Inj Rehabil 2017;23(3):188–206.

82. Connors P. Dietary Guidelines 2015–2020. Journal of Nutrition Education and Behavior 2016;48(7):518.

83. Clinical practice guidelines: spinal cord medicine, 2018. Paralyzed Veterans of America. Available at: https://pva-cdnendpoint.azureedge.net/prod/libraries/media/pva/library/publications/cpg_cardiometabolic-risk_digital.pdf.

84. Daneschvar HL, Aronson MD, Smetana GW. FDA-approved anti-obesity drugs in the United States. Am J Med 2016;129(8):879.e1-6.

85. Kota SK, Jammula S, Kota SK, et al. Nutraceuticals in pathogenic obesity; striking the right balance between energy imbalance and inflammation. Journal of Medical Nutrition and Nutraceuticals 2012;1(2):63.

86. Conroy K, Davidson I, Warnock M. Pathogenic obesity and nutraceuticals. Proc Nutr Soc 2011;70(4):426–38.

87. Najm W, Lie D. Herbals used for diabetes, obesity, and metabolic syndrome. Prim Care 2010;37(2):237–54.

88. Vetter ML, Faulconbridge LF, Webb VL, et al. Behavioral and pharmacologic therapies for obesity. Nat Rev Endocrinol 2010;6(10):578–88.

89. Hollander P. Orlistat in the treatment of obesity. Prim Care 2003;30(2):427–40.

90. Rössner S, Sjöström L, Noack R, et al, European Orlistat Obesity Study. Weight loss, weight maintenance, and improved cardiovascular risk factors after 2 years treatment with orlistat for obesity. Obes Res 2000;8(1):49–61.

91. Torgerson JS, Hauptman J, Boldrin MN, et al. Xenical in the prevention of diabetes in obese subjects (XENDOS) study. Diabetes Care 2004;27(1):155–61.

92. Ioannides-Demos LL, Proietto J, Tonkin AM, et al. Safety of drug therapies used for weight loss and treatment of obesity. Drug Saf 2006;29(4):277–302.

93. Rucker D, Padwal R, Li SK, et al. Long term pharmacotherapy for obesity and overweight: updated meta-analysis. BMJ 2007;335(7631):1194.

94. Garvey WT, Ryan DH, Look M, et al. Two-year sustained weight loss and metabolic benefits with controlled-release phentermine/topiramate in obese and overweight adults (SEQUEL): a randomized, placebo-controlled, phase 3 extension study. Am J Clin Nutr 2012;95(2):297–308.

95. Allison DB, Gadde KM, Garvey WT, et al. Controlled-release phentermine/topiramate in severely obese adults: a randomized controlled trial (EQUIP). Obesity (Silver Spring) 2012;20(2):330–42.

96. Rothman RB, Hendricks EJ. Phentermine cardiovascular safety. Am J Emerg Med 2009;27(8):1010–3.

97. Kang J, Park CY, Kang J, et al. Randomized controlled trial to investigate the effects of a newly developed formulation of phentermine diffuse-controlled release for obesity. Diabetes Obes Metab 2010;12(10):876–82.

98. Greenway FL, Fujioka K, Plodkowski RA, et al. Effect of naltrexone plus bupropion on weight loss in overweight and obese adults (COR-I): a multicentre, randomised, double-blind, placebo-controlled, phase 3 trial. Lancet 2010; 376(9741):595–605.

99. Wadden TA, Foreyt JP, Foster GD, et al. Weight loss with naltrexone SR/bupropion SR combination therapy as an adjunct to behavior modification: the COR-BMOD trial. Obesity 2011;19(1):110–20.

100. Garber AJ, Abrahamson MJ, Barzilay JI, et al. Consensus statement by the American Association of Clinical Endocrinologists and American College of Endocrinology on the comprehensive type 2 diabetes management algorithm–2016 executive summary. Endocr Pract 2016;22(1):84–113.

101. Chamberlain JJ, Herman WH, Leal S, et al. Pharmacologic therapy for type 2 diabetes: synopsis of the 2017 American Diabetes Association Standards of Medical Care in Diabetes. Ann Intern Med 2017;166(8):572–8.

102. Finnie A, Buchholz A, Ginis KM. Current coronary heart disease risk assessment tools may underestimate risk in community-dwelling persons with chronic spinal cord injury. Spinal Cord 2008;46(9):608–15.

103. Ellenbroek D, Kressler J, Cowan RE, et al. Effects of prandial challenge on triglyceridemia, glycemia, and pro-inflammatory activity in persons with chronic paraplegia. J Spinal Cord Med 2015;38(4):468–75.

104. Nash MS, deGroot J, Martinez-Arizala A, et al. Evidence for an exaggerated postprandial lipemia in chronic paraplegia. J Spinal Cord Med 2005;28(4): 320–5.

105. Chopra AS, Miyatani M, Craven BC. Cardiovascular disease risk in individuals with chronic spinal cord injury: prevalence of untreated risk factors and poor adherence to treatment guidelines. J Spinal Cord Med 2018;41(1):2–9.

106. Lieberman JA, Hammond FM, Barringer TA, et al. Adherence with the National Cholesterol Education Program guidelines in men with chronic spinal cord injury. J Spinal Cord Med 2011;34(1):28–34.

107. Stillman M, Aston C, Rabadi M. Mortality benefit of statin use in traumatic spinal cord injury: a retrospective analysis. Spinal Cord 2016;54(4):298–302.

108. Nash MS, Lewis JE, Dyson-Hudson TA, et al. Safety, tolerance, and efficacy of extended-release niacin monotherapy for treating dyslipidemia risks in persons with chronic tetraplegia: a randomized multicenter controlled trial. Arch Phys Med Rehabil 2011;92(3):399–410.

109. La Fountaine MF, Cirnigliaro CM, Hobson JC, et al. Fenofibrate therapy to lower serum triglyceride concentrations in persons with spinal cord injury: a preliminary analysis of its safety profile. J Spinal Cord Med 2019;1–6.

110. La Fountaine MF, Cirnigliaro CM, Hobson JC, et al. A four month randomized controlled trial on the efficacy of once-daily fenofibrate monotherapy in persons with spinal cord injury. Sci Rep 2019;9(1):1–9.

111. James PA, Oparil S, Carter BL, et al. 2014 evidence-based guideline for the management of high blood pressure in adults: report from the panel members appointed to the Eighth Joint National Committee (JNC 8). J Am Med Assoc 2014;311(5):507–20.

112. Qaseem A, Wilt TJ, Rich R, et al. Pharmacologic treatment of hypertension in adults aged 60 years or older to higher versus lower blood pressure targets: a clinical practice guideline from the American College of Physicians and the American Academy of Family Physicians Pharmacologic Treatment of Hypertension in Adults. Ann Intern Med 2017;166(6):430–7.

113. Weber MA, Schiffrin EL, White WB, et al. Clinical practice guidelines for the management of hypertension in the community. J Clin Hypertens 2014;16(1):14–26.

114. Go AS, Bauman MA, King SMC, et al. An effective approach to high blood pressure control. Hypertension 2014;63(4):878–85.

115. Barry W, St Andre J, Evans C, et al. Hypertension and antihypertensive treatment in veterans with spinal cord injury and disorders. Spinal Cord 2013;51(2):109–15.

116. Alaedeen DI, Jasper J. Gastric bypass surgery in a paraplegic morbidly obese patient. Obes Surg 2006;16(8):1107–8.

117. Williams G, Georgiou P, Cocker D, et al. The safety and efficacy of bariatric surgery for obese, wheelchair bound patients. Ann R Coll Surg Engl 2014;96(5):373–6.

118. Wong S, Barnes T, Coggrave M, et al. Morbid obesity after spinal cord injury: an ailment not to be treated? Eur J Clin Nutr 2013;67(9):998–9.

119. Fried M, Yumuk V, Oppert J, et al. Interdisciplinary European guidelines on metabolic and bariatric surgery. Obes Surg 2014;24(1):42–55.

120. Mechanick JI, Youdim A, Jones DB, et al. Clinical practice guidelines for the perioperative nutritional, metabolic, and nonsurgical support of the bariatric surgery patient—2013 update: cosponsored by American Association of Clinical Endocrinologists, the Obesity Society, and American Society for Metabolic & Bariatric Surgery. Obesity 2013;21(S1):S1–27.

121. Aminian A, Andalib A, Khorgami Z, et al. Who should get extended thromboprophylaxis after bariatric surgery?: a risk assessment tool to guide indications for post-discharge pharmacoprophylaxis. Ann Surg 2017;265(1):143–50.

122. Grundy SM, Brewer HB Jr, Cleeman JI, American Heart Association, National Heart, Lung, and Blood Institute. Definition of metabolic syndrome: report of the National Heart, Lung, and Blood Institute/American Heart Association conference on scientific issues related to definition. Circ 2004;109(3):433–8.

123. Grundy SM, Cleeman JI, Merz CN, et al. Implications of recent clinical trials for the National Cholesterol Education Program Adult Treatment Panel III Guidelines. J Am Coll Cardiol 2004;44(3):720–32.

Therapeutic Interventions to Improve Mobility with Spinal Cord Injury Related Upper Motor Neuron Syndromes

Edelle C. Field-Fote, PT, PhD[a,b,c,*]

KEYWORDS

• Practice • Training • Walking • Wheeling

KEY POINTS

- Mobility, regardless of whether achieved by walking or the use of a wheelchair, is essential for quality of life and social participation after spinal cord injury.
- New technologies are evolving in the form of overground robotic exoskeletons, which have the potential to transform upright mobility in the future.
- Practice and training are needed to develop proficiency in whatever form of mobility is most appropriate for the individual with a spinal cord injury.
- Understanding how residual motor function impacts not only walking or propelling a wheelchair, but also maintains sound joint alignment, is key for optimal mobility.

INTRODUCTION

Like beauty, mobility is in the eye of the beholder. For the uninitiated observer, the most obvious consequence of spinal cord injury (SCI) is loss of functional walking ability. For many individuals with SCI, particularly those with more recent injury, restoration of walking ability is a high priority.[1,2] Walking may be a reasonable goal for a proportion of the SCI community. However, for most individuals with SCI, mobility takes the form of a wheelchair for at least some portion of their functional mobility needs.

The literature indicates that the prognosis for independent walking by 1 year after injury is strong for individuals with SCI who, within the first 2 weeks after SCI, demonstrate sufficient sparing of spinal pathways for functional volitional activation of the

[a] Spinal Cord Injury Research, Crawford Research Institute, Shepherd Center, 2020 Peachtree Road Northwest, Atlanta, GA 30309, USA; [b] Department of Rehabilitation Medicine, Emory University School of Medicine, Atlanta, GA, USA; [c] Georgia Institute of Technology, School of Biological Sciences, Atlanta, GA, USA
* Shepherd Center, 2020 Peachtree Road Northwest, Atlanta, GA 30309.
E-mail address: Edee.Field-Fote@Shepherd.org

Phys Med Rehabil Clin N Am 31 (2020) 437–453
https://doi.org/10.1016/j.pmr.2020.04.002
1047-9651/20/© 2020 Elsevier Inc. All rights reserved.

lower extremity muscles.[3,4] However, there are a substantial proportion of individuals who do not meet these criteria early after SCI, but regain volitional control over the course of the first postinjury year and who have the potential for restoration of varying degrees of walking function. Even when walking is not feasible as the primary means of mobility, there may be benefits from training to improve walking ability. For some individuals, the goals of walking are simply to have increased mobility options in the home, whereas others pursue walking for its many physiologic and psychological benefits.[5]

For walking to be a functionally viable means of mobility, particularly for community distances, the individual must have adequate voluntary control over the lower extremities. In the absence of sufficient volitional lower extremity control, slow walking speed makes walking an inefficient form of mobility. Beyond the need to achieve sufficient speeds, the high metabolic demand of walking, pathologic lower extremity movement patterns that risk joint health, and the need for excessive upper extremity weight bearing may also limit walking as a viable means of mobility. Although there are promising indications that in the not-too-distant future overground robotic exoskeletons may become a viable means of community mobility, the present state of development of these devices makes them too slow and cumbersome for community mobility.

For a large proportion of the SCI community, wheeled mobility is the most efficient and functional option currently available and offers a highly efficient and functional way of life. In this article, therapeutic approaches to restoration of mobility are discussed. Because the preponderance of the relevant literature focuses on walking, the coverage of locomotor training and gait training approaches are more extensive. However, walking is not a goal for all individuals with SCI, and in those instances, learning skills in wheelchair use is essential for function and social participation.

RESTORATION OF WALKING FUNCTION AFTER SPINAL CORD INJURY

Two different forms of physical therapeutic intervention, locomotor training and gait training, are used to improve walking function. Ideally, in most cases, outcomes are best when both forms of intervention are used concurrently. Locomotor training involves high numbers of repetition of stepping practice, either overground or on a treadmill, to promote the development of a more fluid movement. Gait training focuses on the pattern of walking and the use of assistive devices to develop the most biomechanically efficient gait. These 2 forms of training are discussed in detail elsewhere in this article. In some cases, the lines between locomotor training and gait training are blurred. For example, electrical stimulation and robotic devices can be used as part of a program of locomotor training, and they can be a valuable adjunct to gait training.

Locomotor Training

Every motor skill requires repetition and practice to optimize the efficiency and quality of movement performance. Use-dependent plasticity is the neural mechanism underlying improvements in performance of all skilled behaviors. Repeatedly engaging the same neural circuits evokes neuroplastic mechanisms such as improved synaptic efficacy and long-term potentiation.[6,7] Although walking is considered an innate behavior, watching a toddler learn to walk clearly shows that the development of functional bipedal locomotion requires repetition and practice. The same is no less true for walking after SCI. Although the basic neural output required to sequence muscle activation for walking exists in the spinal central pattern generators, these spinal circuits must be activated by supraspinal centers.

After SCI, damage to these descending circuits results in a loss of the automaticity that is typically associated with walking. As a result, walking requires a greater level of volitional control. However, with practice and training, walking performance can be improved in those individuals who have sufficient residual lower extremity function. Although in past decades there was much excitement about the possibility of restoring walking solely based on the activation of spinal central pattern generator circuits, in more recent years it has become clear that functional walking depends on the ability of the supraspinal circuits to activate spinal circuits and spinal motoneurons.[8]

There is definitive evidence from preclinical models that practice and training are essential for the restoration of functional movement. Pharmacologic and biologic interventions have little to no value unless paired with skill-related training, a finding that is true for both grasping function and walking function.[9,10] The options for locomotor training after SCI are numerous, with the availability of treadmills, body weight support systems, electrical stimulation systems, robotic exoskeletons, and combinations of these devices. The use of these technologies in combination with practice and training strengthens the neural circuits that underlie walking behavior. Walking speed and timed walking distance are the 2 outcome measures that are typically of greatest interest for outcomes of locomotor training. To date, the evidence for the superiority of one form of locomotor training over others for the improvement of walking speed is mixed[11,12]; however, there is evidence that overground training is superior to treadmill-based training for improvement of walking distance.[12,13]

As with comparisons between overground versus treadmill-based training, the evidence related to the value of higher intensity training is also mixed. Although a case series of 4 individuals with SCI indicated that treadmill walking speed and movement patterns improved to a greater extent in individuals trained at higher intensities, the metrics used to determine intensity suggest that the intensity of training used in the study is considered moderate by most accounts. Further, because kinematics were measured only during treadmill-based walking, it is unclear whether these improvement translate to real-world over ground walking.[14] Conversely, data from a randomized crossover study of 74 individuals with SCI suggested that overground training was associated with greater effects on walking speed and distance despite lower training intensity.[15] Newer evidence from studies of individuals without SCI shows that repeated brief bouts of training facilitate learning a locomotor pattern compared with a single extended training session.[16] These findings may have valuable implications for locomotor training in persons with SCI.

Overground training

Locomotor training in the real-world overground environment offers the opportunity to practice moving the body over the base of support and generating the propulsive forces required for everyday walking. Walking speed has often been considered the gold standard measure of walking function, and a faster walking speed is associated with greater lower extremity muscle strength. The strength of the lower extremities and preferred walking speed are strongly predictive of the amount of daily walking activity people with SCI perform.[17] Walking speeds of 0.44 ± 0.14 m/s are necessary if an individual is to walk in the community and home as their primary means of mobility.[18] Conversely, for functional indoor mobility, significantly lower walking speeds are required, on the order of 0.15 ± 0.08 m/s. Beyond lower extremity strength, upright postural control and balance are requirements for walking to be functional in any environment (**Fig. 1**).

Despite the great emphasis on walking speed, it has been argued that, for people with SCI, the functional value of walking is more likely to be limited by the inability

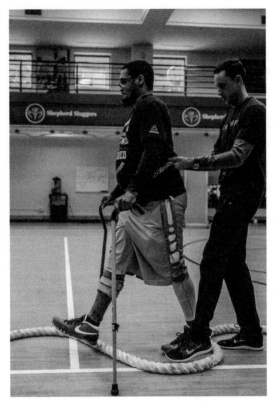

Fig. 1. Overground locomotor training provides the opportunity to practice walking skills in a real-world environment.

to walk longer distances rather than by the speed of walking.[13] As noted, there is some evidence to suggest that overground training has a greater impact on improvements of walking distances compared with treadmill-based training.[13] Because locomotor training involves high numbers of step repetitions, longer stretches of open space are needed. When overground training is augmented by body weight support devices, the space requirements are further increased. Overground training typically incorporates elements of gait training. Upper extremity support devices are usually used for balance, and lower extremity orthotics are used to compensate for weak muscles and protect joints. In some cases where there is sufficient muscle control to avoid joint damage, electrical stimulation can be used to augment muscle activity as a part of overground locomotor training. Although it is possible for therapists to provide manual assistance for stepping in the overground environment, such training often requires more than 1 therapist or the use of a body weight support device to ensure safety.

Treadmill-based training

The treadmill is a valuable technology for locomotor training, providing an environment wherein stepping can be practiced with high numbers of repetitions with nominal space requirements. Because stepping practice occurs within the boundaries of a defined space, the treadmill offers the opportunity for the therapist to provide manual assistance with achieving limb advancement. Preclinical studies of treadmill-based locomotor training in animal models of SCI laid the foundations for our current understanding of the neurophysiologic basis for use-dependent plasticity.[19–22]

For treadmill-based training to be of greatest value, practice involves more than simply performing a high number of repetitions. Practice must include maintaining an upright posture over the moving belt and, when balance is sufficient, incorporating reciprocal arm swing into the training advances the goals of improved upright mobility. When the treadmill technical capabilities allow for slope walking, early evidence suggests that the eccentric muscle control associated with downslope walking may facilitate improved neural activation during stepping.[23]

Despite the value of treadmill-based training and its facility for use in the clinic because of the low space requirements, treadmill-based training does have drawbacks. Anyone with experience running on a treadmill can attest that although the kinematics are the same as walking overground, it does not "feel" the same as walking overground—the nervous system senses that the environment is different. There is evidence to indicate that the motor learning that occurs on the treadmill does not transfer completely to the overground environment and, even when transfer occurs, it may be short lasting.[24]

Gait Training

Although locomotor training focuses on high numbers of stepping repetitions, gait training stresses the importance of the most normal possible walking pattern along with appropriate timing between lower extremity stepping and upper extremity assistive device placement. Prescription of optimal lower extremity orthotic devices, that maximize both function and joint protection, along with upper extremity assistive devices that offer stability and upper extremity weightbearing are prerequisites for optimal outcomes of gait training.

The development of a gait training program begins with an analysis of gait kinematics. By identifying the key gait components that the patient is and is not able to accomplish, the therapist can prescribe the most appropriate assistive device. Although motion capture of 3-dimensional gait kinematics is the gold standard, the instrumentation and technical requirements often put this form of analysis out of reach for clinical use. However, validated observational gait analysis tools, specific for persons with SCI, are available for clinical use.[25] These tools can assist with identification of gait impairments to target during training, as well as offering a means to track training-related progress.

Therapist feedback and the use of mirrors for visual cuing are essential to the development of the individual's internal reference of correctness of the walking pattern. Although gait training emphasizes the development of the optimal individual-specific biomechanical pattern of walking using prescribed assistive devices, which can be a goal in itself, gait training is often paired with locomotor training. In fact, locomotor training that emphasizes only repetitions of movement, without attention to the kinematics of that movement, risks the development of faulty motor patterns that are biomechanically less efficient than they could be, or worse put the individual at risk for joint damage. For that reason, gait training is an important aspect of a sound locomotor training program.

Assistive Technologies to Augment Locomotor Training or Gait Training

These days with assistive technologies in the form of electrical stimulation and robotic exoskeletons, the options for therapeutic interventions for restoration of walking are growing exponentially. Electrical stimulation approaches include both the traditional functional electrical stimulation approaches, peripheral nerve stimulation to evoke reflex stepping, and the more recent advent of transcutaneous spinal stimulation to activate spinal circuits in support of walking function. Robotics can be used as a form of locomotor training, and as an assistive device in gait training applications.

Body weight support

Walking requires sufficient lower extremity extensor muscle strength to support the weight of the body during the stance phase of gait, as well as adequate lower extremity flexor muscle strength to advance the limb during the swing phase. For individuals with SCI who lack sufficient lower extremity strength to support the body in stance phase, body weight support devices are available to provide partial support of body weight during either overground training or treadmill-based training (**Fig. 2**). These devices provide a harness-based suspension system with adjustable levels of support for body weight, and are available in the forms of both mobile device that roll overground, or fixed ceiling-mounted devices. As discussed elsewhere in this article, beyond the traditional lower extremity orthotic devices, electrical stimulation devices can assist those who have insufficient flexor muscle strength to achieve foot clearance and limb advancement during stepping.

Mobile body weight support devices (eg, Andago, Hocoma, Volketswil, Switzerland; LiteGait, Mobility Research, Tempe AZ; NxStep, Biodex, Shirley NY; Lode BWSS,

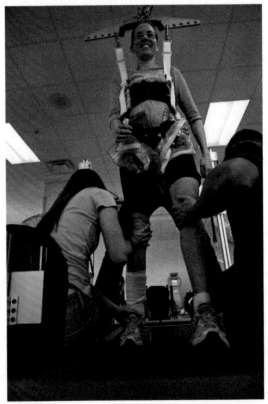

Fig. 2. Treadmill-based locomotor training with body weight support is performed within the boundaries of a defined space. The treadmill offers the opportunity for the therapist(s) to provide manual assistance with achieving limb advancement.

Lode, Groningen, the Netherlands) consist of an overhead lift supported by a wheeled frame that is attached to a user-worn harness. The assembly allows partial support of body weight to be provided for overground walking, during which the user or the therapist moves the device over fixed ground. In addition, some models of mobile body weight support devices have sufficiently high ground clearance to be rolled over a low-profile treadmill, allowing support to be provided during treadmill walking. Mobile body weight support devices have the advantage of allowing the user to walk anywhere, provided the ground is level and there is sufficient space to accommodate the device. The disadvantage of these devices is that the user cannot practice using upper extremity arm swing owing to the need to either push the device while walking, or to use upper extremity assistive devices for balance support while the therapist pushes the device.

Beyond the mobile body weight support systems, there are fixed, ceiling-mounted body weight support systems available (eg, ZeroG, Aretech, Ashburn, VA; Vector, Bioness Inc, Valencia, CA). These devices provide motorized, low-inertia support that moves with the user. Ceiling-mounted devices represent advanced technologies, with support that can be adjusted as specified by the therapist based on the goals of training. The patient has the opportunity to practice the use of various upper extremity assistive devices for balance while being safeguarded against falls.

Body weight support devices provide a safe environment to practice upright mobility activities. The ceiling-mounted devices can be used in any indoor environment, including walking up slopes and stairs, and are limited only by the space in which they are mounted. A possible drawback of these devices is that, in supporting the trunk, the individual may have little opportunity to practice the postural righting and balance responses that are necessary for real-world walking. For this reason, body weight support devices may be most appropriate in the early stages of locomotor training, when transitioning to new assistive devices, or when practicing advanced upright mobility skills.

Electrical simulation

Functional electrical stimulation The use of functional electrical stimulation was among the first technologies to promote improved walking function in persons with SCI. Its first application was in individuals with stroke, wherein stimulation was used to remedy drop foot by activating the dorsiflexors. These days there are commercial devices available to activate dorsiflexion during stepping (eg, WalkAide, Innovative Neurotronics, Reno NV; L300, Bioness Inc). Stimulation can be triggered by either pressure sensors in the shoe that are activated at heel strike or by tilt sensors that sense the ankle of the shank during stepping. These devices are most useful for individuals who have relatively good control of the muscles about the hip and knee and need assistance mostly with dorsiflexion for foot clearance.

More extensive muscle activation can be achieved by multielectrode systems that activate muscles according the phase of the gait cycle. Because of the high computational requirements for appropriately timing muscle activation and the high metabolic demand associated with extracellular activation of muscles, these devices have not achieved commercial viability and remain relegated to the research domain.[26] The Parastep system (Sigmedics Inc., Fairborn, OH) is the sole multielectrode system that has achieved commercial availability. The design of this device incorporates user control of stimulation via an instrumented walker, and makes use of the unique features of the reflex control of muscle to achieve stepping. Electrodes on the hip and knee extensor muscles are tonically activated when the device is in operating mode, providing support in the stance phase of gait. Electrodes overlying the common peroneal nerves are activated by the user to initiate the swing phase of walking. The brief, high-intensity train of stimulation to the common peroneal nerve activates the flexor reflex–crossed extension response. This response simultaneously elicits ankle dorsiflexion along with flexion of the hip and knee on the stimulated side (via the flexor reflex response), as well as contributing to whole limb extension on the contralateral limb (via the crossed extension response). These reflex responses engage the spinal reflex arcs, which are preserved after SCI in individuals with lesions at the cervical and thoracic levels. The high intensity of stimulation required to elicit robust muscle activation and reflex responses means that the stimulation is noxious, and for that reason these systems are typically used only be persons with little or no sensory function in the lower extremities.

For locomotor training purposes, electrical stimulation to trigger a reflex stepping response via the flexor reflex — crossed extension response has been used in conjunction with experimental treadmill-based training approaches in persons with relatively intact sensation.[13] However, perhaps because of the high stimulation intensity, and associated risk for falls when walking in the overground environment, this technique has not been used in commercial applications. Functional electrical stimulation-assisted walking provides a way for the individual's own nervous system to contribute to stepping; beyond its functional value, stimulation has beneficial effects on use-dependent plasticity and motor learning as evidenced by improved independent joint control with a decreased need for stimulation,[27] and contributes to more normal modulation of the spinal reflex activity underlying spasticity.[28]

Epidural and transcutaneous spinal stimulation Spinal stimulation is an approach that originated almost 4 decades ago,[29,30] but which has recently garnered renewed interest and attention. These devices comprise the same epidural stimulation technology that was originally referred to as "dorsal column stimulation," and used for the management of pain. Although often referred to as "spinal cord stimulation," the evidence indicates that the dura is highly nonconductive and for that reason the effects of stimulating electrodes placed over the spinal vertebrae are in truth primarily owing to activation of the spinal nerve roots. For this reason, both the invasive surgical implantation of electrodes over the dura and the noninvasive transcutaneous placement of electrodes have their effects via the same mechanisms.[31] Evidence for the value of spinal stimulation comes from case studies wherein stimulation has been combined with long-term locomotor training and practice of upright control activities.[32,33]

Robotic locomotor exoskeletons

Treadmill-based robotic exoskeletons The high personnel demands of treadmill-based locomotor training led to the development of robotic exoskeletons (eg, Lokomat, Hocoma) that are capable of producing a standardized walking pattern via computer-controlled gait orthosis. The hip and knee joints are powered with the capability of providing variable amounts of assistance as determined by the therapist, while the ankle joints are passively supported with spring and strap mechanisms. Locomotor training using treadmill-based robotic exoskeletons have the advantage that they can be used early in the rehabilitation process when the individual with SCI may have experienced minimal motor return in the lower extremities. However, there is some evidence to suggest that, for individuals who have the ability to take steps overground, the transfer of training from the treadmill-based locomotor exoskeleton to the overgound environment may be limited.[13] This limited transfer may be due in part to the restricted opportunity to learn through trial and error within the set walking pattern of the device,[34] as well as the lack of a need to generate the propulsive forces that are needed for real-world walking (**Fig. 3**).

Overground robotic exoskeletons The last decade has seen exponential progress in the realm of overground robotic exoskeletons for persons with SCI. These technologies offer the opportunity for intensive overground locomotor training, even when the individual has significant impairment of lower extremity motor function.[35] Given the relatively early stage of their development, the evidence for the value of overground robotic exoskeletons as a locomotor training approach for improving real-world walking is as yet limited.[36,37] However, there is early evidence from quasi-experimental (pre–post) studies that prolonged and consistent training in these devices is associated with improvements in bone density,[38] muscle mass in the lower extremities,[38] regularity of bowel movements,[35] sleep, and feelings of well-being.[39] In addition, there are reports that use of overground robotic exoskeletons is associated with decreased pain and spasticity.[35,40]

Although the literature contains no randomized studies to directly compare outcomes of overground robotic exoskeletons with other locomotor training approaches, a published systematic review of the available literature on robotic overground exoskeletons compared the outcomes using these devices to other rehabilitation approaches. When considering the primary outcome measure of post-training change in walking speed, the relative value of robotic overground exoskeletons was not greater than conventional approaches.[37]

In the United States, device approval by the Food and Drug Administration is required for the use of overground robotic exoskeletons in rehabilitation. Four devices currently have this approval, of these three device (ie, Ekso, Ekso Bionics, Richmond, CA; Indego, Parker Hannifin Corp., Cleveland, OH; and ReWalk, ReWalk Robotics Ltd, Yokneam, Israel) have class II medical device approval. One additional device (ie, Rex Rex Bionics, Melbourne, Australia) is approved as a class I medical device. At the present time, these devices are available in adult sizes only, with use limited to persons who fit defined anthropometric criteria (**Fig. 4**).

With the current state of technology, robotic overground exoskeletons have primarily been used as rehabilitation devices. Although some devices are approved for personal use, they are accompanied by the requirement for availability of a support person in the event of a fall or other emergency. This, along with their slow walking

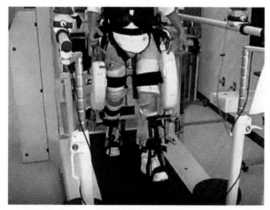

Fig. 3. Treadmill-based robotic gait orthoses enable high repetitions of stepping within the treadmill environment for individuals with minimal lower extremity function.

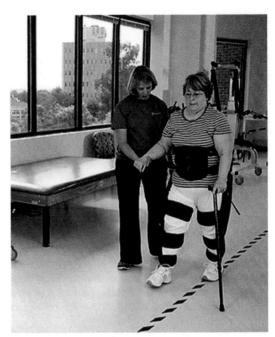

Fig. 4. Overground robotic exoskeletons represent a rapidly advancing technology. Although currently primarily used as a rehabilitation tool, the potential exists for these devices to develop into mobility devices.

speed, limits in the terrain over which they can be used, the need to use the hands for balance, the time required for donning and doffing, and the activities that cannot be performed while in the devices (eg, sitting for prolonged periods, driving or riding in a car) are current barriers to the usefulness of these devices for daily life.[41] However, these technologies are advancing at a rapid pace, and it seems likely that technical limitation can be overcome to make them feasible as mobility devices in the foreseeable future.

Rehabilitation and technology-based approaches for improving walking function continue to be an area of focus in research. In the clinical realm, collaborative goal planning between the individual with SCI and the therapist are essential. The goals related to walking can range from physiologic benefits, to the achievement of defined functional or recreational tasks, to being a primary means of mobility. Regardless of the goal, the selection of optimal lower extremity orthotics, upper extremity stability aids, and training approach can maximize available function and preserve joint health (**Figs. 5** and **6**).

WHEELED MOBILITY

For many individuals with SCI, walking is not a practical goal. Even for those who have some walking function, limited walking speeds and having the hands occupied with an upper extremity assistive device makes walking slow and cumbersome as a means of mobility. For these individuals, skilled wheelchair use is essential to independence. As with locomotor training, skilled wheelchair use requires practice, the development of biomechanically efficient techniques to propel the wheelchair, the development of dynamic balance to negotiate the wheelchair safely and efficiently, and the development

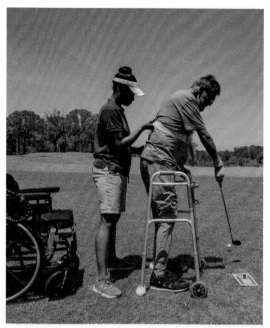

Fig. 5. Beyond being a means of functional mobility, walking and upright control make recreational activities possible.

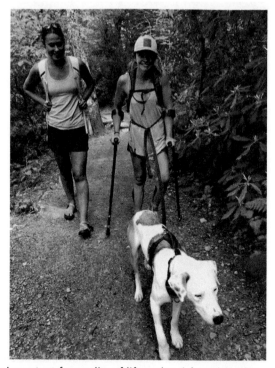

Fig. 6. Mobility is important for quality of life and social participation.

of an intuitive sense of biomechanical leverage to navigate the body between the wheelchair and other surfaces. With practice and training, individuals can attain exceptional skill in wheeled mobility (**Fig. 7**).

Importance of Manual Wheelchair Propulsion Techniques

For manual wheelchair users, efficient and biomechanically sound wheelchair propulsion skills are essential not only for mobility, but also for preservation of upper extremity joint health. Although wheelchair propulsion does not require the prolonged high force levels that are experienced during surface-to-surface transfers, the high number of repetitions involved in wheelchair propulsion can pose a threat to upper extremity joint health. Wheelchair selection (including optimal postural support) and training in push mechanics for efficient propulsion are fundamental to maximizing efficient wheelchair mobility while minimizing joint forces.

On level surfaces, push mechanics are most efficient when all joints are working in the middle range of available motion. Efficiency is optimized by a circular propulsive motion, wherein the hand contacts the push rim during the forward swing of the arms, and drops below the push rim on recovery.[42] When the wheelchair is lightweight and well-tuned, there is a period of hands-free glide between push strokes, with only light contact needed when necessary to correct the direction of wheelchair motion. Although stresses on the shoulder during propulsion receive a great deal of attention in the literature, the other upper extremity joints are at risk with faulty push mechanics as well. For example, the deleterious habit of gripping and releasing the handrim with every stroke results in excessive stress on the wrist joint. Repeated gripping and

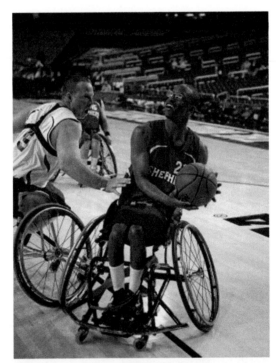

Fig. 7. Wheeled mobility skills, like other skilled motor behavior, can be developed to a high level with practice and training.

releasing also decreases the biomechanical efficiency of propulsion by reducing the forward momentum at the end of the propulsive stroke. Smooth propulsion is best achieved by pushing the rim with the wrist in neutral, and the fingers relaxed so that the hand is slightly open. Gripping the push rim is best reserved for situations, such as inclines or curbs, wherein more forceful propulsion is required.

Push mechanics can often be optimized through wheelchair configuration, particularly as it relates to the position of the rear axle. For example, in the horizontal plane, a more forward position of the rear axle focuses the arc of propulsion on the posterior upper quadrant of the wheel. This configuration decreases the forces on the shoulder joint[43] and can be beneficial in individuals with limited or absent triceps function in whom biceps and the anterior deltoid are needed to provide the propulsive forces. However, such modifications can come with a tradeoff, in this case making the wheelchair less stable to the rear. Vertical plane position of the axle (ie, seat height) also affects push mechanics, and there seems to be a tradeoff between improvement in the temporal aspects of propulsion with lower seat height, with an accompanying increase in shoulder abduction and nonpropulsive forces.[44] Finally, loading on the shoulder joint does not seem to be influenced to a meaningful extent by changes in seat tile angle or backrest angle, provided that these changes do not alter the relative position of the shoulder and rear axle.[45]

Training to Protect Joint Health

Beyond the value of proper wheelchair propulsion mechanics for preserving upper extremity joint health, a well-designed home exercise program has an essential place. Evidence indicates that a home-based program directed at movement optimization, strengthening, and stretching in combination with expert pointers on optimal performance of propulsion, transfers, and unloading raises can have a meaningful impact on shoulder pain.[46] A major limitation of the available studies related to the impact of an exercise program on upper extremity joint health is that study inclusion has mostly been restricted to individuals with paraplegia, in whom the upper extremities have full innervation. Although there have been no studies to assess the impact of exercise for protection of joint health in persons with tetraplegia, there is evidence that physical therapy interventions clearly improve upper extremity strength in paretic upper extremity muscles.[47] Therefore, by extension, exercise and training directed at strengthening the muscles that support the upper extremity joints is of value for individuals with tetraplegia, as it is for those with paraplegia.

Power assist wheels are an excellent option for many manual wheelchair users. The lower force and energy requirements made possible by the motor assist make this technology particularly useful for individuals with tetraplegia. Power assist wheels may offer mobility access to new recreational activities and terrains; however, there is a related mobility-related trade-off because they can be difficult to transport.[48] The additional training needed to learn to use power assist wheels is minimal.[49]

Wheelchair Skills Training

Skilled wheelchair mobility expands the navigable world for the wheelchair user. There is a strong body of literature supporting the value of skills training for improving wheelchair mobility in manual wheelchair users.[50] Among the most robust of these studies is a randomized, double-masked multicenter trial involving 4 SCI model systems centers that enrolled 114 participants in standardized wheelchair skills program course.[51] The outcomes of this study demonstrated that wheelchair skills training was most valuable for improving performance of more advanced wheelchair

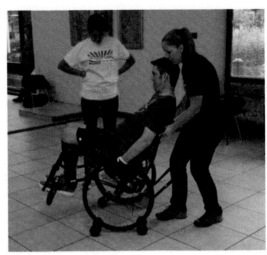

Fig. 8. Wheelchair skills training can make a meaningful difference in the performance of advanced wheelchair activities and broaden the range of opportunities for social participation.

skills, such as negotiating curbs, rolling over soft surfaces, and turning while in a wheelie position. Conversely, mobility training did not result in a significant difference between the trained and control group in basic indoor and community wheelchair mobility. Those with lower baseline skill levels made the greatest gains in mobility, suggesting that there may have been ceiling effects in those with higher baseline wheelchair mobility skills. Not surprisingly, greater gains were also observed in those who attended a greater proportion of the six 90-minute training sessions indicating that, just as with locomotor training, repetition and practice are essential to skill development (**Fig. 8**).

Just as with manual wheelchairs, skill in the use of powered wheelchairs also improves with practice and training. The wide variability in residual motor control in individuals with SCI necessitates a broad range of drive controls for powered chairs. From joysticks and finger controls to sip-and-puffs to tongue drives, the possibilities for drive control continue to advance in step with technology and computing capacity. The assessment of an individual's proficiency in wheelchair use is important for determining the impact of a wheelchair skills program. There are a number of wheelchair skills test available, some of which entail a standardized course over which skills are tested.[52]

SUMMARY

Mobility, regardless of whether it is achieved by walking or the use of a wheelchair, is essential for quality of life and social participation after SCI. In the realm of walking function, new technologies are evolving in the form of overground robotic exoskeletons, which may have the potential to transform upright mobility in the future. Practice and training are needed to develop proficiency in whatever form of mobility is most appropriate for the individual with SCI. Understanding how residual motor function impacts not only the ability to step or to propel the wheelchair, but also to maintain biomechanically sound joint alignment is key for optimal lifelong mobility.

DISCLOSURE

The authors have nothing to disclose.

REFERENCES

1. Ditunno PL, Patrick M, Stineman M, et al. Who wants to walk? Preferences for recovery after SCI: a longitudinal and cross-sectional study. Spinal Cord 2008;46: 500–6.
2. Lo C, Tran Y, Anderson K, et al. Functional priorities in persons with spinal cord injury: using discrete choice experiments to determine preferences. J Neurotrauma 2016;33:1958–68.
3. van Middendorp JJ, Hosman AJ, Donders AR, et al. A clinical prediction rule for ambulation outcomes after traumatic spinal cord injury: a longitudinal cohort study. Lancet 2011;377:1004–10.
4. Hicks KE, Zhao Y, Fallah N, et al, RHSCIR Network. A simplified clinical prediction rule for prognosticating independent walking after spinal cord injury: a prospective study from a Canadian multicenter spinal cord injury registry. Spine J 2017; 17:1383–92.
5. Hicks AL, Ginis KAM. Treadmill training after spinal cord injury: it's not just about the walking. J Rehabil Res Dev 2008;45:241–8.
6. Berghuis KMM, Veldman MP, Solnik S, et al. Neuronal mechanisms of motor learning and motor memory consolidation in healthy old adults. Age (Dordr) 2015;37:9779.
7. Rosenkranz K, Kacar A, Rothwell JC. Differential modulation of motor cortical plasticity and excitability in early and late phases of human motor learning. J Neurosci 2007;27:12058–66.
8. Field-Fote EC, Yang JF, Basso DM, et al. Supraspinal control predicts locomotor function and forecasts responsiveness to training after spinal cord injury. J Neurotrauma 2017;34:1813–25.
9. García-Alías G, Barkhuysen S, Buckle M, et al. Chondroitinase ABC treatment opens a window of opportunity for task-specific rehabilitation. Nat Neurosci 2009;12:1145–51.
10. Torres-Espín A, Forero J, Fenrich KK, et al. Eliciting inflammation enables successful rehabilitative training in chronic spinal cord injury. Brain 2018;141: 1946–62.
11. Yang JF, Musselman KE, Livingstone D, et al. Repetitive mass practice or focused precise practice for retraining walking after incomplete spinal cord injury? A pilot randomized clinical trial. Neurorehabil Neural Repair 2013;28:314–24.
12. Mehrholz J, Harvey LA, Thomas S, et al. Is body-weight-supported treadmill training or robotic-assisted gait training superior to overground gait training and other forms of physiotherapy in people with spinal cord injury? A systematic review. Spinal Cord 2017;55:722–9.
13. Field-Fote EC, Roach KE. Influence of a locomotor training approach on walking speed and distance in people with chronic spinal cord injury: a randomized clinical trial. Phys Ther 2011;91:48–60.
14. Holleran CL, Hennessey PW, Leddy AL, et al. High-intensity variable stepping training in patients with motor incomplete spinal cord injury: a case series. J Neurol Phys Ther 2018;42:94–101.
15. Field-Fote E, Lindley S, Sherman A. Locomotor training approaches for individuals with spinal cord injury: a preliminary report of walking-related outcomes. J Neurol Phys Ther 2005;29:127–37.

16. Day KA, Leech KA, Roemmich RT, et al. Accelerating locomotor savings in learning: compressing four training days to one. J Neurophysiol 2018;119: 2100–13.

17. Stevens SL, Fuller DK, Morgan DW. Leg strength, preferred walking speed, and daily step activity in adults with incomplete spinal cord injuries. Top Spinal Cord Inj Rehabil 2013;19:47–53.

18. van Hedel HJA, EM-SCI Study Group. Gait speed in relation to categories of functional ambulation after spinal cord injury. Neurorehabil Neural Repair 2008;23:343–50.

19. Wolpaw JR. Operant conditioning of primate spinal reflexes: the H-reflex. J Neurophysiol 1987;57:443–59.

20. JR W, Wolpaw JR. Adaptive plasticity in the primate spinal stretch reflex: reversal and re-development. Brain Res 1983;278:299–304.

21. Wolpaw J, Carp JS. Adaptive plasticity in spinal cord. Adv Neurol 1993;74: 163–74.

22. Wolpaw JR, O'Keefe JA, Noonan PA, et al. Adaptive plasticity in primate spinal stretch reflex: persistence. J Neurophysiol 1986;55:272–9.

23. Basso DM, Lang CE. Consideration of dose and timing when applying interventions after stroke and spinal cord injury. J Neurol Phys Ther 2017;41(Suppl 3): S24–31.

24. Reisman DS, Block HJ, Bastian AJ. Interlimb coordination during locomotion: what can be adapted and stored? J Neurophysiol 2005;94:2403–15.

25. Field-Fote E, Fluet G, Schafer S, et al. The spinal cord injury functional ambulation inventory (SCI-FAI). J Rehabil Med 2001;33:177–81.

26. Triolo RJ, Bailey SN, Foglyano KM, et al. Long-term performance and user satisfaction with implanted neuroprostheses for upright mobility after paraplegia: 2- to 14-year follow-up. Arch Phys Med Rehabil 2018;99:289–98.

27. Street T, Singleton C. A clinically meaningful training effect in walking speed using functional electrical stimulation for motor-incomplete spinal cord injury. J Spinal Cord Med 2018;41:361–6.

28. Mirbagheri MM, Ladouceur M, Barbeau H, et al. The effects of long-term FES-assisted walking on intrinsic and reflex dynamic stiffness in spastic spinal-cord-injured subjects. IEEE Trans Neural Syst Rehabil Eng 2002;10:280–9.

29. Dimitrijevic MM, Dimitrijevic MR, Illis LS, et al. Spinal cord stimulation for the control of spasticity in patients with chronic spinal cord injury: I. Clinical observations. Cent Nerv Syst Trauma 1986;3:129–44.

30. Dimitrijevic MR, Illis LS, Nakajima K, et al. Spinal cord stimulation for the control of spasticity in patients with chronic spinal cord injury: II. Neurophysiologic observations. Cent Nerv Syst Trauma 1986;3:145–52.

31. Hofstoetter US, Freundl B, Binder H, et al. Common neural structures activated by epidural and transcutaneous lumbar spinal cord stimulation: elicitation of posterior root-muscle reflexes. PLoS One 2018;13:e0192013.

32. Angeli CA, Boakye M, Morton RA, et al. Recovery of over-ground walking after chronic motor complete spinal cord injury. N Engl J Med 2018;379:1244–50.

33. Wagner FB, Mignardot J-B, Le Goff-Mignardot CG, et al. Targeted neurotechnology restores walking in humans with spinal cord injury. Nature 2018;563:65–71.

34. Emken JL, Reinkensmeyer DJ. Robot-enhanced motor learning: accelerating internal model formation during locomotion by transient dynamic amplification. IEEE Trans Neural Syst Rehabil Eng 2005;13:33–9.

35. Miller LE, Zimmermann AK, Herbert WG. Clinical effectiveness and safety of powered exoskeleton-assisted walking in patients with spinal cord injury: systematic review with meta-analysis. Med Devices (Auckl) 2016;9:455–66.

36. Bach Baunsgaard C, Vig Nissen U, Katrin Brust A, et al. Gait training after spinal cord injury: safety, feasibility and gait function following 8 weeks of training with the exoskeletons from Ekso Bionics. Spinal Cord 2018;56:106–16.

37. Fisahn C, Aach M, Jansen O, et al. The effectiveness and safety of exoskeletons as assistive and rehabilitation devices in the treatment of neurologic gait disorders in patients with spinal cord injury: a systematic review. Glob Spine J 2016;6:822–41.

38. Karelis AD, Carvalho LP, Castillo MJ, et al. Effect on body composition and bone mineral density of walking with a robotic exoskeleton in adults with chronic spinal cord injury. J Rehabil Med 2017;49:84–7.

39. Gagnon DH, Vermette M, Duclos C, et al. Satisfaction and perceptions of long-term manual wheelchair users with a spinal cord injury upon completion of a locomotor training program with an overground robotic exoskeleton. Disabil Rehabil Assist Technol 2019;14(2):138–45.

40. Stampacchia G, Rustici A, Bigazzi S, et al. Walking with a powered robotic exoskeleton: subjective experience, spasticity and pain in spinal cord injured persons. NeuroRehabilitation 2016;39:277–83.

41. Heinemann AW, Jayaraman A, Mummidisetty CK, et al. Experience of robotic exoskeleton use at four spinal cord injury model systems centers. J Neurol Phys Ther 2018;42:256–67.

42. Boninger ML, Koontz AM, Sisto SA, et al. Pushrim biomechanics and injury prevention in spinal cord injury: recommendations based on CULP-SCI investigations. J Rehabil Res Dev 2005;42:9–19.

43. Boninger ML, Baldwin M, Cooper RA, et al. Manual wheelchair pushrim biomechanics and axle position. Arch Phys Med Rehabil 2000;81:608–13.

44. Kotajarvi BR, Sabick MB, An K-N, et al. The effect of seat position on wheelchair propulsion biomechanics. J Rehabil Res Dev 2004;41:403–14.

45. Desroches G, Aissaoui R, Bourbonnais D. Effect of system tilt and seat-to-backrest angles on load sustained by shoulder during wheelchair propulsion. J Rehabil Res Dev 2006;43:871–82.

46. Mulroy SJ, Thompson L, Kemp B, et al, Physical Therapy Clinical Research Network (PTClinResNet). Strengthening and optimal movements for painful shoulders (STOMPS) in chronic spinal cord injury: a randomized controlled trial. Phys Ther 2011;91:305–24.

47. Aravind N, Harvey LA, Glinsky JV. Physiotherapy interventions for increasing muscle strength in people with spinal cord injuries: a systematic review. Spinal Cord 2019;57:449–60.

48. Giacobbi PR, Levy CE, Dietrich FD, et al. Wheelchair users' perceptions of and experiences with power assist wheels. Am J Phys Med Rehabil 2010;89:225–34.

49. Sawatzky B, Mortenson WB, Wong S. Learning to use a rear-mounted power assist for manual wheelchairs. Disabil Rehabil Assist Technol 2018;13:772–6.

50. Tu C-J, Liu L, Wang W, et al. Effectiveness and safety of wheelchair skills training program in improving the wheelchair skills capacity: a systematic review. Clin Rehabil 2017;31:1573–82.

51. Worobey LA, Kirby RL, Heinemann AW, et al. Effectiveness of group wheelchair skills training for people with spinal cord injury: a randomized controlled trial. Arch Phys Med Rehabil 2016;97:1777–84.e3.

52. Fliess-Douer O, Vanlandewijck YC, Lubel Manor G, et al. A systematic review of wheelchair skills tests for manual wheelchair users with a spinal cord injury: towards a standardized outcome measure. Clin Rehabil 2010;24:867–86.

Nerve and Tendon Transfers After Spinal Cord Injuries in the Pediatric Population

Clinical Decision Making and Rehabilitation Strategies to Optimize Function

Joshua A. Vova, MD[a],*, Loren T. Davidson, MD[b,c]

KEYWORDS

- Pediatric • Spinal cord injury • Rehabilitation • Nerve transfer • Tendon transfer
- Tetraplegia

KEY POINTS

- The goal of rehabilitation following loss of upper extremity function caused by tetraplegia is to maximize function and independence. Previous studies cite that regaining arm and hand function remains the highest priority for patients recovering from tetraplegia. However, a very low percentage of eligible patients get referred for reconstructive surgery.
- This article focuses on the 2 most commonly used surgical strategies to restore upper extremity function: upper extremity tendon transfer and nerve transfer. Both tendon transfer and nerve transfer have advantages and disadvantages that should be taken into account when determining the appropriate surgical intervention.
- Physicians should understand the role of examination, patient selection, timing, and the rehabilitation process in tendon transfers and nerve transfers. Pediatric patients have unique characteristics that should be taken into account in order to ensure a successful outcome.

It is estimated that approximately 3% to 5% of the spinal cord injuries (SCIs) that occur in the United States each year involve children less than 15 years old.[1] Pediatric SCIs, although less frequent than in the adult population, have some unique characteristics. Children less than 8 years of age are thought to be more vulnerable to cervical SCI because of the anatomy of the developing spine. Notably, in children, the primary

[a] Department of Physical Medicine and Rehabilitation, Children's Healthcare of Atlanta, 1001 Johnson Ferry Road, Northeast, Atlanta, GA 30342, USA; [b] Department of Physical Medicine and Rehabilitation, University of California Davis Health System, 4860 Y Street, Suite 3850, Sacramento, CA 95817, USA; [c] Shriners Hospitals for Children, Northern California, USA
* Corresponding author.
E-mail address: Joshua.vova@choa.org

Phys Med Rehabil Clin N Am 31 (2020) 455–469
https://doi.org/10.1016/j.pmr.2020.04.006
1047-9651/20/© 2020 Elsevier Inc. All rights reserved.

fulcrum of motion at the neck is C2-C3, as opposed to C5-C6 in adults, and C2 does not completely fuse until approximately 12 years of age.[2] Pediatric patients are typically associated with higher risk of cervical SCI because of incomplete ossification of the cervical spine, large head to body ratio, horizontal arrangement of the facets, weak neck musculature, and elastic ligaments and support structures.[3] They are also at risk for nontraumatic causes, such as tumors, or infections, such as transverse myelitis and acute flaccid myelitis. Childhood skeletal dysplasia, trisomy 21, and juvenile rheumatoid arthritis also place them at increased risk of cervical SCIs.[4] Despite these unique causes of SCI, cervical SCI in the pediatric population seems to have a similar incidence to SCI in adults, and there is no evidence to suggest that the recovery trajectory is any different. There are significant variations in mortality in individuals with SCI, based on level of injury and ventilator requirement.[5–7] However, children have the potential to live into adulthood and would benefit from opportunities to acquire more independence. Functional use of the upper extremities is important in improving community activities and performing independent activities of daily living (ADLs). Previous studies cite that regaining arm and hand function remains the highest priority for patients recovering from tetraplegia.[8] Even a partial recovery can make a big impact on independence, the ability to use adaptive equipment, and success in adopting compensatory strategies.

When considering the potential for function-restoring upper extremity surgery in a patient with tetraplegia, there are several factors to consider. Physiatrists must be familiar with the indications for, and appropriate timing of, referral for upper extremity surgery because it can have significant ramifications on the outcome. Once patients are medically stable, including spine stabilization surgery when indicated, they are usually transferred to a rehabilitation service for further recovery and education about SCI. The rehabilitation facility may be part of the same hospital, at a different hospital, or a freestanding rehabilitation facility. However, a rehabilitation team with surgical expertise in function-restoring upper extremity surgery is not universal and may require advocacy and planning by the physiatrist. Patients who are potential surgical candidates for upper extremity reconstruction may never be referred for evaluation or referred late, which may limit reconstructive options. Early rehabilitation treatment goals and education must include a focus on preservation of range of motion by optimizing splinting, spasticity management, and tissue mobilization in order to not limit potential for neurologic recovery or surgical reconstruction.

Traditionally, tendon transfers have been the pillar of reconstructive surgical strategy to restore function, control, and strength in tetraplegia.[9] The transfer of a muscle results in either loss of the donor muscle's original function or, more commonly, weakening of a movement the donor muscle participated in owing to redundancy of muscles contributing to a given joint movement in the upper extremity. In patients with cervical tetraplegia, there may be few available donor muscles, especially with high cervical injuries. Injuries above the C5 motor level generally lack available donor muscles for reconstruction. Tendon transfer postoperative risks may include tendon rupture and tenodesis failure.[10] There is also a risk that the transfers or tenodesis may lose strength because of progressive stretching over time, especially in growing pediatric patients. In turn, this may change the biomechanical advantage.[10]

In recent years, nerve transfers have been revisited as an option for the treatment of tetraplegia, especially when innervated donor muscle and tendon units are not available distal to the elbows. Nerve transfers allow direct reinnervation of the target muscle originally intended to perform a task. Although nerve transfers do require sacrificing a nerve, thoughtful donor selection using nerves with inherent redundancy or that subserve a less important function is done to minimize the residual donor deficit. A single nerve has the potential to reinnervate multiple muscles and, in theory, restore multiple functions.[11] Nerve transfers have been well described in pediatric literature in the setting of birth-related and traumatic brachial plexopathies. Recent literature, especially in pediatrics, has explored this intervention in pediatric patients with acute flaccid myelitis (AFM).[12–15] In addition, advancements in microsurgical instrumentation have allowed surgeons to separate different branches of nerves; for example, the wrist flexors from the finger flexors in the median nerve.[16] However, nerve transfers have some disadvantages as well. Nerve transfers are time sensitive and require the surgeon to sacrifice intact neural structures.

Given distinct advantages and disadvantages to both tendon transfer and nerve transfers, it is important for rehabilitation physicians to be familiar with both options. Tendon transfers typically require weeks of immobilization postoperatively, whereas nerve transfers do not require strict immobilization. Tendon transfers have the distinctive advantage of not being time sensitive and they can be performed once the normal motor recovery has reached a plateau. Children may expect miracles and emotionally not be ready to proceed with further surgical interventions after the initial injury. The additional time allows the patient and family to process the implications of SCI and accept that further recovery may not occur, making the decision to proceed with surgical upper extremity reconstruction more palatable. Although there are cases in the literature of nerve transfers being performed many years after injury, standard consensus is that they are best performed between 6 and 12 months after the injury. Following nerve transfer, the nerve must regenerate from the coaptation site to the target muscle in a length-dependent fashion at a rate of approximately 2.5 cm/mo (1 inch/mo). Thus, clinical evidence of muscle reinnervation and functional strength following nerve transfer may take 6 to 12 months or more,[16] and success rates are not as established as for tendon transfers. Both procedures come at the expense of sacrificing all or a portion of a donor muscle or nerve, respectively.

PATIENT SELECTION AND TIMING OF REFERRAL

Injury to the cervical spinal cord resulting in tetraplegia can result from trauma, infection, immune-mediated attack, tumor, or ischemia. The prognosis for recovery differs significantly based on the cause, and this must be considered when contemplating restorative upper extremity reconstruction. In general, recovery from traumatic SCI may occur for up to 2 years; however, the most significant changes occur in first 6 months.[17] In contrast, patients with AFM have a recovery pattern that plateaus during the first 6 to 9 months[18–21] and have a worse prognosis for spontaneous recovery than traumatic SCI. Given the critical time period in complete SCI when nerve transfers are most successful, upper extremity reconstruction should be contemplated at the point where there has not been significant appreciable change over the previous 3 months. Patients with incomplete SCI, or tendon transfer candidates, do not have such a critical timetable.

Given the variability of patients with tetraplegia, it is useful to categorize the neurologic injury by the extent of injury and the remaining innervated segments that may serve as potential donors for muscle or nerve transfer. Upper extremity muscle innervation in patients with tetraplegia caused by SCI can be divided in to 3 categories.[22] The first category are muscle groups that are innervated by the spinal cord segment above the level of injury, remain under volitional control, and thus have nerves and muscle that can be used as donors for transfer. The second group of muscles are ones that are directly affected by the spinal cord level of injury. At this level, the SCI produces more focal injury resulting in a predominantly lower motor neuron (LMN) injury, but it may have some upper motor neuron (UMN) involvement as well. The last category is the group of muscles that are innervated below the segment of the SCI. If the patient has a complete SCI, these muscles remain anatomically connected to the anterior horn cells; however, they are disconnected from the descending motor tracts, which results in upper motor dysfunction.[22]

Injury patterns in SCI may be an isolated loss of UMN function or a combination of upper and lower motor dysfunction. Conditions that have a predilection for damage to the anterior horn cell and result in a LMN injury such as AFM or spinal cord ischemia, portend a less favorable prognosis for spontaneous recovery than UMN injury. The concept behind a nerve transfer is to circumvent the damaged spinal cord area and regain muscle function by restoring UMN control. The concomitant lower motor injury in SCI can cause muscles to become significantly atrophied or fibrotic.[23] In order for the nerve transfer to be successful, surgery should occur before the target muscle is permanently damaged, which is why nerve transfers or targeted reinnervation is time sensitive. End-plate motor changes and loss of neurotrophic support for nerve regeneration is a process that occurs in denervated motor units, and it is theorized by some that this happens within the first year of injury.[22] Muscle groups that have intact LMNs but damaged UMNs may have the opportunity for intervention beyond 12 months of injury.[24] Bertelli and Ghizoni[25] reported functional success with nerve transfers performed after 18 months. However, it is generally accepted that surgical intervention should be between 6 and 12 months. Muscles that remain completely paralyzed at 1 year after injury are not likely to regain function.[22] However, reinnervation of muscles emanating from the infralesional segment are not time dependent and have greater flexibility in determining surgical intervention.

Evaluation

Before considering surgical intervention in a pediatric patient, a multidisciplinary approach is recommended. Input must be considered from a variety of specialties, including therapists, physiatrists, surgeons, and parents. The team must also consider the patient's ability to participate and follow instructions. The child and the parent's ability to follow postoperative care plans, participate in preoperative and postoperative therapy, and continue a home exercise care plan is crucial to supporting a successful operative procedure. Setting realistic short-term and long-term goals with the family and child is important because restoration of normal function is often the expectation initially. Children may interpret every potential intervention as a cure. It may be difficult for younger children to conceptualize the difference small changes may make for improving future independence. For example, improvement of wrist extension from trace volitional contraction to antigravity can augment tenodesis function and the ability to pinch and grip small, light items (food, utensils, and urinary catheters).

Children's maturity level may affect their ability to participate in therapy sessions. Younger children have poorer inherent fine-motor skills and decreased attention spans compared with older children and adults. In addition, children need repetition in their routines as well as educated and motivated caregivers that can continue to reinforce their home exercise programs. Emotionally, children may also be reluctant to undergo more surgical interventions because of fear of pain and may exhibit emotional or behavioral regression. Nerve transfers, in particular, have a critical period in which they can be performed and this may not afford sufficient time for emotional adjustment. Some children may still be grieving their loss of function and not have the patience to undergo many more months of rehabilitation. Psychological support from a counselor/therapist in conjunction with a skilled occupational therapist is necessary in guiding recovery. In some cases, a coexisting traumatic brain injury also affects the patient's ability to perform in therapy. The incidence of concomitant traumatic brain injuries in patients who have sustained SCIs has been reported in the adult literature to be 25% to 74%.[26–29]

Examination

Detailed motor and sensory examination of the upper extremities can be challenging in pediatric patients. Age and emotional maturity often determine the child's ability to follow directions for a manual muscle examination, as well as the ability to generate significant resistance to the examiner. For example, it may be difficult for an examiner to distinguish between grade 4 and 5 strength by the British Medical Research Council (MRC) grading system (https://mrc.ukri.org/research/facilities-and-resources-for-researchers/mrc-scales/mrc-muscle-scale/). However, generally grade 4 or greater is considered functional. Previous work by Mulcahey and colleagues[30] found that the neurologic classification of SCI was unreliable in children less than the 6 years of age. The International Standards for Neurological Classification of Spinal Cord Injury (ISNCSCI), published by the American Spinal Injury Association (ASIA), is well known to physiatrists and is used to quantify the neurologic impairment resulting from SCI. However, the ISNCSCI examination is not specific enough for use in planning either nerve or tendon transfers. The key muscles used to determine an intact motor level for the purposes of the ISNCSCI examination are innervated by multiple nerve roots, and individual patients may have variable innervation patterns. For these reasons, the International Classification for Surgery of the Hand (ICSHT) was initially developed and continues to be revised.[31] The ICSHT (https://www.researchgate.net/figure/International-classification-for-surgery-of-the-hand-in-tetraplegia_tbl1_51390925) includes muscles below the elbow, and thus tendon transfer reconstruction of elbow extension and proximal movements including shoulder abduction are considered separately.

When performing a clinical examination, if possible, the child should be seated with trunk supported. Children may not have the attention to sit through a detailed clinical examination and it may have to be done in more than 1 session, or incorporated into therapy sessions so that a full assessment can be obtained and confirmed for surgical planning. Areas that should be assessed include shoulder and scapular stability and range of motion, elbow flexion and extension, forearm supination and pronation, wrist flexion and extension, hand flexion, hand extension, and intrinsic hand muscles. It is important to palpate muscle activation when possible, such as the anterior, middle, and posterior deltoid. Elbow flexion should be assessed with the forearm in neutral, supination, and pronation to distinguish between the brachioradialis, biceps brachii, and brachialis, respectively. However, it is difficult to grade the brachioradialis because it is an elbow flexor and difficult to fully isolate from the biceps brachii and brachialis muscles. In general, it is tested by palpation of its belly during elbow flexion, but this is only an indirect measure of strength. Identify whether all 3 heads of the triceps are functioning. If the child is unable to overcome gravity, reposition the limb to determine whether the child can generate the motion with gravity eliminated. When examining the digits, make sure that movement in the wrist is eliminated. Evaluate joint stability. The evaluation of the upper extremity should include both active and passive range of motion. It is also important that pinch and grip strength measurements be assessed if possible. Pinch and grip dynamometers may be used for objective quantifiable assessment and also to monitor recovery. Assess for areas of spasticity as well as muscle atrophy, scar, and skin breakdown. In addition, it is important to note how the child uses prehensile patterns as well as adaptive compensations to perform ADLs.

Electrodiagnostic testing is crucial in preoperative planning. It is useful in determining upper and LMN patterns as well as determining suitable nerves for transfer. Electrodiagnosis can be challenging in pediatric patients and is best performed by experienced clinicians. Compound muscle action potentials are lower in pediatric patients and increase as children age; however, they do not reach adult values until end of the first decade.[32] Sensory nerve action potentials may have 2 peaks because of differences in maturation between nerve fibers. Conduction velocity trends toward adult values between the ages of 3 and 5 years as peripheral nerve fibers reach their maximum diameter and the nodes of Ranvier reach their peak internodal distances.[32] Age-appropriate tables are available.

It is reasonable to consider initial electrodiagnostic testing 4 to 6 months after initial injury.[23] Motor nerve studies provide information on the degree of injury of LMNs. Electromyography can further identify the health of muscles along a nerve distribution and localize the level of injury. Reduced or absent motor action potentials on nerve conduction study or fibrillations and positive sharp waves on electromyogram (EMG) indicate lower motor nerve injury that may require time-sensitive intervention. Reduced or absent activation indicates UMN injury. Electrodiagnostics are also important in determining which muscles or nerves can be sacrificed as donors. Sensory nerve conduction study results are reviewed to assess for superimposed peripheral nerve abnormalities (such as brachial plexus injury or cubital tunnel syndrome). EMG should be performed on both recipient and donor muscles preoperatively. Some investigators also advocate intraoperative retesting of recipient and donor muscles as well.[16] LMN injuries can be identified by large and fast-firing motor unit potentials, as well as a reduction in the interference pattern. Although there is software available that can count motor units, quantification can be performed objectively and with alterations to the filter settings. Mandeville and colleagues[33] define a nerve to be an excellent donor if it shows 7 or more motor units and a fair donor if it has 5 or 6. They caution that muscle size alone may not be a reliable assessment of LMN injury because of collateral reinnervation. Collateral innervation may obscure the relationship between innervation and recorded compound muscle action potential. Within the first year of injury, the motor endplates in the recipient nerve remain intact. However, to consider a nerve transfer beyond this time frame, then the clinician may consider quantifying the number and characteristics of the motor units in the recipient nerve as well.[33]

The use of ultrasonography may aid EMG evaluation by identifying nerves, atrophied muscle, or deep muscles for direct needle examination. This information may be particularly relevant in the forearm, where muscles are overlapping and potentially difficult to isolate, or in distinguishing between individual finger flexors. Ultrasonography may also help reduce the dilemma of coactivation of muscle agonists during nerve stimulus by facilitating selective stimulation of a branch of the nerve close to the target. An example is testing the flexor pollicis longus by direct stimulation of the anterior interosseous nerve as opposed to the median nerve at the elbow.[33] Ultrasonography may also provide examiners with a direct visualization of muscle quality and composition, revealing pathologic changes such as fatty infiltration and fibrosis. It may also provide an objective measure of changes to muscle thickness over time to quantify muscle hypertrophy or atrophy.[34] Ultrasonography is also capable of identifying muscle fasciculations.[34]

Some surgeons advocate the use of direct nerve stimulation during the procedure in conjunction with intraoperative evoked potentials in order to verify cortical activation.[22,35] Although paralyzed muscles respond to direct stimulation, they may not show response with cortical activation. This possibility may be particularly important in areas where the boundaries are indistinct between supralesional and infralesional segments,[35] and it also provides intraoperative confirmation of distal muscle innervation in the infralesional segment.[35,36] In addition, direct stimulation can help in fascicular identification without dissecting the nerve proximally and distally.[22]

SURGICAL CONSIDERATIONS

The level of function and independence that can be achieved based on the neurologic level of injury is well described. As shown in https://www.sci-info-pages.com/spinal-cord-injury-functional-goals/, the restoration of even 1 level of motor function distal to the lesion has huge dividends with regard to independence. The prioritization of upper extremity function to be restored via tendon transfer is well established in traditional SCI with a discrete level of cervical injury. In order for a muscle to be considered as a potential donor, it must have at least antigravity strength and preferably a 4 to 5 out of 5. Algorithms have been published based on the ICSHT with regard to tendon transfer reconstruction options distal to the elbow (**Fig. 1**). Nerve transfers may also provide additional options (**Table 1**).

Proximal motor movements of the upper extremity, such as shoulder abduction and elbow flexion, are generally not amenable to tendon transfer as a reconstructive option because of lack of sufficient donor muscle proximally. The most common level of tetraplegia is at the C5/6 spinal segment in children more than 12 years of age, which results in preservation of shoulder movements and elbow flexion, and the impairment of elbow extension and distal function below the elbow.[37] Elbow extension

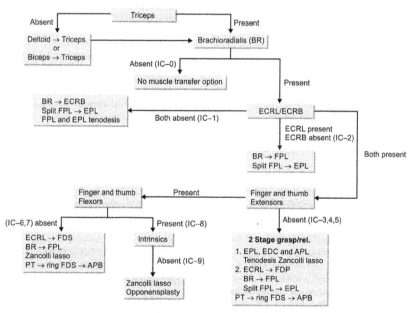

Fig. 1. Algorithm for tendon transfer. APB, abductor pollicis brevis; APL, abductor pollicis longus; ECRB, extensor carpi radialis brevis (wrist extensor); ECRL, extensor carpi radialis longus; EPL, extensor pollicis longus; FDP, flexor digitorum profundus; FDS, flexor digitorum superficialis; FPL, flexor pollicis longus; IC, International Classification; PT, pronator teres. (*From* Bielicka DL, Kwan LE, James MA. Upper Extremity in Tetraplegia. In: Chapman MW, James MA, eds. Chapman's Comprehensive Orthopaedic Surgery. 4th ed. New Dehli, India: Jaypee Brothers Medical Publishers (P) Ltd.; 2019: 1953-1969; with permission.)

Table 1
Summary of nerve transfers for spinal cord injury

Function	Donor	Recipient
Elbow extension	Selected deltoid branch of axillary nerve Teres minor branch of axillary nerve	Triceps branch of radial nerve
Wrist extension	Brachialis branch of musculocutaneous nerve Supinator branch of radial nerve	Extensor carpi radialis longus Extensor carpi ulnaris
Finger flexion	Brachialis branch of musculocutaneous nerve Brachioradialis nerve Extensor carpi radialis brevis nerve	Flexion branches of median nerve (anterior interosseous nerve), anterior interosseous, flexor carpi radialis, flexor digitorum profundus Flexion branches of median nerve (anterior interosseous nerve), anterior interosseous, flexor carpi radialis flexor digitorum profundus Flexion branches of median nerve (anterior interosseous nerve), ranterior interosseous, flexor carpi radialis flexor digitorum profundus
Finger extension	Supinator branch of radial nerve	Posterior interosseous nerve Extensor carpi ulnaris

Data from Hill EJR, Fox IK. Current Best Peripheral Nerve Transfers for Spinal Cord Injury. *Plast Reconstr Surg.* 2019;143(1):184e-198e.

is arguably the most important function to restore because it allows the patients to extend their reach away from the body for feeding and ADLs, allows prop sitting, improves transfers, and facilitates propulsion of a manual wheelchair through a full arc of motion, which is far more efficient than propelling solely with elbow flexors and anterior shoulder muscles. In addition, reconstruction of hand function is aided by active elbow extension because the length tension curve for transferred donor muscle/tendon units is optimized with the elbow in extension.

The surgical reconstruction priorities below the elbow for children mirror those for adults. The ability to manipulate objects requires acquisition, grasp, manipulation, and release. Wrist extension is the first priority and provides a tenodesis grip even in the absence of innervated finger flexors. The second priority is lateral or key pinch for object manipulation during ADLs such as holding a fork, toothbrush, or a pen. Grasp is the third priority and requires brachioradialis and both wrist extensors (extensor carpi radialis brevis/extensor carpi radialis longus). Restoration of grasp allows holding a cup and potentially pulling up pants. **Fig. 1** shows further reconstructive options via tendon transfer to include opponensplasty when additional distal muscles are present. Inalterable joint contractures, indoctrinated substitutions and patterns of upper extremity use, and the lack of adequate and expendable motor nerve donors may also make surgery to improve upper extremity function contraindicated.

Rehabilitation

It is important to have a therapist who is familiar with both nerve and muscle transfer precautions to guide mobilization postoperatively. Because nerve transfers are done without tension, there is less need for immobilization postoperatively. However, there are limitations in repetitive movements at the surgical site to avoid seroma formation.[16] The duration of immobilization following tendon transfer varies depending on the procedure but averages about 4 weeks, at which time the patient begins active and passive mobilization. With nerve transfer, full activity can be resumed at 4 weeks postoperatively, at which time motor reeducation can be instituted.[16] Exercises should focus on overfiring the donor, donor-recipient cocontracture, and detecting early innervation. Note that rehabilitation following nerve transfer is a lengthy endeavor. The nerve must regenerate from the coaptation site to reinnervate the muscle, and different donors have different time courses. For example, a supinator branch of the radial nerve to posterior interosseous nerve transfer may start to show distal reinnervation in 4 to 6 months, whereas using the brachialis branch of the musculocutaneous nerve to help reinnervate finger flexors may take more than a year.[38] In addition, there must be the opportunity for cortical remodeling to take place and adapt to the new rewired patterns. Neuroplasticity and cortical remodeling must also occur following tendon transfer but there is no need to await peripheral nerve regeneration and thus active movement is seen more immediately.

While awaiting reinnervation following nerve transfer, therapists must focus on maintaining range of motion of all the affected joints. Patient education and encouragement is particularly important in the early phase of recovery. Both parents and children must be educated and kept motivated to continue the home exercise programs even in the absence of clinically evident progress. Once successful reinnervation is confirmed, the process of motor reeducation begins. Initially, motor reeducation starts when cocontracture of the donor can activate fasciculation in the recipient muscle. At this stage, the patient is working on improving cortical representation and maintaining range of motion. The next step is to focus on muscle strengthening. During this stage, the patient is working on isolating and strengthening the recipient muscle. Ideally, the goal is to achieve MRC grade 3 or better. Successful cortical remapping depends on teaching the patient to appropriately recruit the reinnervated muscle and perform task-specific functions and compensatory strategies.[39]

Functional electrical stimulation (FES) may serve an important role in both preoperative evaluation and postoperative rehabilitation following nerve and muscle transfers. Diagnostically, electrical stimulation can be used to discern UMN versus LMN injury. The threshold for producing an action potential across a neuron is much smaller than directly stimulating the muscle. In 1976, Peckham and colleagues[40] determined that a pulse duration of 300 microseconds to achieve a muscular contraction requires an intact LMN from the anterior horn cell. In contrast, muscle excitation requires 10 milliseconds of pulse duration.[41]

FES may also be used for prehabilitation before surgery by helping to strengthen donor or recipient muscles. FES can be used to improve muscle torque and output on donor muscles[42] before surgery and even possibly to improve the quality of muscle donor candidates. This process is done by keeping the frequency between 20 and 50 Hz and the pulse width between 250 and 400 microseconds. The amplitude should titrated to stimulate as many motor units as possible.[41] Training should start at least 3 months before surgery, 3 times a week in 30-minute sessions.[41] The donor muscle should be positioned against resistance or gravity and the recipient muscle should be functional. In the postoperative period, the upper extremity FES bike can be initiated without resistance 4 weeks postoperatively and, after 2 to 4 additional weeks, resistance may be added.

Motor learning is initiated using the hands-on/hands-off principles that were initially designed for stroke rehabilitation.[43] The first stage is the cognitive stage, where the patient first learns the motor task. During this stage the therapist has a "ands-on role in assisting the patient perform the task. The second stage is the associative phase. During this stage, the patient is able to learn to perform the skill independently and refine the skill. The last phase is the the autonomous phase, in which the patient can perform the task independently. FES may play a role in that FES triggers a task-specific muscle contraction and afferent nerves transmit that information via the spinal cord to the motor cortex. If a muscle function is not performed, its representation on the motor cortex disappears.[44] After surgery, the patient has to learn new functions with a muscle that was previously used for a different function. For example, after transferring the brachioradialis muscle to the extensor carpi radialis brevis, the patient must learn to extend the wrist without elbow flexion. Furthermore, FES may help improve coordination with other functioning muscles. There are several commercially available products that are able to deliver sequenced stimulation in order to perform task-specific functions.

OUTCOMES

Tendon transfer surgical reconstruction of the upper extremity began after World War II when tetraplegic patients began to survive past their acute injuries and thus have a long history. Building on early reports of tendon transfers, Zancolli[45] and Moberg[46] in the early 1970s revolutionized this approach to surgical management of patients with tetraplegia caused by SCI. Outcomes of tendon transfer surgeries may be defined in the technical domain by efficacy in achieving surgical objectives, effect on functional independence measures, patient satisfaction, and quality of life. Numerous reports in the adult literature have documented improved function following tendon transfer, including Lamb and Chan[47] in 1983 reporting that 83% of 41 patients achieved good to excellent improvement, which was sustained at greater than 7-year follow-up. In the same study, 75% of individuals undergoing lateral pinch reconstruction were able to self-catheterize, which correlated with an improved quality of life.

The supporting evidence for upper extremity reconstruction in tetraplegia using nerve transfer is limited primarily to case studies and small case series. Pino and colleagues[14] published a retrospective case analysis of 15 pediatric patients whose age ranged from 4 months to 12 years, with a median age of 5 years. Nerve transfers to restore elbow function had excellent results, which they defined as greater than 50% of motion against gravity, 87% of the time. Nerve transfers to the elbow had excellent results 67% of the time.[14] However, shoulder function was more difficult to restore with, only half of the cases achieving excellent shoulder external rotation, but 90% of their cases did have resolution of shoulder pseudosubluxation following nerve transfer to the suprascapular nerve.[14]

Although many case reports and series report MRC grade 3 or better, the success rates of MRC grade 4 and 5 are extremely variable among case studies. Although some investigators' case series show rates exceed 90%,[48,49] most studies reviewed cite success rates that range between 50% and 76%[24,50,51] for finger flexor restoration but 60% and 100% for finger extension.[51] The variability in reports and techniques between investigators highlights the need for research to be done on improving and standardizing elements such as timing after injury,[52–54] incorporation of electrodiagnostics,[33,55] electrical stimulation, and even intraoperative axonal counts,[56] which may improve outcomes. Moreover, axonal regeneration over long coaptation sites may also play a role in variable outcomes.[48,57]

Several investigators recommend strategies combining tendon transfers and nerve transfers.[9,16,57,58] In a recent prospective case series by van Zyl and colleagues,[57] the researchers showed statistically significant functional improvements after early nerve transfers that were comparable with those of tendon transfers. However, when they compared the results of grasp and pinch reconstruction following tendon transfers with nerve transfers after 24 months, both grasp and pinch strength were greater in the patients that had undergone tendon transfers. They did note improved grasp strength with distal nerve grafts, presumably caused by the shorter distance between coaptation site and target muscle. They also reported that patients who received supinator branch of the radial nerve to the posterior interosseous nerve transfer to restore hand opening were more satisfied than patients whose hand opening was reconstructed by tendon transfer. It was also noted that there is not always a direct correlation between improvement in function and patient satisfaction. The investigators speculated that, because nerve transfers occur earlier in the recovery phase, patients may not recognize the changes that occurred as a result of the surgery. Although the surgical results around nerve transfers are encouraging, most studies are case reports and small case series, which carry the risk of selection bias and selection reporting bias.[51]

Outcome success in pediatric patients differs from that in the adult population in that it depends on family support, emotional response to the surgical process, and developmental maturity. Children who are younger have short attention spans and require more repetition and reinforcement. Successful surgeries require both the child and the parent's ability to participate in the therapy program. Finding pediatric hand therapists who are adept in techniques to mobilize tendon transfers can also be a significant challenge. The development of a good relationship between a therapist and child is crucial in determining whether the child will be able to participate in a prescribed program postoperatively. Although nerve transfers are time dependent, muscle transfers are not. Some experts may delay surgery until a child is of school age and able to better participate in a prescribed program.[59] However, in the study by Pino and colleagues[14] described earlier, 43% of the subjects were younger than school age at the time of the procedure and outcomes were equivalent to those of the older participants. Pediatric procedures differ from those in the adult population in that they require longer periods of follow-up to address changes in growth and development.[60] However, long-term longitudinal studies in the pediatric population are needed. It is unknown how interventions ultimately change growth and development. Growth deformity is a significant concern in the pediatric population. In 1 study, 86% of patients with brachial plexus injuries had some degree of deformity.[61] The associations between timing of surgical interventions, deformity, and functional outcomes are still being determined.[62–64]

Psychologically, children have different expectations than the adult population. Peljovich and colleagues[60] note that children may not fully comprehend the procedures that they are agreeing to or the rehabilitation process. Children are often very critical of the process and difficult to satisfy. Children may also be fearful of the hospital because of the prolonged hospitalization associated with the initial injury. Peljovich and colleagues[60] recommend performing surgeries in outpatient centers or in rehabilitation centers to minimize stress. Also, procedures that fulfill the child's need to gain social acceptance by reducing the need for orthosis, correcting deformities, and improving social contact are better accepted. Upper limb reconstruction may reduce the need for adaptive equipment and allow children to require less effort to complete tasks and, in turn, gain better independence.[59] Improvement in dexterity may lead to improvement in keyboard/computer skills that may allow for more independence and potential for academic achievements with less adaptive modification.

SUMMARY

Despite positive surgical outcomes for both muscle and nerve transfers in patients with tetraplegia, less than 10% of eligible candidates undergo surgery.[65] Underuse of surgical reconstruction of the upper extremity is multifactorial and includes patient, provider, and health care systems barriers to care. It is physiatrists' job to advocate for optimization of function in patients with SCI. Thoughtful evaluation and surgical intervention, coupled with a comprehensive rehabilitation program, can have a profound impact on the quality of life and development of pediatric patients with tetraplegia. Both nerve and tendon transfer surgeries have been well documented in the literature to improve function in patients with SCI.

DISCLOSURE

The authors have nothing to disclose.

REFERENCES

1. Vogel LC, Betz RR, Mulcahey MJ. Spinal cord injuries in children and adolescents. Handb Clin Neurol 2012;109:131–48.
2. Lustrin ES, Karakas SP, Ortiz AO, et al. Pediatric cervical spine: normal anatomy, variants, and trauma. Radiographics 2003. https://doi.org/10.1148/rg. 233025121.
3. Hornyak JE, Wheaton MW, Nelson VS. Chapter 16: spinal cord injuries. In: Alexander M, Matthews DJ, editors. Pediatric rehabilitation: principles and practice. 5th edition. New York: Demos Medical Publishing; 2015. p. 412–28.
4. Wills BPD, Dormans JP. Nontraumatic Upper Cervical Spine Instability in Children. J Am Acad Orthop Surg 2006;14(4):233–46.
5. Savic G, Devivo MJ, Frankel HL, et al. Long-term survival after traumatic spinal cord injury: A 70-year British study. Spinal Cord 2017;55(7):651–8.
6. Devivo MJ, Savic G, Frankel HL, et al. Comparison of statistical methods for calculating life expectancy after spinal cord injury. Spinal Cord 2018;56(7): 666–73.
7. Frontera JE, Mollett P. Aging with Spinal Cord Injury: An Update. Phys Med Rehabil Clin N Am 2017;28(4):821–8.
8. Anderson KD. Targeting recovery: Priorities of the spinal cord-injured population. J Neurotrauma 2004;21(10):1371–83.
9. Bednar MS, Woodside JC. Management of Upper Extremities in Tetraplegia. J Am Acad Orthop Surg 2018;26(16):e333–41.
10. Fridén J, Gohritz A. Tetraplegia management update. J Hand Surg Am 2015; 40(12):2489–500.
11. Tung TH, Mackinnon SE. Nerve transfers: indications, techniques, and outcomes. J Hand Surg Am 2010;35(2):332–41.
12. Saltzman EB, Rancy SK, Sneag DB, et al. Nerve transfers for enterovirus D68-associated acute flaccid myelitis: a case series. Pediatr Neurol 2018;88:25–30.
13. Madaan P, Saini L. Nerve transfers in acute flaccid myelitis: a beacon of hope. Pediatr Neurol 2019;93:68.
14. Pino PA, Intravia J, Kozin SH, et al. Early results of nerve transfers for restoring function in severe cases of acute flaccid myelitis. Ann Neurol 2019;607–15.

15. Nath RK, Somasundaram C. Functional improvement of upper and lower extremity after decompression and neurolysis and nerve transfer in a pediatric patient with acute flaccid myelitis. Am J Case Rep 2019;20:668–73.

16. Fox IK, Miller AK, Curtin CM. Nerve and tendon transfer surgery in cervical spinal cord injury: Individualized choices to optimize function. Top Spinal Cord Inj Rehabil 2018;24(3):275–87.

17. Waters RL, Sie IH, Gellman H, et al. Functional hand surgery following tetraplegia. Arch Phys Med Rehabil 1996;77(1):86–94.

18. Van Haren K, Ayscue P, Waubant E, et al. Acute flaccid myelitis of unknown etiology in California, 2012-2015. JAMA 2015;314(24):2663–71.

19. Messacar K, Schreiner TL, Van Haren K, et al. Acute flaccid myelitis: A clinical review of US cases 2012–2015. Ann Neurol 2016;80(3):326–38.

20. Martin JA, Messacar K, Yang M, et al. Outcomes of Colorado children with acute flaccid myelitis at 1 year. Neurology 2017;89:129–37.

21. Andersen EW, Kornberg AJ, Freeman JL, et al. Acute flaccid myelitis in childhood: a retrospective cohort study. Eur J Neurol 2017;24(8):1077–83.

22. Senjaya F, Midha R. Nerve transfer strategies for spinal cord injury. World Neurosurg 2013;80(6):e319–26.

23. Hill EJR, Fox IK. Current best peripheral nerve transfers for spinal cord injury. Plast Reconstr Surg 2019;143(1):184e–98e.

24. Khalifeh JM, Dibble CF, Van Voorhis A, et al. Nerve transfers in the upper extremity following cervical spinal cord injury. Part 2: Preliminary results of a prospective clinical trial. J Neurosurg Spine 2019;1–13. https://doi.org/10.3171/2019.4.spine19399.

25. Bertelli JA, Ghizoni MF. Single-stage surgery combining nerve and tendon transfers for bilateral upper limb reconstruction in a tetraplegic patient: Case report. J Hand Surg Am 2013;38(7):1366–9.

26. Macciocchi S, Seel RT, Thompson N, et al. Spinal cord injury and co-occurring traumatic brain injury: assessment and incidence. Arch Phys Med Rehabil 2008;89(7):1350–7.

27. Em H, Ge E, Rekand T, et al. Traumatic spinal cord injury and concomitant brain injury: a cohort study. Acta Neurol Scand Suppl 2010;122(190):51–7.

28. MacCiocchi S, Seel RT, Warshowsky A, et al. Co-occurring traumatic brain injury and acute spinal cord injury rehabilitation outcomes. Arch Phys Med Rehabil 2012;93(10):1788–94.

29. Sharma B, Bradbury C, Mikulis D, et al. Missed diagnosis of traumatic brain injury in patients with traumatic spinal cord injury. J Rehabil Med 2014. https://doi.org/10.2340/16501977-1261.

30. Mulcahey MJ, Gaughan JP, Chafetz RS, et al. Interrater reliability of the international standards for neurological classification of spinal cord injury in youths with chronic spinal cord injury. Arch Phys Med Rehabil 2011;92(8):1264–9.

31. Moberg E, McDowell CL, House JH. Third International conference on Surgical Rehabilitation of the upper limb in tetraplegia (quadriplegia). J Hand Surg Am 1989;14(6):1064–6.

32. Mcdonald CM. Electrodiagnosis in Pediatrics. In: Alexander M, Matthews DJ, editors. Pediatric rehabilitation: principles and practice. 5th edition. New York: Demos Medical Publishing; 2015. p. 113–52.

33. Mandeville RM, Brown JM, Sheean GL. A neurophysiological approach to nerve transfer to restore upper limb function in cervical spinal cord injury. Neurosurg Focus 2017;43(1):1–9.

34. Pillen S, van Alfen N. Skeletal muscle ultrasound. Neurol Res 2011;33(10): 1016–24.
35. Brown J. Nerve transfers in tetraplegia I: Background and technique. Surg Neurol Int 2011;2(1):121.
36. Mackinnon SE, Yee A, Ray WZ. Nerve transfers for the restoration of hand function after spinal cord injury: Case report. J Neurosurg 2012;117(1):176–85.
37. DeVivo MJ, Vogel LC. Epidemiology of spinal cord injury in children and adolescents. J Spinal Cord Med 2004;27(Suppl 1). s4–10.
38. Fox IK. Nerve transfers in tetraplegia. Hand Clin 2016;32(2):227–42.
39. Hahn J, Cooper C, Flood S, et al. Rehabilitation of supinator nerve to posterior interosseous nerve transfer in individuals with tetraplegia. Arch Phys Med Rehabil 2016;97(6):S160–8.
40. Peckham PH, Mortimer JT, Marsolais EB. Upper and lower motor neuron lesions in the upper extremity muscles of tetraplegics. Paraplegia 1976;14(2):115–21.
41. Bersch I, Fridén J. Role of functional electrical stimulation in tetraplegia hand surgery. Arch Phys Med Rehabil 2016;97(6):S154–9.
42. Coupaud S, Gollee H, Hunt KJ, et al. Arm-cranking exercise assisted by functional electrical stimulation in C6 tetraplegia: A pilot study. Technol Health Care 2008;16(6):415–27.
43. Carr JH, Shepherd RB. Enhancing physical activity and brain reorganization after stroke. Neurol Res Int 2011;2011. https://doi.org/10.1155/2011/515938.
44. Ramachandran VS. Behavioral and magnetoencephalographic correlates of plasticity in the adult human brain. Proc Natl Acad Sci U S A 1993;90(22): 10413–20.
45. Zancolli E. Functional restroratin of the upper limbs in traumatic quadriplegia. In: Structural and Dynamic Bases of Hand Function. Philadelphia, PA: JB Lippincott Company; 1978.p.229.
46. Moberg E. Surgical treatment for absent single-hand grip and elbow extension in quadriplegia. Principles and preliminary experience. J Bone Joint Surg Am 1975; 57(2):196–206.
47. Lamb DW, Chan KM. Surgical reconstruction of the upper limb in traumatic tetraplegia. A review of 41 patients. J Bone Joint Surg Br 1983;65(3):291–8.
48. Bertelli JA, Ghizoni MF. Nerve transfers for restoration of finger flexion in patients with tetraplegia. J Neurosurg Spine 2017;26(1):55–61.
49. Bertelli JA, Ghizoni MF. Nerve transfers for elbow and finger extension reconstruction in midcervical spinal cord injuries. J Neurosurg 2015;122(1):121–7.
50. Fox IK, Davidge KM, Novak CB, et al. Nerve transfers to restore upper extremity function in cervical spinal cord injury: Update and preliminary outcomes. Plast Reconstr Surg 2015;136(4):780–92.
51. Khalifeh JM, Dibble CF, Van Voorhis A, et al. Nerve transfers in the upper extremity following cervical spinal cord injury. Part 1: Systematic review of the literature. J Neurosurg Spine 2019;1–12. https://doi.org/10.3171/2019.4.spine19173.
52. Cain SA, Gohritz A, Fridén J, et al. Review of upper extremity nerve transfer in cervical spinal cord injury. J Brachial Plex Peripher Nerve Inj 2015;10(1):e34–42.
53. Fu SY, Gordon T. Contributing factors to poor functional recovery after delayed nerve repair: Prolonged axotomy. J Neurosci 1995;15(5 II):3886–95.
54. Fu SY, Gordon T. Contributing factors to poor functional recovery after delayed nerve repair: Prolonged denervation. J Neurosci 1995;15(5 II):3886–95.
55. Fox IK, Novak CB, Krauss EM, et al. The use of nerve transfers to restore upper extremity function in cervical spinal cord injury. PM R 2018;10(11):1173–84.e2.

56. Wang W, Kang S, Coto Hernández I, et al. A rapid protocol for intraoperative assessment of peripheral nerve myelinated axon count and its application to cross-facial nerve grafting. Plast Reconstr Surg 2019;143(3):771–8.

57. van Zyl N, Hill B, Cooper C, et al. Expanding traditional tendon-based techniques with nerve transfers for the restoration of upper limb function in tetraplegia: a prospective case series. Lancet 2019;394(10198):565–75.

58. Titolo P, Fusini F, Arrigoni C, et al. Combining nerve and tendon transfers in tetraplegia: a proposal of a new surgical strategy based on literature review. Eur J Orthop Surg Traumatol 2019;29(3):521–30.

59. Kozin SH. Pediatric Onset Spinal Cord Injury: Implications on Management of the Upper Limb in Tetraplegia. Hand Clin 2008;24(2):203–13.

60. Peljovich A, Gillespie B, Bryden AM, et al. Rehabilitation of the Hand and Upper Extremity in Tetraplegia. In: Skirven T, Osterman A, Fedorczyk J, et al, editors. Rehabilitation of the hand and upper extremity. 6th edition. Philadelphia: Elsevier Mosby; 2011. https://doi.org/10.1016/j.optmat.2011.11.002.

61. Waters PM, Smith GR, Jaramillo D. Glenohumeral deformity secondary to brachial plexus birth palsy. J Bone Joint Surg Am 1998;80(5):668–77.

62. Bain JR, Dematteo C, Gjertsen D, et al. Limb Length Differences after Obstetrical Brachial Plexus Injury: A Growing Concern. Plast Reconstr Surg 2012;130(4):558e–71e.

63. Larson EL, Santosa KB, Mackinnon SE, et al. Median to radial nerve transfer after traumatic radial nerve avulsion in a pediatric patient. J Neurosurg Pediatr 2019;24(2):209–14.

64. Gosk J, Wnukiewicz W, Urban M. The effect of perinatal brachial plexus lesion on upper limb development. BMC Musculoskelet Disord 2014;15(1). https://doi.org/10.1186/1471-2474-15-116.

65. Punj V, Curtin C. Understanding and overcoming barriers to upper limb surgical reconstruction after tetraplegia: The need for interdisciplinary collaboration. Arch Phys Med Rehabil 2016;97(6):S81–7.

Hand Reconstruction in Children with Spinal Cord Injury

Allan Peljovich, MD, MPH[a,b,c,d,*]

KEYWORDS

- Tetraplegia • Spinal cord injury • Tendon transfer • Nerve transfer • Hand

KEY POINTS

- Optimizing hand and upper extremity function in children with traumatic tetraplegia is as much a pillar of their rehabilitation as it is for adults.
- Indications for surgical reconstruction in children, primarily in the form of tendon transfers, are similar to those for adults.
- The unique challenges to planning and executing surgery in children include smaller anatomy, open growth plates, spasticity, and rehabilitation protocols.
- When indicated, surgical outcomes are positive, and lifelong; however, the effect of growth may necessitate revisions in select children.
- The application of nerve transfers in children is a newer technique that has the potential to help augment traditional surgical strategies.

INTRODUCTION

Tetraplegia in children is rare. Children 18 years old or younger at the time of injury represented approximately 13% of all those with a spinal cord injury (SCI) in 2018, and 5.4% of all newly injured in 2017 were 16 years old and younger.[1] Cervical-level spinal injury seems to vary between 20% and 30% of all spinal injury, with some investigators finding the prevalence as high as 85%.[2–6] Most report that approximately 25% to 35% of cervical-level injuries result in SCI, with varying degrees of neurologic impairment.[2,3,6,7]

Children who sustain a significant cervical-level SCI at 10 years of age can anticipate an average lifespan of an additional 42 years.[1] Although this lifespan is shorter than for children with lower-level injuries (49 years), children with cervical-level SCI

[a] The Hand & Upper Extremity Center of Georgia, Suite 1020, 980 Johnsons Ferry Road, Atlanta, GA 30342, USA; [b] Hand & Upper Extremity Program, Children's Healthcare of Atlanta, Atlanta, GA, USA; [c] Orthopaedic Surgery Residency Program, Atlanta Medical Center, Atlanta, GA, USA; [d] Hand & Upper Extremity Program, Shepherd Center
* The Hand & Upper Extremity Center of Georgia, Suite 1020, 980 Johnsons Ferry Road, Atlanta, GA 30342.
E-mail address: drp@handcenterga.com

Phys Med Rehabil Clin N Am 31 (2020) 471–498
https://doi.org/10.1016/j.pmr.2020.04.008
1047-9651/20/© 2020 Elsevier Inc. All rights reserved.

on average live longer with their impairment than any adult age group.[1] Any treatment that improves their quality of the life, therefore, is of paramount importance. Treatment directed to the hand and upper extremity should begin early in the acute phase of care and should incorporate more than exercise, splinting, and braces when appropriate. Hanson and Franklin[8] studied adult patients with SCI to determine what they perceived as their greatest functional losses. Among both tetraplegic patients (76%) and caregivers (64%), hand and upper extremity function was considered the most important function to be restored. These concepts have been reinforced in recent studies, where people with tetraplegia continue to place great importance in improving hand and upper extremity function.[9-13] Robert Waters,[14] a surgeon from Ranchos Los Amigos, noted "…the greatest potential for improvement of quality of life lies in rehabilitation and maximal restoration of upper extremity function."

The basic tenets that apply to management of SCI in adults also apply to children, but special attention must be paid to the additional stress that SCI places on the psychological development of children and its consequence on rehabilitation compliance; the unique nature of the relationship between affected children and their caregivers, which are usually the parents; as well as more physiologic components such as remaining growth. Only limited literature is available to guide the treating health care providers in the care of the hand for pediatric patients with SCI; however, a team approach that takes into account the cognitive and psychosocial development of the child is pivotal for treatment success.

Barriers

Despite the reliability of surgical restoration of the tetraplegic hand, studies continue to demonstrate underuse of resources and treatment.[12,15-18] There seem to be too few surgeons and not enough physiatrists paying attention to the hand and upper extremity. The traditional pillars of SCI rehabilitation that most centers emphasize (ie, bowel/bladder care, skin care, sexual reproduction, and ambulation) seem difficult to break into. Because this surgery is practiced in numbers only in a few centralized SCI model centers, and only sporadically elsewhere, most surgeon-trainees are not exposed or trained in these techniques. There is thus a lack of momentum for interdisciplinary associations between surgeons and physiatrists. In part, misconceptions persist that people with SCI tend to be noncompliant with treatment and lack the resources and support to perform rehabilitative protocols in an outpatient setting. In addition, there is misperception, or frank ignorance, regarding patients' understanding of the availability and reliability of such procedures.

What Is it that Makes Children Different?

Children experience cervical SCI different than their adult counterparts. For example, violence and sports are a substantially more prevalent mechanism of injury.[4,19-21] The upper cervical spine, especially in the youngest of children, is a frequent location of the injury, as opposed to the C5/C6 level of adults. A child's SCI occasionally masks behind normal radiographs, known as SCIWORA (SCI without radiographic abnormality), which most often occurs in the cervical spine.[19] Children also navigate their injuries differently. Children are compelled to be trusting in a complex process they may not fully understand or consent to. They rely on their parents and family networks for medical and surgical decision making. Children may be less tolerant of failure than adults. They are sharp critics and good observers of true progress. They are hard to satisfy. Many children expect miracles or immediate gratification and lack tolerance for months of rehabilitation. Younger children have short attention spans, may not be fully compliant with delicate rehabilitation proto-cols, and need reinforcement and repetition in their training. Older children and ad-olescents are distracted by their social needs and conscious of cosmetic appearance, incisions, braces, and hardware. They want to be physically and visibly normal. Reconstruction that incorporates correction of paralytic posture, removes wrist braces, or improves social contact is well received.

NONOPERATIVE MANAGEMENT

Early therapy, ideally initiated at the acute care hospital, is used to obtain/maintain joint mobility and maximize the strength, endurance, and the balance of voluntary muscles. Orthotics are initially used to help mold the resting hand positions needed for tenodesis grasp (**Fig. 1**). Children learn to use their hands and arms as they recover from SCI with a combination of therapy, functional orthotics, and creative strategizing that could fool the casual observer into believing they had good control

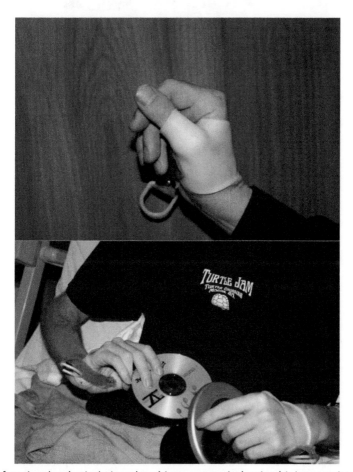

Fig. 1. A functional orthotic designed to this teenager pinch using his intact wrist tenodesis function. This hand-based orthotic does not interfere with wrist extension and places the thumb carpometacarpal (CMC) joint in opposition for best pinch position. The thumb's metacarpophalangeal and interphalangeal joints are free to move by tenodesis positioning.

of their elbow and hands when they are lacking in these abilities but have found ways to compensate. There are a variety of commercially available orthotics/prostheses designed to aid individuals with particular functions (**Fig. 2**), but most individuals do not use them and generally prefer to be brace free.[22] Moreover, older children and adolescents tend to be self-conscious regarding braces and hardware. Simply stated, despite excellent nonoperative management, individuals with tetraplegia remain severely impaired compared with the able-bodied upper extremity.

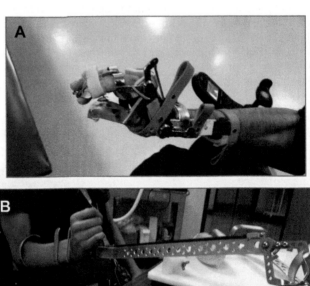

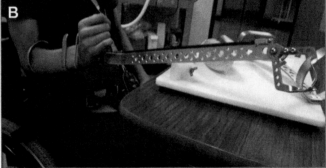

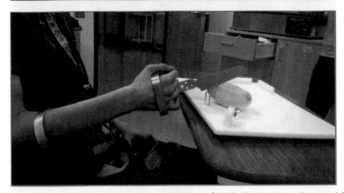

Fig. 2. Various prosthetics exist to assist in activities of daily living in patients with tetraplegia. (*A*) A tenodesis hinge brace creates functional grasp and pinch powered by active wrist extension and gravity-assisted wrist flexion. (*B*) Two different prosthetics designed to help with specific daily living tasks; that is, retrieving objects at a distance, and cutting/preparing food.

SURGICAL MANAGEMENT

The results of surgical reconstruction in children can be very rewarding in the automatic way they adjust to new capabilities, the generally good results they experience with surgery, and the joy to the health care team for changing their lives. However, children are not small adults. There are psychosocial challenges because many children dread the return to the sick role, and many have bad memories of the time they spent in the hospital at the acute injury. The therapist often has the key role in preparing, and guiding the child, contributing the subjective support and continuity to recovery. Surgical challenges include the technical considerations associated with smaller muscles, tendons, nerves; the presence of growth plates within the bones; and contractures and secondary bone changes associated with children, especially around the elbow, forearm, and digital metacarpophalangeal (MCP) joints. Otherwise, surgical priorities, procedures, and decision making are identical to those in adults.[23] Muscle spasticity is common in children with cervical SCI, and must be accounted for in surgical planning.[24] Postoperative care follows the same protocols as for adults except that protocols may need to be prolonged to accommodate smaller tendons and weaker tendon transfer coaptation sites, and longer-term monitoring is required to assess the effects of growth and development.

Only with a thorough evaluation of an individual with tetraplegia at various points in time can clinicians determine the appropriate goals of rehabilitation and reconstruction.[14,22,25–38] Consideration for surgical intervention requires that the child and primary caregivers understand their reconstructive options, including advantages and disadvantages. For example, tendon transfer surgery means that, for a short period of time, the individual will be more impaired as the arm is temporarily immobilized and then progressively "given back" to them over a couple of months during therapy. Nerve transfer surgery often takes many months at a minimum before there is any sign of innervation, then up to another 1 to 2 years for maximal strength. Children must have a good support system in place to assist them through what is a trying time for themselves and their assistants/families.

Not all children with tetraplegia benefit from surgical reconstruction because of adherence to strict criteria designed to ensure that those who will undergo surgery are likely to experience a successful outcome (**Box 1**). These criteria have been developed and distilled over decades of experience. The most critical factors are realistic expectations and firm goals. Patients with specific functional goals in mind (school, home, daily living activities) are most likely to be satisfied with the results and will remain motivated throughout the process to devote the time needed to "learn" their reconstructed hands.[39–41] In addition, the child's medical and physical condition must be stable in order to undergo surgery and so as not to interfere in the postoperative rehabilitation program. Children plagued with frequent hospitalizations, urinary tract infections, and problems with skin care find their potential recovery continuously interrupted to their detriment. Nonambulatory children should be easily transferable to a wheelchair, have good trunk support, and adequate seating so they can take full advantage of their upper extremities.

The physical prerequisites to successful procedures include supple joints and sufficient strength/neural integrity of the donor muscle and/or nerve. Children with functionally limiting joint contractures are treated with formal physiotherapy, or surgical release; otherwise, they will be poor candidates for a complete restorative program. Poorly controlled spastic muscles cannot serve as effective donors in tendon transfers. Nerve transfers cannot succeed if the recipient muscle is either chronically denervated or will become so by the time the donor nerve reaches the recipient muscle's motor endplate;

Box 1
Prerequisites for surgery

1. Physical
   a. Neurologic
      i. Stability: no further expectation of meaningful recovery
         1. For nerve transfer, sound expectation that target muscle will not become voluntary
         2. For nerve transfer, no impending denervation
      ii. Control of, or absence of, spasticity of critical donor muscles/nerves
   b. Robust health and systems: likely to remain healthy throughout the recovery
      i. Skin
      ii. Cardiorespiratory system
         1. Control of postural hypertension
      iii. Urologic systems
   c. Stable and comfortable in wheelchair
   d. Functional passive range of motion to shoulder, elbow, wrist, fingers
      i. Ideally good passive wrist tenodesis grasp/release
   e. Physical examination meets criteria for tendon transfers or nerve transfers
   f. For nerve transfer, target muscles that remain peripherally innervated and viable

2. Mental health
   a. Acceptance of the injury
   b. Desire and motivation
   c. Individual has reasonable goals for surgery
   d. Sufficient cognition to learn tendon and/or nerve transfers

3. Resources
   a. Family/friend support
      i. Nurse/aide availability
   b. Transportation
   c. Access to qualified therapist

---

it is vital to evaluate the innervation of the potential recipient muscle using a combination of functional electrical nerve stimulation (FES) and neurodiagnostic studies.[42,43]

The final consideration in surgery is timing. Surgical reconstructions are traditionally undertaken once an individual's neurologic recovery is deemed complete or chronic. This chronic phase of SCI was, and still generally is, the earliest that surgical restoration should be considered and performed for any tendon transfer and most nerve transfers.[44] It is commonly accepted that complete injuries plateau by 1 year postinjury; however, data support the notion that children with complete injury often plateau by 6 months.[23,45–47] However, many people are not emotionally prepared to consider surgery at this early a juncture, and it is also important to wait until the individual is ready. The incomplete injury is a different situation because recovery may continue longer than 1 year. There is no maximum time within which to consider intervention because even individuals years from their injuries can benefit from surgery.[41] Nerve transfers add another consideration because not all desired recipient muscle remains peripherally innervated, especially in the setting of associated peripheral nerve injury, which is common for muscles innervated within the zone of injury. Nerve transfers for these intralesional, or denervated, recipients must occur before the permanent fibrosis that occurs around 18 months from injury. Nerve transfer in these cases must be completed before full recovery in the acute phase of injury, if at all.

Types of Procedures

The great difficulty in hand restoration is that it is not possible with currently available techniques to completely restore upper extremity function to the able-bodied state.

Upper extremity function must be distilled into its most fundamental elements to maximize gains. Surgical strategies have traditionally relied primarily on tendon transfer–based restoration, with some research centers performing FES neuroprosthesis–based restoration.[22,30,35,48–55] Recently, the application of nerve transfer techniques in tetraplegia have proved that these surgical procedures can augment current strategies and may help improve reconstructions.[43,56–58]

A tendon transfer procedure is one in which a functioning muscle and its tendon are detached from their normal insertion and rerouted into a different muscle that helps perform the function that needs restoration (**Fig. 3**). In this way, when the donor muscle contracts, it will power a new and desired motion. For tendon transfer–based restoration, the number of functions and joints that can be restored is directly proportional to the distal level of injury because more muscles are left under voluntary control as the injury moves caudally in the spine. Compromise and creativity form the basis of planning surgery for individuals, but there are traditional compromises and priorities that exist based on experience gained in treating individuals with paralysis of all forms. Recovering a tendon transfer does require a period of immobilization, but newer and biomechanically stronger suturing techniques have shortened this time to a few weeks at most (see **Fig. 3**). In some cases, formal physiotherapy, with the extremity otherwise splinted, is initiated within a week of surgery.

A nerve transfer procedure, in concept, is very similar to a tendon transfer. A motor fascicle/branch innervating a functioning and voluntarily controlled muscle, typically from a major peripheral nerve, is cut and coapted into the motor fascicle/branch of a paralyzed muscle (**Fig. 4**). As with tendon transfers, there are specific criteria that need to be met before a particular transfer can be effective; that is, the muscle to innervate is still viable. In addition, as with tendon transfers, the original function of the donor nerve (or muscle) is lost for the sake of a newer and more desired function, so the function of the donor must be either functionally unimportant or duplicative. Among its greatest potential advantages is the lack of immobilization required postoperatively. Further, there is an idea that a single donor nerve could innervate as many muscles as the recipient nerve would normally innervate. Patients with limited resources or without access to therapy who would normally fail to meet criteria for tendon transfer could still consider surgical reconstruction via nerve transfers. Potential disadvantages include the length of time for functional strength to develop in successful transfers, which ranges from 6 months to 2 years, and failure rates that can approach 40% depending on the specific transfer. By the nature of the procedure, a failed nerve transfer means that both the donor muscle and the recipient muscle may become irreversibly denervated by the time a failure is apparent.

The author considers children and adults with SCI to be a population in which any surgeries to improve function must work all or nearly all of the time because they are already functioning at the edge of ability and cannot tolerate failures that result in loss of further function compared with able-bodied individuals who otherwise function with little to no disability.

Nerve transfer for SCI is in its nascent stage of development. To date, the results of fewer than 100 adults undergoing nerve transfer for tetraplegia have been published.[59–61] These studies have generally focused on efficacy in case reports and series. Unlike research concerning tendon transfers over the last several decades, the recent application of nerve transfers for SCI does not yet answer best applications or indications. Some transfers involve important muscles (ie, the brachialis), and studies do not address the implications of using the brachialis or whether the biceps alone truly substitute over the lifetime of the individual given the rotator cuff issues that are so common over time in people with tetraplegia. The author thus thinks

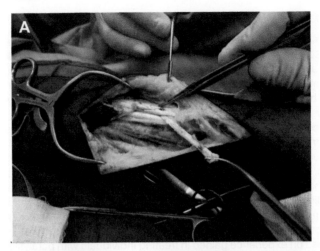

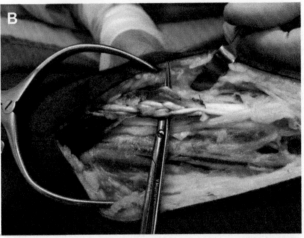

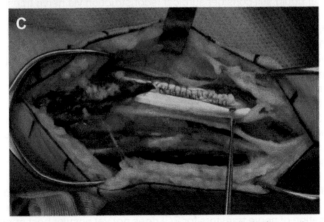

Fig. 3. (*A*) Tendon transfer coaptation with the brachioradialis (BR) sewn into the extensor carpi radialis brevis (ECRB) tendon for wrist extension reconstruction. The BR tendon is weaved in and out of the ECRL and (*B*) then sewn together once tension is set. (*C*) The modified side-side coaptation technique is shown with the same BR to ECRB transfer. This method of coaptation confers even greater mechanical strength to the transfer, allowing very early mobilization and therapy.

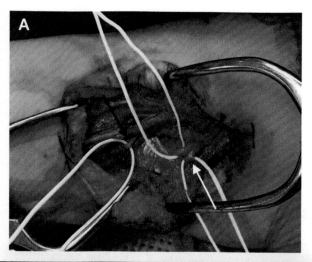

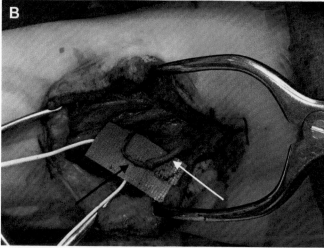

Fig. 4. A nerve transfer for elbow extension performed in the underarm area. (*A*) The axilla is on the right, and the elbow is toward the left. The black arrow is pointing toward the long head triceps branch of the radial nerve. The white arrow is pointing to the posterior division of the axillary nerve. The third looped nerve is the anterior division of the axillary nerve. (*B*) In the same child, the nerve ends are now prepared for coaptation. The posterior division of the axillary nerve is transected as distally as possible and mobilized distally toward the long head branch of the radial nerve, which has been transected as proximally as possible so that the coaptation is under no tension.

that tendon transfer–based reconstructions continue to form the basis of surgical restoration. Nerve transfers are currently suited to augment tendon transfers, such as creating voluntary thumb/finger extension, as opposed to forming the basis of reconstruction (**Fig. 5**). Continued research and technique modifications continue and, as knowledge accrues and indications become more refined, the author believes that nerve transfers will assume a greater and more reliable role for some individuals, including those with high-level tetraplegia who lack sufficient donor muscles for tendon transfer.

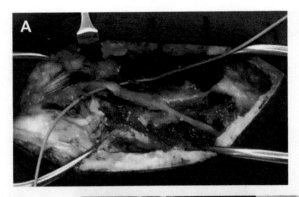

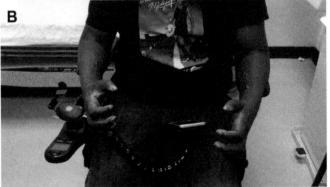

Fig. 5. Example of an International Classification for Surgery of the Hand in Tetraplegia (ICT) 5 individual who underwent staged reconstruction with a nerve transfer for digital and thumb extension, and tendon transfers for pinch and grasp flexion. (*A*) The orientation is proximal/left and distal/right, showing the 2 motor branches of the supinator (running on either side and parallel to the posterior interosseous nerve under the vessel loop), innervated primarily through C6 and under voluntary control as they are ready to be transected and coapted to a transected posterior interosseous nerve (large nerve under the vessel loop) distal to the takeoff of the supinator branches. The distal motor fibers to innervate the finger and thumb extensors are primarily innervated by C7-C8 and are not under voluntary control. (*B*) The result of the procedure in its early stages. The patient activates the nerve transfer with supination to generate active digital extension, and powers pinch and grasp via tendon transfers.

Surgical Classification in Tetraplegia

Although useful for the general examination and classification of SCI, the International Standards for Neurological Classification of SCI (ISNCSCI) and the American Spinal Injury Association Impairment Scale (AIS) are not precise enough from the standpoint of hand reconstruction. Critical to categorizing someone's arm and hand when considering surgery is to understand the number of potential donor muscles/nerves available to use in the restoration of lost function. This need served as the impetus for the International Classification for Surgery of the Hand in Tetraplegia (ICSHT), first created in 1984, and since modified (**Table 1**).[62,63] The ICSHT takes advantage of the consistent innervation order of forearm and hand muscles associated with a caudal direction in the cervical spine. The ICSHT is based on 2 variables: sensation and voluntarily controlled muscles. Sensation is binary (2-point discrimination <10 mm in the

Table 1	
International Classification for Surgery of the hand in tetraplegia	
Group	**Muscle at Grade 4 Strength**
0	No muscles below the elbow have strength
1	Brachioradialis
2	Extensor carpi radialis longus
3	Extensor carpi radialis brevis
4	Pronator teres
5	Flexor carpi radialis
6	Extensor digitorum communis and finger extensors
7	Extensor pollicus longus and thumb extensors
8	Finger flexors
9	All except intrinsics
0	Exceptions
T+ or T−	Triceps at grade 4

From Peljovich AE, Gillespie BT, Bryden AM, et al. Rehabilitation of the Hand and Upper Extremity in Tetraplegia. In: Skirven TM, Osterman AL, Fedorczyk J, Amadio PC, Felder S, Shin EK eds. Rehabilitation of the Hand and Upper Extremity. 7th ed. Philadelphia, PA: Elsevier; 2021:1582-1604; with permission.

index finger and thumb): cutaneous (Cu) if present, and ocular (O) if absent. Motor classification depends on greater than or equal to ≥M4 strength. This information (those muscles with a strength of ≥4) supplies physicians with the number of candidate donor muscles eligible for tendon transfer. The ICSHT is currently the accepted classification used by most surgeons performing hand surgery in patients with tetraplegia. There is no current formal system that is designed for nerve transfers, and there is a need to account for the 3 zones of SCI (supralesional, intralesional, infralesional).

Reconstructive Priorities

It is useful to think of the hand as the universal tool for manipulation, and the shoulder, elbow, and forearm as the crane transporting the hand in space and positioning it for function. The fundamental functions to be restored, in order of traditional priority, include elbow extension, wrist extension, lateral pinch and release, and palmar grasp and release.[14,26,31–33,36,44,64–68] Elbow extension is extremely important and can translate to functional abilities such as self-care, hygiene, wheelchair propulsion, and transferring (critical to creating functional independence, and a priority for surgical intervention in these individuals).[13,69–72]

The basis for hand function in most individuals is the wrist tenodesis effect, the key to which is voluntary wrist extension. Wrist extension activates the natural tenodesis grasp pattern and serves as the foundation on which finger function is activated and restored (**Fig. 6**). Surgical restoration of hand function builds on the wrist tenodesis pinch and grasp by providing strength and stability to the pinch and grasp postures. Because lateral pinch is used more often for activities of daily living, this form of grasp is generally prioritized over palmar grasp when both cannot be restored.[73] A limitation to surgical restoration is that, to date, sensation cannot be reliably restored, but some clinicians have explored the use of nerve transfer.[74,75]

The sequelae of the initial trauma are so varied and multifactorial that patients are unique in their presentations. Surgical protocols that are rigidly set to the level of injury

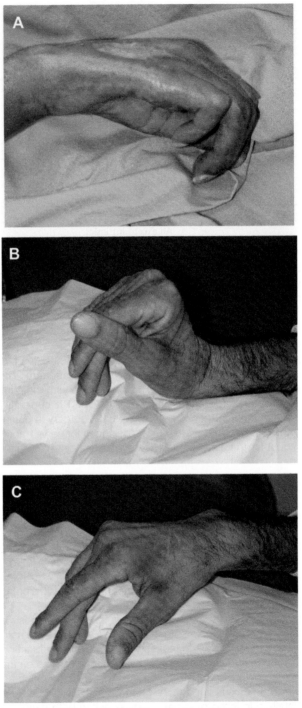

Fig. 6. The wrist tenodesis effect. (*A*) A stiff hand with intrinsic minus posturing. Despite a flexed wrist, the fingers remain flexed, especially at proximal interphalangeal joints. The thumb remains opposed as well. (*B*) As the individual extends the wrist, the fingers and thumb assume a flexed lateral pinch posture because of the passive properties of the extrinsic digital flexors. (*C*) In wrist flexion, the passive properties of the extrinsic extensor create extension of the fingers and thumb to release a held object.

will fail in many patients if these issues are not considered early in the surgical planning. The child's goals and desires inform the rationale that surgical planning must be both flexible and creative. Surgeons should be aware of and experienced with various treatment modalities and surgical reconstructive techniques in order to match the treatment strategy to the patient.

Specific surgical procedures

The specific types of tendon and nerve transfers that can be performed in children are reviewed here. As stated earlier, tendon transfer reconstruction forms the basis of surgical procedures currently and forms the current status quo of hand/upper extremity reconstruction in children and adults.

Elbow extension

Eric Moberg,[67] a pioneering SCI orthopedic surgeon, stressed the importance of restoring active elbow extension for patients with tetraplegia. Restoring elbow extension confers intrinsic stability to the elbow joint through the provision of moment forces in all of the joint's axes of motion. From a technical perspective, restoring elbow extension also improves the outcomes of the more distal tendon transfers used to restore hand function.[67] Pinch strength following brachioradialis (BR) to flexor pollicis longus (FPL) tendon transfer increases by 150% when the elbow is stabilized by tendon transfer.[76] Additional beneficial effects of active elbow extension include the ability to reach objects easily by increasing an individual's work space, push a wheelchair, self-transfer, write, and stretch out the arm while supine.[70] Adults and children most often cite active elbow extension as their favorite new function achieved with surgery. Two tendon transfer procedures, as well as 2 nerve transfer procedures, may now be used to restore active elbow extension. Two studies have compared the results of tendon transfers, but none have evaluated the relative efficacy of the nerve transfers.[77,78]

Posterior deltoid to triceps transfer

Restoring elbow extension using the deltoid as a donor muscle was first advocated by Moberg[79] in 1975. The function of the triceps is restored by using the posterior one-third to one-half of the deltoid as a donor muscle. The intrinsic biomechanics of the deltoid muscle result in contractile forces of 20% to 50% of the average triceps,[80] which is consistent with the observed outcomes of the procedure in that it rarely provides more than good antigravity strength.[81–83] There are 2 aspects of the posterior deltoid to triceps procedure that merit mentioning: the short length of the gross muscle requires a bridging tissue graft to allow attachment into the triceps, and the postsurgical rehabilitation protocol is very demanding to avoid stretching and weakening (**Fig. 7**).[33,67,84–89] Newer postsurgical protocols that include early mobilization of the transfer result in improved elbow mobility and elbow extension strength.[90]

Biceps to triceps transfer

The first published description of using biceps brachii to provide elbow extension appeared in 1954, but this technique gained momentum as an alternative to the deltoid transfer in the 1990s.[77,91–93] It has become the primary mode of surgically restoring elbow extension in many centers (**Fig. 8**). Research indicates that the biceps proves as strong as, if not stronger than, the deltoid as a donor for elbow extension.[77,92] The loss of elbow flexion strength is nonimpairing, and the functional gains associated with the provision of strong elbow extension more than compensate for the reduction in elbow flexion strength.[77,93] Although the transfer seems nonsynergistic,

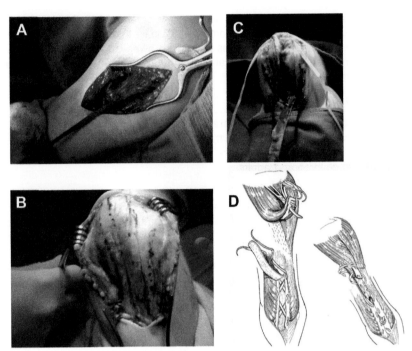

Fig. 7. The deltoid to triceps transfer restores elbow extension using the posterior deltoid and some form of bridging tendon graft. Use of the central one-third triceps tendon turn-up graft is shown. (*A*) The posterior one-third to one-half of the deltoid is exposed and mobilized through the interval between the deltoid and lateral triceps. (*B*) The triceps insertion is exposed via a separate more distal incision; the central portion of the tendon that will serve as the graft is marked. (*C*) The central one-third triceps turn-up graft mobilized. (*D*) The attachment between the deltoid and triceps using Dacron as a graft material to augment the coaptation. ([*D*] *From* Hoyen H, Gonzalez E, Williams P, et al. Management of the paralyzed elbow in tetraplegia. Hand Clin. 2002;18(1):113-33; with permission.)

the biceps is primarily a forearm supinator and this is what allows patients to rehabilitate the transfer. Critical advantages of this procedure include an easier and less cumbersome rehabilitation, and its applicability even in the setting of an elbow flexion contracture.

Nerve transfers restoring active elbow extension
The feasibility of reinnervating the triceps muscle using either the motor branch to the teres minor or the motor branch to the deltoid muscle, both of which are part of the axillary nerve, and coapting them to a nerve branch innervating either the medial or long head of the triceps was confirmed in a cadaveric study (**Fig. 9**).[94] The advantage of using the teres minor to triceps nerve transfer to restore elbow extension is the preservation of the posterior deltoid muscle as a tendon transfer should the nerve transfer prove ineffective. Only 3 publications report on the results of 5 or more people.[61,95,96] Although the biceps to triceps transfer routinely provides M4 strength, the nerve transfers, as reported, provide that level to perhaps one-third of its recipients, with nearly another third experiencing no or weak results.[70,77,78,92,96-99] The combined results of nerve transfers for elbow extension perform just less than that of the posterior deltoid transfer.

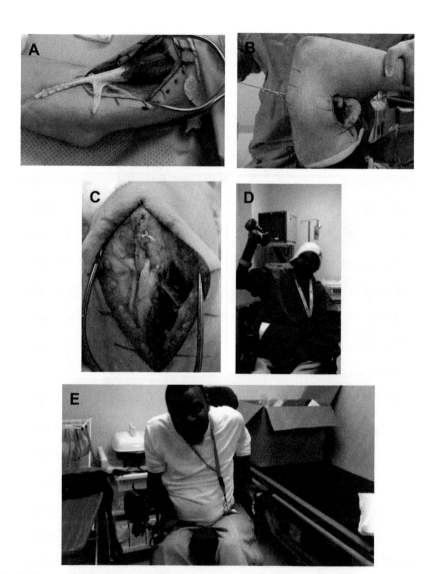

Fig. 8. Example of biceps to triceps transfer. (*A*) The biceps tendon is detached, and the tendon and muscle are both mobilized via an anterior incision. (*B*) The biceps is then routed around the medial side of the upper arm (*C*) and then weaved into the triceps tendon and anchored directly into the bone of the olecranon. (*D*) The transfer provides M4 strength allowing even weight shifts (*E*).

Wrist extension Moberg[79] pointed out that, in individuals with higher levels of injury, namely those who are under International Classification 0 or 1, voluntary wrist extension is either absent or weak; therefore, the primary goal of surgical restoration of the hand is the provision of wrist extension. If this can be achieved, then an automatic/passive lateral tenodesis pinch can be constructed with a series of secondary procedures to augment the strength of natural tenodesis pinch. When considering tendon transfers for weak ICSHT 1 (extensor carpi radialis longus [ECRL] <M3) individuals, the BR is the donor muscle into the extensor carpi radialis brevis (ECRB) (**Fig. 10**).

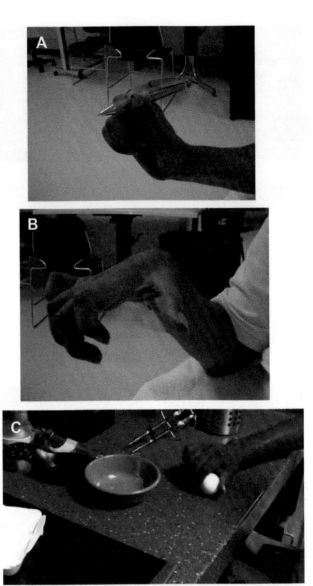

Fig. 9. The (A) grasp and (B) release phases of the lateral pinch following tendon transfer reconstruction. This individual powers his pinch using a pronator teres to flexor pollicis longus transfers. His thumb CMC joint opposition was secured using a brachioradialis mediated flexor digitorum superficialis ring opponensplasty. Notice how his thumb rests against the radial side of his index at about P2/distal interphalangeal while holding a pen. The interphalangeal joint is stabilized using the flexor pollicis longus split transfer to keep the joint from hyperflexing when activated by the pronator teres. By flexing his wrist, his fingers and thumb extend to release. (C) A patient using the reconstructed lateral pinch to break an egg.

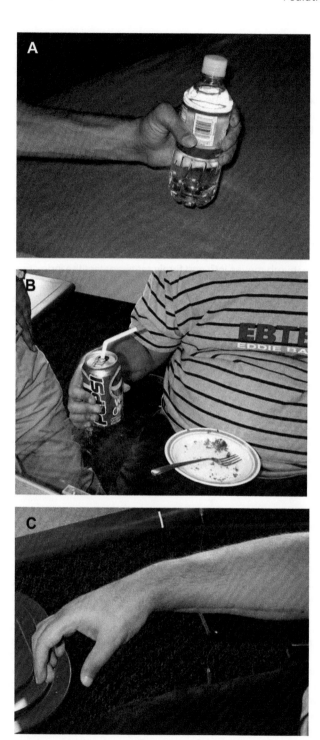

Fig. 10. Palmar grasp involves composite finger flexion with the thumb opposed while acquiring larger objects. (*A* and *B*) Acquisition of objects; (*C*) composite release with gravity-induced, or flexor carpi radialis–powered wrist flexion.

Strong ICSHT 1 (ECRL ≥ 3) individuals, and all those with higher grades, do not require this transfer. A brachialis to ECRL nerve transfer is a surgical alternative to restore wrist extension. The brachialis muscle is innervated by the musculocutaneous nerve from a single motor fascicle that can be transferred to the motor branch supplying the ECRL, which arborizes from the radial nerve. In the author's experience, either procedure provides sufficient stability to the wrist so that a patient no longer requires a universal wrist cuff, but they inconsistently provide enough wrist extension to power an effective tenodesis pinch and grasp.

Lateral pinch The active lateral pinch provides the ability to secure small objects with useful force. The result is the enhancement of activities of daily living functions, including self-catheterization, writing, and feeding. Pinch/grasp can be understood as the ability to open the fingers/thumb and then secure an object with sufficient strength until the task is completed, and then let it go (open the finger/thumb) (see **Fig. 6**).[75] In the case of lateral pinch, object acquisition depends on the thumb extending sufficiently with gravity-powered wrist flexion. A secure grasp is best achieved as the thumb moves into and firmly rests against the index finger with force. The grasp must be secure enough that the individual can maintain it with minimal fatigue while an object is handled, and then the person must be able to easily release the object. In most individuals with C5 to C6 tetraplegia, the number of muscles remaining under voluntary control is insufficient to replace the many paralyzed hand and forearm muscles involved in the lateral pinch function of able-bodied individuals.[100] Therefore, the challenges of this procedure are to recreate a meaningful pinch, as well as achieve precise digital positioning by distilling this complex set of motions into its most fundamental elements. This outcome can be achieved with activation of a single muscle, the FPL, whether through passive tenodesis or active tendon transfer using the BR. Active pinch reconstruction requires sufficiently strong voluntary wrist extension, so this procedure is only performed in strong ICSHT (≥1) in which wrist extension strength is M4 or greater.[101] All of the other aspects of lateral pinch are recreated using ancillary procedures that include fusions, tenodeses, and joint stabilization; in this way, the complexity of lateral pinch is mimicked by 1 tendon transfer.

Nerve transfer for lateral pinch
Rather than dividing the various phases of lateral pinch into actions performed by a multitude of individual muscles, it can also be thought of as the function of mostly 2 nerves: the posterior interosseous nerve (PIN) for object acquisition and release as well as the anterior interosseous nerve (AIN) for pinch and hold (see **Fig. 5**). Restoration of AIN and PIN function via nerve transfers is therefore, at least conceptually, a strategy. The motor branch to the brachialis is part of the musculocutaneous nerve, serves as the donor for the AIN, and is harvested above the elbow, where it is then coapted into the AIN fascicles within the median nerve. This proximal coaptation of the brachialis and AIN fascicles has the downside of requiring a long recovery period (about 12 months) because nerves regenerate at a rate of about 1 mm/d, but, when successful, it restores function to the FPL and the index finger flexor profundus, creating rudimentary pinch function. To create the release phase, as an alternative to the tenodesis of the extensor pollicus longus (EPL), the motor branches to the supinator muscle can be coapted into the PIN with an expectation of restoring finger and thumb extension within about 6 to 9 months. This last option is only available in children with voluntary wrist extension and as long as the biceps is not going to be used or needed to restore elbow extension; otherwise, all voluntary forearm supination would

be lost. Ancillary procedures can also be used to stabilize and position the thumb as with tendon transfers.

There is a presumption, based on published studies and surgeon experience, that the nerve transfer pinch does not have the same strength as tendon transfer–based pinch. The former also requires sacrificing all, or part, of the brachialis muscle, which is the primary elbow flexor. Therefore, the biceps cannot be used for elbow extension should the child need it (AIS<C7). The long-term effect of relying on the biceps for primary elbow flexion is unclear and of concern in light of the frequency of rotator cuff issues that confound many patients in wheelchairs over the course of time. Are there long-term problems with biceps tendinitis in this situation? Would it affect arm strength? At the same time, the dexterity of the nerve transfer is likely superior to that of the tendon transfer. However, again, does that make a functional difference? Further study is required.

Palmar grasp Palmar grasp allows individuals to manipulate larger objects than they would be capable of with just pinch alone. The presence of sufficient donor muscles (at least 2) is required to reconstruct both lateral pinch and palmar grasp (ICSHT $\geq$ 3) in order to preserve an active, strong wrist extensor.[102] In general, the results of the procedure are better in individuals with lower cervical levels of injury (IC $\geq$ 4) where more potential donor muscles are available for more versatile reconstructions.[103] As with pinch, able-bodied individuals use a multitude of muscles during normal palmar grasp for opening, grasping, and manipulating; these functions are distilled into combined flexor digitorum profundus for flexion, combined extensor digitorum communis (EDC) and EPL for extension, and tenodeses for intrinsic function (keeping the fingers balanced). Finger extension must be powered by tenodesis, tendon transfer, or nerve transfer in order to avoid longer-term finger flexion contractures (3 $\leq$ ICSHT<6). Surgically activating finger extension when not already present (ICSHT<6) is a critical component of palmar grasp reconstructions. The problem is that, for children and adults whose ICSHT is between 3 and 6, these procedures have traditionally required 2 surgeries: 1 to create the finger extension and 1 to create the flexion. The postoperative care required to rehabilitate the extensor transfers would jeopardize the integrity of the transfers for flexion if they were performed simultaneously, and vice-versa. Fridén and colleagues,[104] in Europe, have since offered newer techniques and rehabilitative strategies to successfully animate both pinch and grasp in 1 single operation.[104,105] This innovative strategy, coined the alphabet procedure, incorporates all of the steps of standard pinch and grasp procedures, but, instead of activating digital extension by activating the extrinsic extensor tendons (EPL, EDC), it relies on the intrinsic activation to achieve sufficient hand opening. The magnitude of digital extension, or opening, is reduced in the alphabet procedure because the MCPs stay flexed while the interphalangeal joints extend. Single-stage pinch and grasp is the norm for stronger individuals (ICSHT $\geq$ 6) with favorable results.[106]

Creating and Initiating Surgical Plans

In general, as a child's functional level moves caudally, and as the ICSHT grade improves, the number of strong voluntary donor muscles and nerves in the forearm available for transfer increases. Although any child who lacks voluntary elbow extension qualifies for an elbow extension reconstruction, the numbers of donor muscles and nerves determine the possibilities for hand reconstruction. For high-level children, ICSHT 0, an elbow extension transfer is performed if the individual has a particularly strong deltoid or biceps, but only nerve transfers are available for distal reconstruction. In such rare cases, the goals are elbow and wrist extension, with remote possibility of pinch. At ICSHT 1, a wrist extension transfer and possibly a subsequent passive pinch or grasp transfer are possible. However, if elbow extension is provided using the posterior deltoid instead of the biceps, or the nerve to the teres minor, active pinch can be accomplished by transferring the BR into the ECRB, and a branch of the brachialis nerve into the AIN. These presentations are less common. Typically, children and adults present with at least ICSHT 2 level tetraplegia (BR, ECRL), and it is when these hand reconstructions are powered by tendon transfers and become more effective.[103] As the ICSHT jumps to 3 or greater, muscles are available and both lateral pinch and palmar grasp can be reconstructed. As the ICSHT motor score continues to improve to a score of 4 or greater and more donor muscles become available, both flexion and extension can be powered without requiring tenodeses, and opposition of the thumb can be powered as well in the reconstruction of lateral pinch. As the levels continue to increase beyond ICSHT 6, some functions, such as digital extension, no longer require reconstruction. At each level, with increasing donor muscles come increasing potential donor nerves for nerve transfer–based reconstruction.

Bilateral Upper Extremity Reconstruction

Many children and their parents desire reconstruction of both upper extremities. There are no fundamental differences in surgical strategy when reconstructing both limbs, but there are a few considerations. The surgeon in concert with the patient can choose alternative methods of treating the carpometacarpal (CMC) joint when reconstructing lateral pinch in each hand. In one, the thumb CMC joint is treated with an arthrodesis, which confers strength and frees one of the donor muscles to some other function, such as powered finger extension. In the other, an opponensplasty is created for the thumb to add dexterity provided the child's ICSHT is greater than or equal to 4. There is the timing of bilateral reconstructions. The advantage of simultaneous bilateral reconstruction is the obvious time saved in the completion of surgeries and total rehabilitation time. There are many personal reasons for this choice. The author has found that individuals needing to return to school or home (distant location), for example, cite this as a prime motivator. These individuals must be carefully counseled to understand how the additional arm temporarily changes the degree of their disability, dependence, and need for constant assistance. Any doubts and questions should push the individual to staged reconstructions.

Incomplete Spinal Cord Injury

Children with an incomplete injury may present with any combination of function that is not concordant to their level of injury. The procedures required to achieve pinch and grasp are often modified to consider functions that may already be present; for example, elbow extension in an individual with incomplete C6 level injury or single-stage pinch and grasp restoration in an individual with incomplete C6 level injury who presents with intact digital and thumb extension. Hence, the ICSHT reserves the special label of X for those with incomplete SCI. Surgeons must creatively alter reconstructive goals and procedures to accommodate these presentations.

OUTCOMES

A well-selected, comprehensive program of hand and upper extremity rehabilitation has a reliably beneficial impact on people's lives. These benefits can and have been measured in terms of improved strength of grasp and pinch, increased number of different daily living activities performed without braces, increased independence, and a reduction in full-time assistant care. As early as 1972, investigators reported results from surgical restoration that extended beyond simply measuring improved voluntary motion.[32] House and colleagues[29,107] documented independent bowel and bladder care along with other daily living activities. In 1983, Lamb and Chan[31] reported that 83% of 41 patients with greater than 7-year follow-up experienced excellent outcomes with improved function. Hand restoration facilitated the development of personal interests and hobbies along with the ability to self-catheterize, and better quality of life.[108] In Freehafer and colleagues'[109] experience with treating 68 patients, none were worse, and only 4 remained unimproved.[109] Ejeskar and Dahllof[110] noted improvements in 35 of 43 patients. In 1992, Mohammed and colleagues[111] presented their results of surgical restoration using tendon transfers in a heterogeneous group of 57 patients, with 84% reporting an improved quality of life. About two-thirds noted independence in eating, writing and typing, using a telephone, and improvements in self-care. The long-term benefit of surgery was confirmed in this same group of patients when they were reevaluated 10 years later.[112] Lo and colleagues,[113] in 1998, found that all of the 9 patients with C6 motor-level tetraplegia benefited from surgical reconstruction both objectively and subjectively, and would have the surgery again.[11,43] Paul, and colleagues[83] reported that, in addition to improvements in activities of daily living, many patients were able to become brace free. Recent studies exploring long-term outcomes of reconstruction confirm that both patient satisfaction and positive functional benefits persist with little evidence of any deterioration.[114–118]

The greatest benefit may be on the patients' psyches, with dramatic improvements in their self-image, confidence, and overall quality of life.[119,120] As stated by Sterling Bunnell many years ago, "if you have nothing, a little is a lot."[33] Two recent studies explored long-term outcomes of reconstruction and confirmed excellent patient satisfaction and positive functional benefits with little evidence of any deterioration.[114,115] A recent Swedish study examined individual functional goals, finding that individuals in their cohort were able to perform 78% of desired activities after surgery compared with only 36% before surgery.[121] Two studies from the Netherlands reported improved functional ability in more than 81% of individuals after surgery, and up to 90% of individuals would be willing to undergo surgery again given their higher degrees of independence with less need for attendant care and functional aids.[116,122] In addition, importantly, these benefits prove consistent and reliable over the individuals' lifetimes.[118] Elbow extension provided significant improvements in wheelchair maneuverability, transfers, and notably, the ability to write and reach out for objects.[70,72] Pinch reconstructions dramatically improved bladder care, with 75% of patients gaining the ability to self-catheterize following surgery.[123]

To date, publications concerning nerve transfers have been focused on technique and efficacy rather than outcomes. Two studies have investigated a series of patients undergoing multiple simultaneous nerve transfers; otherwise, most publications are case studies.[57,60,94,96,124–127] Nonetheless, these studies are beginning to document improvements in ability and independence as well.[61]

SUMMARY

A comprehensive program for children with SCI that includes the optimization of hand and upper extremity function along with traditional pillars of rehabilitation helps to improve their overall quality of life and offers increased independence. Although surgery in children involves some unique psychosocial and technical issues that differentiate them from adults, the benefits are nonetheless significant. For those children who would meet surgical criteria, such reconstructions have, over time, repeatedly shown their efficacy and should be offered when appropriate.

DISCLOSURE

The authors have nothing to disclose.

REFERENCES

1. 2016 Annual Report - public version. Birmingham (AL): University of Alabama at Birmingham; 2017.
2. Bilston L, Brown J. Pediatric spinal injury type and severity are age and mechanism dependent. Spine 2007;32:2339–47.
3. Falavigna A, Righesso O, Guarise da Silva P, et al. Epidemiology and management of spinal trauma in children and adolescents <18 years old. World Neurosurg 2018;110:e479–83.
4. Kim C, Vassilyadi M, Forbes JK, et al. Traumatic spinal injuries in children at a single level 1 pediatric trauma centre: report of a 23-year experience. Can J Surg 2016;59:205–12.
5. Hofbauer M, Jaindl M, Hochtl LL, et al. Spine injuries in polytraumatized pediatric patients: characteristics and experience from a Level I trauma center over two decades. J Trauma Acute Care Surg 2012;73:156–61.
6. Piatt J, Imperato N. Epidemiology of spinal injury in childhood and adolescence in the United States: 1997-2012. J Neurosurg Pediatr 2018;21:441–8.
7. Polk-Williams A, Carr BG, Blinman TA, et al. Cervical spine injury in young children: a National Trauma Data Bank review. J Pediatr Surg 2008;43:1718–21.
8. Hanson RW, Franklin MR. Sexual loss in relation to other functional losses for spinal cord injured males. Arch Phys Med Rehabil 1976;57:291–3.
9. Anderson KD. Targeting recovery: priorities of the spinal cord-injured population. J Neurotrauma 2004;21:1371–83.
10. Snoek GJ, MJI J, Hermens HJ, et al. Survey of the needs of patients with spinal cord injury: impact and priority for improvement in hand function in tetraplegics. Spinal Cord 2004;42:526–32.
11. Snoek GJ, MJI J, Post MW, et al. Choice-based evaluation for the improvement of upper-extremity function compared with other impairments in tetraplegia. Arch Phys Med Rehabil 2005;86:1623–30.
12. Curtin CM, Wagner JP, Gater DR, et al. Opinions on the treatment of people with tetraplegia: contrasting perceptions of physiatrists and hand surgeons. J Spinal Cord Med 2007;30:256–62.
13. Ram AN, Curtin CM, Chung KC. Population-based utilities for upper extremity functions in the setting of tetraplegia. J Hand Surg Am 2009;34:1674–16781.e1.
14. Waters RL, Sie IH, Gellman H, et al. Functional hand surgery following tetraplegia. Arch Phys Med Rehabil 1996;77:86–94.
15. Bryden AM, Wuolle KS, Murray PK, et al. Perceived outcomes and utilization of upper extremity surgical reconstruction in individuals with tetraplegia at model spinal cord injury systems. Spinal Cord 2004;42:169–76.
16. Curtin CM, Hayward RA, Kim HM, et al. Physician perceptions of upper extremity reconstruction for the person with tetraplegia. J Hand Surg Am 2005;30:87–93.

17. Curtin CM, Gater DR, Chung KC. Upper extremity reconstruction in the tetraplegic population, a national epidemiologic study. J Hand Surg Am 2005;30:94–9.
18. Punj V, Curtin C. Understanding and overcoming barriers to upper limb surgical reconstruction after tetraplegia: the need for interdisciplinary collaboration. Arch Phys Med Rehabil 2016;97:S81–7.
19. Carroll T, Smith CD, Liu X, et al. Spinal cord injuries without radiologic abnormality in children: a systematic review. Spinal Cord 2015;53:842–8.
20. Brown RL, Brunn MA, Garcia VF. Cervical spine injuries in children: a review of 103 patients treated consecutively at a level 1 pediatric trauma center. J Pediatr Surg 2001;36:1107–14.
21. Babcock L, Olsen C, Jaffe D, et al. Cervical spine injuries in children associated with sports and recreational activities. Pediatr Emerg Care 2018;34:677–86.
22. Stroh Wuolle K, Van Doren CL, Bryden AM, et al. Satisfaction with and usage of a hand neuroprosthesis. Arch Phys Med Rehabil 1999;80:206–13.
23. Kozin SH. Pediatric onset spinal cord injury: implications on management of the upper limb in tetraplegia. Hand Clin 2008;24:203–13.
24. Schottler J, Vogel LC, Sturm P. Spinal cord injuries in young children: a review of children injured at 5 years of age and younger. Dev Med Child Neurol 2012;54: 1138–43.
25. DeBenedetti M. Restoration of elbow extension in the tetraplegic patient using the Moberg technique. J Hand Surg 1979;4:86–9.
26. Freehafer AA, Peckham PH, Keith MW. New concepts on treatment of the upper limb in the tetraplegic. Surgical restoration and functional neuromuscular stimulation. Hand Clin 1988;4:563–74.
27. Gorman PH, Wuolle KS, Peckham PH, et al. Patient selection for an upper extremity neuroprosthesis in tetraplegic individuals. Spinal Cord 1997;35:569–73.
28. Hentz VR, Hamlin C, Keoshian LA. Surgical reconstruction in tetraplegia. Hand Clin 1988;4:601–7.
29. House JH, Gwathmey FW, Lundsgaard DK. Restoration of strong grasp and lateral pinch in tetraplegia due to cervical spinal cord injury. J Hand Surg Am 1976;1:152–9.
30. Keith MW, Peckham PH, Thrope GB, et al. Implantable functional neuromuscular stimulation in the tetraplegic hand. J Hand Surg Am 1989;14:524–30.
31. Lamb DW, Chan KM. Surgical reconstruction of the upper limb in traumatic tetraplegia. A review of 41 patients. J Bone Joint Surg Br 1983;65:291–8.
32. Lamb DW, Landry RM. The hand in quadriplegia. Paraplegia 1972;9:204–12.
33. Moberg E. The upper limb in tetraplegia: a new approach to surgical rehabilitation. Stuttgart (Germany): Georg Thieme Publishers; 1978.
34. Peckham P, Keith M, Freehafer A. Restoration of functional control by electrical stimulation in the upper extremity of the quadriplegic patient. J Bone Joint Surg 1988;70:144–8.
35. Peckham PH, Creasey GH. Neural prostheses: clinical applications of functional electrical stimulation in spinal cord injury. Paraplegia 1992;30:96–101.
36. Zancolli E. Structural and dynamic basis of hand surgery. Philadelphia: JB Lippincott Co.; 1968.
37. Zancolli E. Surgery for the quadriplegic hand with active, strong wrist extension preserved. A study of 97 cases. Clin Orthop 1975;101–13.
38. Zancolli E. Functional restoration of the upper limb in traumatic quadriplegia. Structural and dynamic bases of hand surgery. 2nd edition. JB Lippincott; 1979. p. 229–62.

39. Hay-Smith J, Whitehead L, Keeling S. Getta a good grip on it: people with quadriplegia making decisions about upper limb surgery. Xth International Meeting on Surgical Rehabilitation of The Tetraplegic Upper Limb. Paris, 2010.

40. Tournebise H, Allieu Y. What are elements that help a quadriplegic to decide to have surgery of the upper limb. Xth International Meeting on Surgical Rehabilitation of The Tetraplegic Upper Limb. Paris, 2010.

41. Dunn JA, Hay-Smith EJ, Keeling S, et al. Decision-making about upper limb tendon transfer surgery by people with tetraplegia for more than 10 years. Arch Phys Med Rehabil 2016;97:S88–96.

42. Bryden AM, Hoyen HA, Keith MW, et al. Upper extremity assessment in tetraplegia: the importance of differentiating between upper and lower motor neuron paralysis. Arch Phys Med Rehabil 2016;97:S97–104.

43. Fox IK. Nerve transfers in tetraplegia. Hand Clin 2016;32:227–42.

44. Keith M, Lacey S. Surgical rehabilitation of the tetraplegic upper extremity. J Neuro Rehabil 1991;5:75–87.

45. Ditunno JF Jr, Cohen ME, Hauck WW, et al. Recovery of upper-extremity strength in complete and incomplete tetraplegia: a multicenter study. Arch Phys Med Rehabil 2000;81:389–93.

46. Ditunno JF Jr, Stover SL, Freed MM, et al. Motor recovery of the upper extremities in traumatic quadriplegia: a multicenter study. Arch Phys Med Rehabil 1992;73:431–6.

47. Peljovich AE, Candia J, Kalmer S, et al. Achieving neurological stability in complete traumatic tetraplegia. Tenth International Meeting on Surgical Rehabilitation Of the Tetraplegic Upper Limb. Paris, France, 2010.

48. Peckham PH, Mortimer JT, Marsolais EB. Upper and lower motor neuron lesions in the upper extremity muscles of tetraplegics. Paraplegia 1976;14:115–21.

49. Peckham P, Marsolais E, Moritmer J. Restoration of key grip and release in the C6 tetraplegic patient through functional electrical stimulation. J Hand Surg 1980;5:462–9.

50. Freehafer AA. Tendon transfers in patients with cervical spinal cord injury. J Hand Surg Am 1991;16:804–9.

51. Kilgore KL, Peckham PH, Keith MW, et al. An implanted upper-extremity neuroprosthesis. Follow-up of five patients. J Bone Joint Surg Am 1997;79:533–41.

52. Peckham PH, Keith MW, Kilgore KL, et al. Efficacy of an implanted neuroprosthesis for restoring hand grasp in tetraplegia: a multicenter study. Arch Phys Med Rehabil 2001;82:1380–8.

53. Peckham PH, Kilgore KL, Keith MW, et al. An advanced neuroprosthesis for restoration of hand and upper arm control using an implantable controller. J Hand Surg Am 2002;27:265–76.

54. Kilgore KL, Hoyen HA, Bryden AM, et al. An implanted upper-extremity neuroprosthesis using myoelectric control. J Hand Surg Am 2008;33:539–50.

55. Memberg WD, Polasek KH, Hart RL, et al. Implanted neuroprosthesis for restoring arm and hand function in people with high level tetraplegia. Arch Phys Med Rehabil 2014;95:1201–12011.e1.

56. Tung TH, Mackinnon SE. Nerve transfers: indications, techniques, and outcomes. J Hand Surg Am 2010;35:332–41.

57. Brown JM. Nerve transfers in tetraplegia I: background and technique. Surg Neurol Int 2011;2:121.

58. Senjaya F, Midha R. Nerve transfer strategies for spinal cord injury. World Neurosurg 2013;80:e319–26.

59. Cain SA, Gohritz A, Friden J, et al. Review of upper extremity nerve transfer in cervical spinal cord injury. J Brachial Plex Peripher Nerve Inj 2015;10:e34–42.
60. Bertelli JA, Ghizoni MF. Nerve transfers for restoration of finger flexion in patients with tetraplegia. J Neurosurg Spine 2017;26:55–61.
61. van Zyl N, Hill B, Cooper C, et al. Expanding traditional tendon-based techniques with nerve transfers for the restoration of upper limb function in tetraplegia: a prospective case series. Lancet 2019;394:565–75.
62. McDowell C, Moberg E, House J. The second international conference on surgical rehabilitation of the upper limb in tetraplegia (quadriplegia). J Hand Surg 1986;11A:604–8.
63. LeClercq C, McDowell C. Fourth international conference on surgical rehabilitation of the upper limb in tetraplegia. Ann Chir Main Membre Superievr 1991;10: 258–60.
64. Ejeskar A. Upper limb surgical rehabilitation in high-level tetraplegia. Hand Clin 1988;4:585–99.
65. Freehafer A, Peckham P, Keith M. Surgical treatment for tetraplegia: upper limb. In: Chapman M, editor. Operative orthopaedics. Philadelphia: JB Lippincott; 1988. p. 1459–67.
66. McDowell C, Moberg E, A.G.S.. International conference on surgical rehabilitation of the upper limb in tetraplegia. J Hand Surg 1979;4A:387–90.
67. Moberg E. Helpful upper limb surgery in tetraplegia. In: Hunter J, Schneider L, Mackin E, et al, editors. Rehabilitation of the hand. St. Louis (MO): The CV Mosby Co; 1978.
68. Moberg E. Current treatment program using tendon surgery in tetraplegia. In: Hunter J, Schneider L, Mackin E, editors. Tendon surgery in the hand. St. Louis (MO): The CV Mosby Co.; 1987. p. 496–505.
69. Grover J, Gellman H, Waters R. The effect of a flexion contracture of the elbow on the ability to transfer in patients who have quadriplegia at the sixth cervical level. J Bone Joint Surg 1996;78(A):1397–400.
70. Wangdell J, Friden J. Activity gains after reconstructions of elbow extension in patients with tetraplegia. J Hand Surg Am 2012;37:1003–10.
71. Hoyen H, Gonzalez E, Williams P, et al. Management of the paralyzed elbow in tetraplegia. Hand Clin 2002;18:113–33.
72. Lamberg AS, Friden J. Changes in skills required for using a manual wheelchair after reconstructive hand surgery in tetraplegia. J Rehabil Med 2011;43:714–9.
73. Boelter L, Keller A, Taylor C, et al. Studies to determine the functional requirements for hand and arm prosthesis. Final report to the National Academy of Sciences. University of California, Los Angeles: National Academy of Sciences; 1947. Report No.: Contract VA M-21223.
74. Bertelli JA, Ghizoni MF. Nerve transfer for sensory reconstruction of C8-T1 dermatomes in tetraplegia. Microsurgery 2016;36:637–41.
75. Peljovich AE. Tendon transfers for restoration of active grasp. In: Kozin SH, editor. Atlas of the hand clinics. Philadelphia: W.B. Saunders; 2002. p. 79–96.
76. Brys D, Waters RL. Effect of triceps function on the brachioradialis transfer in quadriplegia. J Hand Surg Am 1987;12:237–9.
77. Mulcahey MJ, Lutz C, Kozin SH, et al. Prospective evaluation of biceps to triceps and deltoid to triceps for elbow extension in tetraplegia. J Hand Surg Am 2003;28:964–71.
78. Peterson CL, Bednar MS, Bryden AM, et al. Voluntary activation of biceps-to-triceps and deltoid-to-triceps transfers in quadriplegia. PLoS One 2017;12: e0171141.

79. Moberg E. Surgical treatment for absent single-hand grip and elbow extension in quadriplegia. Principles and preliminary experience. J Bone Joint Surg Am 1975;57:196–206.

80. Friden J, Lieber RL. Quantitative evaluation of the posterior deltoid to triceps tendon transfer based on muscle architectural properties. J Hand Surg Am 2001;26:147–55.

81. Dunkerley AL, Ashburn A, Stack EL. Deltoid triceps transfer and functional independence of people with tetraplegia. Spinal Cord 2000;38:435–41.

82. Mennen V, Boonzaier A. An improved technique of posterior deltoid to triceps transfer in tetraplegia. J Hand Surg Br 1991;16:197–201.

83. Paul SD, Gellman H, Waters R, et al. Single-stage reconstruction of key pinch and extension of the elbow in tetraplegic patients [see comments]. J Bone Joint Surg Am 1994;76:1451–6.

84. Castro-Sierra A, Lopez-Pita A. A new surgical technique to correct triceps paralysis. Hand 1983;15:42–6.

85. Lacey S, Wilber R, Peckham P, et al. The posterior deltoid to triceps transfer, a clinical and biomechanical assessment. J Hand Surg 1986;11:542–7.

86. Rabischong E, Benoit P, Benichou M, et al. Length-tension relationship of the posterior deltoid to triceps transfer in C6 tetraplegic patients. Paraplegia 1993;31:33–9.

87. Bonds CW, James MA. Posterior deltoid-to-triceps tendon transfer to restore active elbow extension in patients with tetraplegia. Tech Hand Up Extrem Surg 2009;13:94–7.

88. Netscher DT, Sandvall BK. Surgical technique: posterior deltoid-to-triceps transfer in tetraplegic patients. J Hand Surg Am 2011;36:711–5.

89. Friden J, Ejeskar A, Dahlgren A, et al. Protection of the deltoid to triceps tendon transfer repair sites. J Hand Surg Am 2000;25:144–9.

90. Friden J. Early active training of deltoid to triceps transfers: a controlled study. Xth International Meeting on Surgical Rehabilitation of The Tetraplegic Upper Limb. Paris, 2010.

91. Friedenberg Z. Transposition of the biceps brachii for triceps weakness. J Bone Joint Surg 1954;36:656–8.

92. Kuz J, Van Heest A, House J. Biceps-to-triceps transfer in tetraplegic patients; report of the medial routing technique and follow-up of three cases. J Hand Surg 1999;24:161–72.

93. Revol M, Briand E, Servant J. Biceps-to-triceps transfer in tetraplegia: the medial route. J Hand Surg 1999;24B:235–7.

94. Bertelli JA, Tacca CP, Winkelmann Duarte EC, et al. Transfer of axillary nerve branches to reconstruct elbow extension in tetraplegics: a laboratory investigation of surgical feasibility. Microsurgery 2011;31:376–81.

95. Khalifeh JM, Dibble CF, Van Voorhis A, et al. Nerve transfers in the upper extremity following cervical spinal cord injury. Part 2: Preliminary results of a prospective clinical trial. J Neurosurg Spine 2019;1–13.

96. Bertelli JA, Ghizoni MF. Nerve transfers for elbow and finger extension reconstruction in midcervical spinal cord injuries. J Neurosurg 2015;122:121–7.

97. Kozin SH, D'Addesi L, Chafetz RS, et al. Biceps-to-triceps transfer for elbow extension in persons with tetraplegia. J Hand Surg Am 2010;35:968–75.

98. Koch-Borner S, Dunn JA, Friden J, et al. Rehabilitation after posterior deltoid to triceps transfer in tetraplegia. Arch Phys Med Rehabil 2016;97:S126–35.

99. Medina J, Marcos-Garcia A, Jiménez I, et al. Biceps to triceps transfer in tetraplegic patients: our experience and review of the literature. Hand (N Y) 2017;12: 85–90.

100. Johanson ME, Valero-Cuevas FJ, Hentz VR. Activation patterns of the thumb muscles during stable and unstable pinch tasks. J Hand Surg Am 2001;26: 698–705.

101. Ward SR, Peace WJ, Friden J, et al. Dorsal transfer of the brachioradialis to the flexor pollicis longus enables simultaneous powering of key pinch and forearm pronation. J Hand Surg Am 2006;31:993–7.

102. Johanson ME, Murray WM, Hentz VR. Comparison of wrist and elbow stabilization following pinch reconstruction in tetraplegia. J Hand Surg Am 2011;36: 480–5.

103. Hentz VR, Leclercq C. Surgical rehabilitation of the upper limb in tetraplegia. London: W.B. Saunders; 2002.

104. Fridén J, Reinholdt C, Turcsanyii I, et al. A single-stage operation for reconstruction of hand flexion, extension, and intrinsic function in tetraplegia: the alphabet procedure. Tech Hand Up Extrem Surg 2011;15:230–5.

105. Reinholdt C, Friden J. Outcomes of single-stage grip-release reconstruction in tetraplegia. J Hand Surg Am 2013;38:1137–44.

106. Koo B, Peljovich AE, Bohn A. Single-stage tendon transfer reconstruction for active pinch and grasp in tetraplegia. Top Sp Cord Inj Rehab 2008;13:24–36.

107. House JH, Shannon MA. Restoration of strong grasp and lateral pinch in tetraplegia: a comparison of two methods of thumb control in each patient. J Hand Surg Am 1985;10:22–9.

108. Guinet A, Rech C, Even-Schneider A, et al. Self-catheterization acquisition after hand reanimation protocols in C5-C7 tetraplegic patients. Xth International Meeting on Surgical Rehabilitation of The Tetraplegic Upper Limb. Paris, 2010.

109. Freehafer AA, Kelly CM, Peckham PH. Tendon transfer for the restoration of upper limb function after a cervical spinal cord injury. J Hand Surg Am 1984;9: 887–93.

110. Ejeskar A, Dahllof A. Results of reconstructive surgery in the upper limb of tetraplegic patients. Paraplegia 1988;26:204–8.

111. Mohammed K, Rothwell A, Sinclair S, et al. Upper limb surgery for tetraplegia. J Bone Joint Surg 1992;74B:873–9.

112. Rothwell AG, Sinnott KA, Mohammed KD, et al. Upper limb surgery for tetraplegia: a 10-year re-review of hand function. J Hand Surg Am 2003;28:489–97.

113. Lo IK, Turner R, Connolly S, et al. The outcome of tendon transfers for C6-spared quadriplegics. J Hand Surg Br 1998;23:156–61.

114. Carles A, Vincenti P, Floris L, et al. Evaluation of the long term results of functional surgery of the upper limbs in tetraplegic individuals. Xth International Meeting on Surgical Rehabilitation of The Tetraplegic Upper Limb. Paris, 2010.

115. Snoek GJ, Bongers-Janssen H, Nene A. Long term patient satisfaction after reconstructive upper extremity surgery to improve arm-hand function in tetraplegia. Xth International Meeting on Surgical Rehabilitation of The Tetraplegic Upper Limb. Paris, 2010.

116. Jaspers Focks-Feenstra J, Snoek G, Bongers-Janssen H, et al. Long-term patient satisfaction after reconstructive upper extremity surgery to improve arm-hand function in tetraplegia. Spinal Cord 2011;49(8):903–8.

117. Vastamaki M. Short-term versus long-term comparative results after reconstructive upper-limb surgery in tetraplegic patients. J Hand Surg Am 2006;31: 1490–4.

118. Dunn JA, Rothwell AG, Mohammed KD, et al. The effects of aging on upper limb tendon transfers in patients with tetraplegia. J Hand Surg Am 2014;39:317–23.
119. Sinnott KA, Brander P, Siegert R, et al. Life impacts following reconstructive hand surgery for tetraplegia. Top Spinal Cord Inj Rehabil 2009;15:90–7.
120. Wangdell J, Carlsson G, Friden J. Enhanced independence: experiences after regaining grip function in people with tetraplegia. Disabil Rehabil 2013;35: 1968–74.
121. Wangdell J, Friden J. Satisfaction and performance in patient selected goals after grip reconstruction in tetraplegia. J Hand Surg Eur 2010;35:563–8.
122. Gregersen H, Lybaek M, Lauge Johannesen I, et al. Satisfaction with upper extremity surgery in individuals with tetraplegia. J Spinal Cord Med 2015;38: 161–9.
123. Bernuz B, Guinet A, Rech C, et al. Self-catheterization acquisition after hand reanimation protocols in C5-C7 tetraplegic patients. Spinal Cord 2011;49:313–7.
124. Bertelli JA, Mendes Lehm VL, Tacca CP, et al. Transfer of the distal terminal motor branch of the extensor carpi radialis brevis to the nerve of the flexor pollicis longus: an anatomic study and clinical application in a tetraplegic patient. Neurosurgery 2012;70:1011–6 [discussion: 6].
125. Bertelli JA, Ghizoni MF, Tacca CP. Transfer of the teres minor motor branch for triceps reinnervation in tetraplegia. J Neurosurg 2011;114:1457–60.
126. Bertelli JA, Tacca CP, Ghizoni MF, et al. Transfer of supinator motor branches to the posterior interosseous nerve to reconstruct thumb and finger extension in tetraplegia: case report. J Hand Surg Am 2010;35:1647–51.
127. van Zyl N, Hahn JB, Cooper CA, et al. Upper limb reinnervation in C6 tetraplegia using a triple nerve transfer: case report. J Hand Surg Am 2014;39:1779–83.

30 Years After the Americans with Disabilities Act

Perspectives on Employment for Persons with Spinal Cord Injury

Lisa Ottomanelli, PhD[a,b,]*, Lance L. Goetz, MD[c,d],
John O'Neill, PhD[e], Eric Lauer, MPH, PhD[f],
Trevor Dyson-Hudson, MD[g,h]

KEYWORDS

- Spinal cord injury • Disability • Employment • Vocational rehabilitation
- Supported employment • Individual placement and support

KEY POINTS

- Research demonstrates employment is possible for persons with SCI regardless of severity or duration of injury.
- Employment is strongly associated with improvements in multiple life domains. Rehabilitation providers should treat employment as a high priority for the health of their clients with SCI.
- Despite the passage of the Americans with Disabilities Act in 1990, employment rates for persons with SCI, and disabilities in general, remain low. Recent Medical Expenditure Panel Survey (MEPS) data provide a broad view of employment status of persons with SCI and disorders in the United States in relation to several demographic variables.
- Newer paradigms for including effective vocational rehabilitation as part of ongoing SCI care need to be adopted to improve outcomes.

[a] Research Service (151R), James A. Haley Veterans' Hospital and Clinics, 8900 Grand Oak Circle, Tampa, FL 33637, USA; [b] Rehabilitation and Mental Health Counseling Program, Department of Child and Family Studies, College of Behavioral and Community Sciences, University of South Florida, 4202 E. Fowler Ave, Tampa, FL 33620, USA; [c] Spinal Cord Injury and Disorders (128), Department of Veterans Affairs, Hunter Holmes McGuire VA Medical Center, 1201 Broad Rock Boulevard, Richmond, VA 23249, USA; [d] Department of Physical Medicine and Rehabilitation, Virginia Commonwealth University, Richmond, VA, USA; [e] Center for Employment and Disability Research, Kessler Foundation, 120 Eagle Rock Avenue, East Hanover, NJ 07936, USA; [f] Institute on Disability/University Centers for Excellence in Disabilities Education, Research, and Service, College of Health and Human Services, University of New Hampshire, 10 West Edge Drive, Suite 101, Durham, NH 03824, USA; [g] Center for Spinal Cord Injury Research, Kessler Foundation, 1199 Pleasant Valley Way, West Orange, NJ 07052, USA; [h] Department of Physical Medicine and Rehabilitation, Rutgers New Jersey Medical School, Newark, NJ, USA
* Corresponding author.
E-mail address: Lisa.Ottomanelli-Slone@va.gov

Phys Med Rehabil Clin N Am 31 (2020) 499–513
https://doi.org/10.1016/j.pmr.2020.04.007
1047-9651/20/Published by Elsevier Inc.

INTRODUCTION

The Americans with Disabilities Act (ADA) was signed into law by President George H.W. Bush on July 26, 1990. It represented landmark legislation for persons with disabilities by prohibiting discrimination against them in many critical aspects of society, such as housing and employment. For example, employers and builders are required to provide reasonable accommodations to enable access to work places and residences. Since passage of the ADA, physical access to public spaces has increased dramatically, although private residences remain largely unaffected. With respect to employment, however, at the 20-year anniversary of the ADA, the employment rate of persons with disability had worsened; some economists theorized that employers may perceive the cost of accommodations as too high to hire people with disabilities.[1,2]

Disability as defined by the ADA refers to a large array of mental, physical, and other sensory impairments. Persons with spinal cord injury (SCI) represent a small but uniquely complex disability subgroup in that they often have comorbid physical, medical, and sometimes cognitive issues, which create special challenges to their social and vocational integration into society. How did the ADA affect employment of persons with SCI? How does employment of persons with SCI compare with other groups of persons with disability? Are there important differences among persons with SCI that create distinct subgroups? Finally, what is being done or can be done to improve the employment rate in the United States for persons with SCI?

Scope of the Americans with Disabilities Act

The ADA is divided into three major sections, labeled Titles I to III (**Box 1**), and the Civil Rights Division of the Department of Justice hosts a web site dedicated to providing information and technical assistance on all aspects of the ADA.[3] The web site includes resources, such as the following:

- A guide for persons with disabilities seeking employment
- A booklet for returning service members
- A guide to disability rights laws
- Questions and answers related to the ADA and human immunodeficiency virus/ AIDS
- A video, "Ten Employment Myths," aimed at prospective employers and dispelling unfounded myths about persons with disabilities as potential employees

The Employment Myths video notes that the retirement of the Baby Boomers will result in the loss of roughly 20% of the workforce and, thus, a need for 10 to 15 million new workers, and that consumer surveys show they strongly prefer businesses that hire persons with disabilities.

Employment and Persons with Spinal Cord Injury

Despite seemingly comprehensive services for persons with disabilities and a need for them to augment the US workforce, as noted, many barriers limit workforce participation by persons with SCI. Studies with different populations and measures and done at different times consistently report an employment rate of roughly only 35%.[4] Numerous factors may account for this persistently low employment rate. Although architectural barriers have been addressed, employers' attitudes remain a barrier: "When corporate leaders think about diversity, they often think about race, gender, and sexual orientation/identity. They do not think about disability."[5] There is a continued need for more opportunities for education, training, and experience,

---

Box 1
Overview of the Americans with Disabilities Act

Title I: Employment	Title II: State and Local Government	Title III: Public Accommodations and Commercial Facilities
Only applies to employers with 15 or more employees. Prohibits discrimination by private employers, state and local governments, employment agencies, and labor unions in: • Job application procedures • Hiring • Conditions • Compensation • Job training • Privileges of employment • Advancement • Firing • Other terms	"Protects qualified individuals with disabilities from discrimination ... in services, programs, and activities provided by State and local government entities." "Extends the prohibition on discrimination established by section 504 of the Rehabilitation Act of 1973...to all activities of State and local governments regardless of whether these entities receive Federal financial assistance."	Prohibits discrimination in the activities of places of public accommodations, which are businesses that are generally open to the public and fall into 1 of 12 categories listed in the ADA, such as day care facilities, doctors' offices, movie theaters, recreation facilities, restaurants, and schools. Requires compliance with ADA standards for newly constructed or altered public facilities and commercial facilities that are privately owned and nonresidential, such as factories, warehouses, or office buildings.

Data from United States Department of Justice Civil Rights Division. American with Disabilities Act. Available at: https://www.ada.gov/.

---

especially in science, technology, engineering, and math careers. Also, difficulties in navigating complex state vocational agencies persist. Medical problems can limit the number of hours that persons with SCI can work.

Financial concerns and fear of losing benefits are common reasons that people with SCI choose not to return to work.[5,6] Federal benefits, such as Supplemental Security Income and Social Security Disability Insurance, can sometimes be terminated if employment is gained, and making the "money math" work out favorably is daunting. Despite programs, such as Ticket to Work and Work Incentives Planning and Assistance, which provide benefits to employers and employees with disabilities who return to work, persons with disability may fear that benefits could not be quickly reinstated if serious illness recurred and required extended leave or retirement.

Not adequately addressing work as part of health care sentences many people with disabilities to a life of poverty and results in enormous social and financial costs.[5] The independent living movement, which started in the United States in the1960s, emphasized moving persons with disabilities out of nursing homes. An earlier priority, however, may be obtaining financial independence, which gives persons with disabilities more control over their housing situation.

EMPLOYMENT AS A PART OF SPINAL CORD INJURY REHABILITATION

Rehabilitation providers are trained to treat the whole person: physical, mental, avocational, relationship, vocational, and medical needs. The goal of rehabilitation medicine is to improve function and thereby improve quality of life, as evidenced by a past slogan of the American Academy of Physical Medicine and Rehabilitation: "Adding Life to Years." Yet nonmedical needs are often pushed aside by what are perceived to be more pressing concerns.

Rehabilitation for SCI requires involvement of the patient, the family, and an entire team of providers including, but not limited to, rehabilitation nurses, nursing assistants, and physicians; physical, occupational, and recreational therapists; and kinesiologists, social workers, psychologists/sexologists, and ideally, vocational specialists. Providers may be preoccupied with myriad ongoing medical concerns and therefore unfamiliar with advancements in the science of vocational rehabilitation (VR). Employment is often an afterthought, for a variety of reasons, including the possible perception that a person with SCI is too disabled to work. Furthermore, although persons with SCI often perceive themselves as motivated and able to work, they are likely to have many questions about work as they grapple with uncertainty about future employment and the pathway for getting there.[7] During rehabilitation, persons with SCI may ask themselves, "What am I going to do with the rest of my life?" This is a reasonable question, given the dramatic and life-altering physical changes associated with SCI. To understand that going back to productive work is a real possibility can provide an important source of hope and inspiration that can fuel overall rehabilitation efforts. Employment can contribute to meaning, purpose, and relationships, without which a person with SCI is far less likely to care about their medical needs and diligently attend to those needs. Research has clearly shown that employment positively impacts multiple life domains.[8,9] Therefore, all SCI providers should consider employment a part of rehabilitation and familiarize themselves with employment programs available for their SCI rehabilitation clients.

EMPLOYMENT AND SPINAL CORD INJURY: COMPARISON WITH THE GENERAL POPULATION, 1996 TO 2015

A recent analysis of the Medical Expenditure Panel Survey (MEPS) illustrates employment outcomes and health experiences of a nationally representative sample of persons with either SCI or disease (SCI/D). The MEPS sample is particularly relevant to physical medicine and rehabilitation because it includes persons with SCI/D who recently sought medical treatment. Directed by the Agency for Health Care Research and Quality, MEPS is an annual survey of a nationally representative cross-section of noninstitutionalized civilians that is focused on household medical use. Households selected for each MEPS panel are a subsample of households participating in the previous year's National Health Interview Survey conducted by the National Center for Health Statistics. For the analysis, we created a sample of persons with SCI/D and obtained data on their employment and health use (**Table 1**). Our analyses showed that working-age people treated for SCI/D were significantly less likely to be employed than the overall working-age US population. Compared with the overall US employed population, persons with SCI/D who were employed were more likely to (**Table 2**):

- Be older, female, non-Hispanic white, and a veteran
- Have a disability
- Work 1 to 29 hours a week
- Be unable to work for ≥11 days because of disability during the calendar year
- Have a usual source of care
- Have an office-based source of care
- Unable to receive or experience delays in any form of care

Table 1
Medical Expenditure Panel Survey data

Method	Description
Sample source	1996–2015 medical condition and full-year consolidated public-use files for:
	Individuals with spine-related conditions (associated with medical events) typically diagnosed when treating SCI/D and
	Overall sample of the United States
Medical condition identification	3-digit International Classification of Disease, Version 9, Clinical Modification codes 336, 344, 721, 780, 806, 907, and 952
Employment data	Type of job
	Number of jobs held
	Hours/week
	Benefits
	Paid leave to visit a doctor
	Paid sick leave
	Paid vacation
	Pension plans
Health-related data	Health insurance
	Access to care
	Usual source of care
	Ability to receive care and/or delay in care
	Disabilities
	Days unable to work because of disability
	Perceived health status
	Perceived mental health status

Data from Agency for Healthcare Research and Quality. Medical Expenditure Panel Survey (MEPS). Available at: https://www.meps.ahrq.gov/mepsweb/.

- Report health status and mental health status as fair or poor

HEALTH CARE IMPLICATIONS

Although employed persons with SCI/D are thought to be better off than unemployed people with SCI/D, they continue to experience disparities when compared with the overall employed US population. For example, although the SCI/D population is likely receiving SCI/D-related treatment and care and they are more likely to have an office-based source of care, they are also more likely to be unable to receive (or experience delays in) medical care, dental care, and/or prescription medications. Inability to receive or experiencing delays in care are associated with acute health events and worse health outcomes and thus increased risk of hospitalization and increased health costs. Recommendations for preventing these events are consistent with and based on the same principles that underlie an integrated system of specialized care (a form of supported employment [SE]) that has, thus far, proved to be the only evidence-based approach to employment for persons with SCI: the individual placement and support (IPS) model. These recommendations include improvements in care coordination and communication, including provider-to-provider communication. For example, with IPS, an employment specialist can facilitate a physician's learning of a developing health concern. The evidence base for IPS in SCI comprises more than 10 years of data on significantly increased rates of employment of persons with SCI (discussed later).

Table 2
Comparison of sociodemographic and health-related characteristics for the working-age employed population treated for SCI or disease and the overall working-age employed population in the United States, 1996–2015

Characteristic		SCI, % (95% CI)		United States, % (95% CI)	Chi-square
		Overall	Employed	Employed	
		n = 619,859	n = 322,528	n = 143,338,381	
Total		100.0	52.0 (48.1–55.8)	78.6 (78.2–79.0)	271.4[a]
Age, yr	18–44	31.8 (27.9–35.8)	37.3 (31.8–42.7)	62.3 (61.8–62.8)	82.0[a]
	45–64	68.2 (64.2–72.1)	62.7 (57.3–68.2)	37.7 (37.2–38.2)	82.0[a]
Gender	Female	51.8 (47.3–56.3)	55.1 (48.9–61.4)	47.4 (47.2–47.7)	5.7[c]
Race	Non-Hispanic white	73.1 (70.1–76.2)	78.7 (74.7–82.6)	65.5 (64.4–66.6)	33.4[a]
Health insurance	Any private	65.6 (62.0–69.3)	83.2 (79.3–87.2)	80.0 (79.5–80.6)	3.9
	Public only	25.8 (22.5–29.1)	8.6 (5.8–11.4)	4.8 (4.6–5.1)	
	Uninsured	8.6 (6.6–10.6)	8.2 (5.3–11.1)	15.2 (14.7–15.6)	
Education	Less than high school	18.4 (15.1–21.7)	11.3 (7.9–14.6)	12.7 (12.3–13.1)	14.3[b]
	High school	36.1 (32.1–40.1)	34.9 (29.6–40.2)	29.8 (29.2–30.3)	
	Some college or more	45.5 (41.1–49.9)	53.8 (47.9–59.7)	57.5 (56.8–58.2)	
Veteran		14.7 (11.5–17.9)	10.8 (7.2–14.5)	7.5 (7.3–7.7)	4.5[c]
Employment type	Self-employed	15.0 (11.4–18.6)	15.0 (11.3–18.8)	11.8 (11.5–12.1)	3.6
	Temporary	5.1 (2.7–7.5)	4.8 (2.4–7.2)	5.8 (5.6–6.1)	0.6
	Seasonal	3.7 (0.9–6.5)	3.5 (0.7–6.4)	4.0 (3.7–4.2)	0.01
	More than 1 job	9.2 (6.2–12.2)	9.6 (6.4–12.7)	8.5 (8.3–8.7)	0.5
Hours worked	1–29	21.3 (16.5–26.1)	21.0 (15.9–26.0)	14.9 (14.6–15.2)	7.2[b]
	30+	78.7 (73.9–83.5)	79.0 (74.0–84.1)	85.1 (84.8–85.4)	
Benefits	Sick leave for doctor	54.1 (48.3–59.9)	54.1 (48.1–60.2)	54.7 (54.1–55.3)	0.0
	Sick leave	60.8 (55.1–66.4)	60.4 (54.5–66.2)	60.9 (60.3–61.5)	0.0
	Paid vacation	69.0 (63.4–74.6)	69.3 (63.5–75.1)	68.4 (67.9–68.9)	0.1
	Retirement plan	52.7 (46.5–58.9)	53.5 (47.2–59.8)	52.7 (52.1–53.3)	0.1

Usual source of care				
No source of care	9.4 (7.1–11.8)	11.0 (7.3–14.7)	27.6 (27.0–28.2)	38.4[a]
Office-based	73.7 (69.6–77.8)	75.1 (69.3–80.8)	59.2 (58.4–60.0)	23.6[a]
Hospital (not emergency room)	16.8 (13.5–20.2)	13.9 (9.6–18.2)	12.8 (12.2–13.3)	0.3
Emergency room	—	—	0.4 (0.4–0.5)	
Unable to receive or delayed care				
Any	28.4 (25.0–31.7)	25.7 (20.9–30.6)	11.7 (11.4–12.1)	61.2[a]
Medical	15.9 (13.0–18.7)	14.7 (10.7–18.8)	5.3 (5.1–5.5)	54.3[a]
Dental	12.5 (10.2–14.9)	11.5 (8.2–14.8)	6.7 (6.4–6.9)	13.5[a]
Prescription meds	12.7 (10.2–15.3)	9.5 (6.3–12.6)	3.6 (3.4–3.7)	34.1[a]
Health				
Fair or poor	41.4 (37.3–45.5)	23.6 (18.7–28.4)	7.2 (7.0–7.4)	119.2[a]
Mental health				
Fair or poor	22.5 (19.1–25.9)	11.5 (7.8–15.2)	3.9 (3.7–4.0)	46.1[a]
Disability				
Status	69.7 (65.7–73.7)	52.0 (45.9–58.1)	14.6 (14.2–15.0)	312.3[a]
Days unable to work				
0	62.1 (57.1–67.1)	59.7 (54.3–65.1)	79.6 (79.3–80.0)	101.5[a]
1–10	28.0 (23.6–32.5)	32.1 (27.1–37.0)	17.9 (17.6–18.2)	
11+	9.9 (6.9–12.8)	8.3 (5.3–11.2)	2.5 (2.4–2.6)	

Note: Data are from 1996 to 2015 MEPS public use medical condition and full-year consolidated files. MEPS data were not available for the following variables for years noted: veteran status (2005), usual source of care (1996–2001), receipt and delays in care (1996–2001), and disability status (2015). A nonreliable (n <11) number of people with spine-related conditions reported using an emergency room as their usual source of care. All estimates are weighted percentages (%) with 95% CI widths. Statistical inference, comparing employed persons treated for SCI/D and the overall employed US population, was based on Rao-Scott chi-square statistics and took complex survey design effects into account.

[a] Statistical significance: $P<.0005$.
[b] Statistical significance: $P<.005$.
[c] Statistical significance: $P<.05$.

Data from Agency for Healthcare Research and Quality. Medical Expenditure Panel Survey (MEPS). Available at: https://www.meps.ahrq.gov/mepsweb/.

Impact of Employment on Health and Quality of Life

It is now clear from a variety of sources that employment has positive impacts on multiple life domains. A focus group of employed persons with SCI reported benefits in the following areas[10]:

- Salary and what it can support
- Health insurance and other fringe benefits
- Promotions and recognition
- Job satisfaction and enjoyment from working
- Making a difference and helping others
- Social connection and support
- Psychological and emotional health

Other research corroborates that persons with SCI who are employed have better status than those who are unemployed,[11,12] such as improved physical health and longevity.[13]

VOCATIONAL REHABILITATION FOR PERSONS WITH SPINAL CORD INJURY: STATE OF THE ART

Over the last decades, a groundswell of research has advanced the evidence and practice of VR in SCI. This began in 2005, with the first randomized clinical trial of VR in the field, which tested the IPS model of SE, and continues with recent studies of resource facilitation (RF) and other applications of early vocational intervention. Overwhelming evidence supports adopting new paradigms to effectively address employment as an integrated part of SCI rehabilitation. Collectively, this body of research supports abandoning older work readiness models of VR, which were based largely on clinical judgment, and instead adopting newer, more effective evidence-informed practices that incorporate employment services into SCI rehabilitation. Application of older VR approaches in SCI resulted in the clinical notion that a person with SCI is too catastrophically disabled to go directly back to work following SCI. Furthermore, those prevocational, step-wise approaches to VR occurred independently of SCI rehabilitation and were delayed until acute care was completed. Such a paradigm has proved to be less effective because, in this scenario, vocational specialists do not have access to the skills and expertise of the SCI team, which is needed to address work barriers that are unique to persons with SCI. The new SE and related models use innovative and rigorously standardized practices to address employment, one critical practice being integrating vocational services into SCI rehabilitation. These practices effectively lead to competitive employment in the community of persons with SCI. A comparison of specific vocational services in SCI between the use of an older and the newer SE model of VR has identified the practices in conventional VR that are less effective in helping persons with SCI than the newer practices (**Table 3**).[13]

FOUNDATIONAL PRINCIPLES IN STATE-OF-THE-ART VOCATIONAL REHABILITATION

Although the application, context, staffing, and resources may vary by setting, there are common principles that guide effective vocational services in SCI rehabilitation. Core principles comprise the following[14]:

- Competitive integrated employment is the primary outcome. The goal is full or part-time work where the person with SCI and those without disability at the work place:
  - Receive similar wages and opportunities for advancement.

Approach to Vocational Rehabilitation	Conventional Vocational Rehabilitation	Evidence-Based Supported Employment Model
Table 3		
Vocational services associated with likelihood of employment		
Likelihood of employment	Less	More
Timing	Referral to VR after acute SCI rehabilitation VR initiated after functional independence goals reached	Employment services delivered concurrent with SCI rehabilitation and medical care Rapid engagement in job search
Clinical involvement	Separate vocational agency or provider Little or no connection to SCI health care team	Integrated into acute SCI rehabilitation Clinical team involvement continued after employment obtained
Goal	Prepare person to be "ready" to work	Help person achieve a competitive job in the community of their choosing
Strategies or components	Stepwise approaches Independent living programs Skills training Prevocational training Transitional employment	Job development Job placement Community-based services Negotiation with employers Ongoing supports in the workplace

Data from Ottomanelli L, Barnett SD, Goetz LL, Toscano R. Vocational rehabilitation in spinal cord injury: what vocational service activities are associated with employment program outcome? Top Spinal Cord Inj Rehabil. 2015;21(1):31-39.

- o Are fully integrated as coworkers.
- Vocational services and other rehabilitation and health care services are integrated.
  - o Vocational services and other clinical care are delivered concurrently.
  - o A vocational expert cotreats and works in collaboration with other members of the SCI interdisciplinary care team.
  - o The SCI interdisciplinary team is actively engaged in helping to address vocational issues, such as accommodations and schedule recommendations.
- Client-centered choices determine job development. The person with SCI is the driver of the job search and determines the type of job, the hours, and the work setting to pursue.
- Ongoing support (also called follow-along support) is provided after employment begins. These are any services or resources that are used or created to help maintain employment and find employment. For example, benefits counseling and job accommodations are essential to pursuing and sustaining employment.

MODELS OF EFFECTIVE EMPLOYMENT SERVICES IN SPINAL CORD INJURY REHABILITATION
Individual Placement and Support

Multiple randomized controlled trials[15–17] and other studies[18–21] of persons with serious mental illness or substance use disorders have provided abundant data on the IPS model of SE. This model is also referred to as evidence-based SE, which reflects the body of work demonstrating its efficacy over prior standard care approaches. In IPS for SCI, the VR counselor or VR specialist is a full-fledged member of the interdisciplinary team and, as such, is considered equally important as the physician, psychologist, physical therapist, and other health professionals. The integration of the VR professional into health care allows optimal collaboration with the team to achieve employment as a part of SCI rehabilitation. Along with other critical principles (**Table 4**), the goal of IPS is competitive employment in the community in a job that matches the talents, abilities, and lifestyle needs of the person with SCI.[14]

According to systematic reviews, the IPS model of SE has the strongest evidence to date as an effective VR intervention for persons with SCI.[22,23] A randomized clinical trial of IPS in SCI showed it was 2.5 times more likely to result in competitive employment than conventional VR with employment rates of 29% versus 11%, respectively.[24] In a follow-up longitudinal study, 43% of inpatients and outpatients with SCI enrolled in a 24-month program of IPS achieved a competitive employment position.[25] Furthermore, among a subsample of persons with SCI enrolled as outpatients who had no prior history of traumatic brain injury, the rate of employment exceeded 50%. The impact of employment was increases in quality of life, social integration, and ability to access the community.[26,27]

Effective implementation of IPS within the SCI continuum of care required commitment from formal and informal team leaders, integration of vocational and clinical services, and a dedicated vocational expert on the SCI interdisciplinary team.[28,29] Physician and psychologist team leaders who actively embraced and advocated for the principle that anyone with SCI can return to work with the right supports were instrumental in advancing implementation of IPS in their facility to help as many

Table 4
Overview of effective models of SCI employment interventions

Principles and Practices	Individual Placement and Support	Resource Facilitation	Early Intervention Models
Zero exclusion[a]	X		
Job development	X		
Benefits counseling	X		
Rapid job search approach	X		
Competitive employment focus	X	X	X
Integrated care: VR specialist is member of team	X	X	X
Consumer-driven job search/patient-centered approach	X	X	X
Follow-up job supports	X	X	X
Early intervention: services start during inpatient rehabilitation		X	X
Transitions from inpatient to outpatient care		X	X
Linkage with state or governmental VR agencies		X	
Vocational peer support groups		X	
Career coaching			X
Job-seeking skills training			X

[a] Eligibility for services based solely on a person's desire to work.

Modified from O'Neill J, Ottomanelli L. Vocational rehabilitation for individuals with spinal cord injury. In: Kirshblum S, Lin VW, eds. *Spinal Cord Medicine*. 3rd ed. New York, NY: Demos Medical Publishing; 2019:776-788; with permission.

persons with SCI as possible to obtain employment. As reflected in health economic evaluations, use of IPS in SCI resulted in better employment and quality of life outcomes than standard VR care and the cost of IPS per patient was not greater. Hence, SCI rehabilitation program leadership should view implementation of IPS as a reliable way to improve quality of care, consumer choice, and meaningful outcomes.

Resource Facilitation

RF is a promising intervention for delivering vocational services to persons with a new SCI. Starting during inpatient care and continuing after discharge, RF provides systematic and assertive employment service coordination with the goal of competitive employment. Based on the Vocational Case Coordinator model,[30] which was developed for persons with acquired brain injury, the efficacy of RF was demonstrated in three prospective studies at the Mayo Clinic that, collectively, served more than 330 persons with acquired brain injury.[31,32] Competitive employment outcomes ranged between 41% and 56% at 1-year follow-up. The RF protocol emphasized early employment intervention for inpatients with a vocational resource facilitator (VRF) assisting the patient with self-directed vocational plans and networks of medical center and community services.

Early intervention, work trials, use of existing community services, temporary or long-term SE, and employer education are fundamental features of the RF model. Through enhanced early intervention services, efforts are made to maximize an SCI patient's early buy-in to participate in employment support services. A VRF serves as the key staff member who works with program participants throughout to develop a network of medical center and community services. In addition to providing patients with SCI with a single point of contact for vocational and follow-along services, the VRF also ensures that a patient-centered planning philosophy is followed for all proposed services and interventions.

Inpatient phase

The VRF becomes integrated into treatment teams, which consist of physiatrists, occupational therapists, physical therapists, psychologists, nurses, SCI educators, and case managers, and participates in team meetings to promote greater visibility of employment issues and to increase contact with treating clinicians. The VRF also attends treatment team meetings, team meetings with families, and discharge planning meetings. Throughout this phase, the VRF assesses vocational interests, skills, and aptitudes of patients to highlight their strengths and career potential and assists treatment teams to integrate employment goals with rehabilitation therapy goals. For those who had been employed on admission, a return-to-work plan is developed that addresses such issues as hours worked, the work environment, and compensation. Services can focus on returning to the same job or shifting to another career goal, even if remaining with the preadmission employer, which may involve additional training and preparation.

The benefits of VR services are emphasized by the VRF in meetings with patients and family members to encourage participation. The VRF also ensures that, in as many cases as possible, a state VR agency (SVRA) counselor meets with patients before discharge from the hospital to complete or at least start the referral process for SVRA services.

Outpatient phase

During this phase, to prevent former patients, now clients, from drifting away from proposed plans/recommendations made during the inpatient phase, the VRF maintains close, supportive, hands-on contact. In addition, SVRA program staff work directly with the VRF to improve community agency linkages and to develop a team approach that facilitates smooth transitions from medical- to community-based services. Psychosocial and health barriers are identified and addressed via referrals to appropriate community-based services, and family members and significant others continue to be incorporated into each client's person-centered employment plan.

Employment services vary depending on the career trajectory, skills, and preferences of each client. The VRF works with patients, family members, and employers on accessible work environments and necessary accommodations. Based on vocational strengths and interests, some clients with SCI are provided temporary or longer-term SE services. Throughout the outpatient phase, the VRF provides education about SCI to employers, coworkers, and community service providers. Also, the VRF develops vocational support groups for employed persons with SCI living in the community, who present information on their journey to competitive employment and how they overcame obstacles.

Experience with resource facilitation for persons with spinal cord injury

From June 2016 through September 2019, 95 persons with SCI began RF at Kessler Institute for Rehabilitation. Although still inpatients, 41 (43%) returned to work, 13 (54%) with nontraumatic SCI and 28 (39%) with traumatic SCI, which compares favorably with the Kessler Foundation/Kessler Institute for Rehabilitation Model System 1-year follow-up employment rate of 21%.[33] To evaluate the impact of VR we used several 1-year postinjury benchmarks: (1) Spinal Cord Injury Model Systems (SCIMS) employment rate for all centers across all years (12%), (2) SCIMS employment rate for all centers from 2011 to 2016 (16%), and (3) SCIMS employment rate for Northern New Jersey from 2011 to 2016 (21%). At 1-year postdischarge, RF participants with traumatic SCI had a 34% employment rate, which was substantially greater than all three SCIMS benchmark rates.

EARLY INTERVENTION: A WINDOW OF POSSIBILITY

Reports from abroad (New Zealand/Australia)[34,35] on the use of IPS, RF, and other new models of VR using early intervention demonstrate that employment services during rehabilitation lead to positive vocational outcomes. Hence, VR seems to be most potent when delivered early on and as a part of rehabilitation. Research[36] and clinical experience highlight that this early period after injury is a crucial window of intervention for several reasons:

- Likelihood of return to a previous employer is greater when the employment relationship is intact and preinjury skills have not faded.
- Connection to the SCI interdisciplinary team, which is critical to address employment barriers, is strongest during rehabilitation.
- Motivation to maintain or seek employment is higher before social disenfranchisement or reliance on disability benefits develops.
- The ability to leverage existing social and business networks to maintain or find new employment is greater.
- The opportunity to create and capitalize on hope and positive expectancy on the part of the person with the SCI is greater.
- A trusted physician conveying the message that work is possible and making a VR referral (ie, prescribing work) is reported as determining factors to engaging in meaningful post-SCI employment by many successful people with SCI.

- Pursuing employment goals during rehabilitation fuels participation in other reha-bilitation therapies and increases adherence to SCI care and management, which are essential to optimize health that ultimately makes return to work possible.

SUMMARY

The opportunities afforded persons with SCI by the passage of the ADA remain incom-pletely fulfilled. Providers who care for these persons can help them realize opportu-nities by emphasizing the well-established benefits of employment and implementing current VR best practices during rehabilitation.

DISCLOSURE

Contents of this article do not represent the views of the Department of Veterans Af-fairs or the United States Government. The authors have no conflicts of interest to report. Funding for this study was provided by the Rehabilitation Research and Training Center on Employment Policy and Measurement at the University of New Hampshire, which is funded by the National Institute on Disability, Independent Living, and Rehabilitation Research, in the Administration for Community Living, at the US Department of Health and Human Services (DHHS) under cooperative agreement 9ORT5037-02-00. The contents do not necessarily represent the policy of DHHS and you should not assume endorsement by the federal government (EDGAR, 75.620 [b]).

REFERENCES

1. Barnow B. The employment rate of people with disabilities. Mon Labor Rev 2008;44–50.
2. Hastings R. Has the Americans with Disabilities Act made a difference?. 2010. Available at: https://www.shrm.org/ResourcesAndTools/hr-topics/behavioral-competencies/global-and-cultural-effectiveness/Pages/HastheADAMadeaDifference.aspx. Accessed December 9, 2019.
3. Civil Rights Division, U.S. Department of Justice. Information and technical assis-tance on the Americans with Disabilities Act. ADA.gov. Available at: https://www.ada.gov/index.html. Accessed December 9, 2019.
4. Ottomanelli L, Lind L. Review of critical factors related to employment after spinal cord injury: implications for research and vocational services. J Spinal Cord Med 2009;32(5):503–31.
5. Appelbaum L. 27 years after ADA, employment for people with disabilities still too low. Respectability. 2017. Available at: https://www.respectability.org/2017/07/27-years-ada-employment-people-disabilities-still-low/. Accessed December 10, 2019.
6. Krause JS, Terza JV, Saunders LL, et al. Delayed entry into employment after spi-nal cord injury: factors related to time to first job. Spinal Cord 2010;48(6):487–91.
7. Krause JS, Reed KS. Barriers and facilitators to employment after spinal cord injury: underlying dimensions and their relationship to labor force participation. Spinal Cord 2011;49(2):285–91.
8. Meade MA, Forchheimer MB, Krause JS, et al. The influence of secondary con-ditions on job acquisition and retention in adults with spinal cord injury. Arch Phys Med Rehabil 2011;92(3):425–32.

9. Krause JS, Edles PA. Injury perceptions, hope for recovery, and psychological status after spinal cord injury. Rehabil Psychol 2014. https://doi.org/10.1037/a0035778.

10. Meade M, Reed K, Saunders L, et al. It's all of the above: benefits of working for individuals with spinal cord injury. Top Spinal Cord Inj Rehabil 2015;21(1):1–9.

11. Hess D, Meade M, Forchheimer M, et al. Psychological well-being and intensity of employment in individuals with a spinal cord injury. Top Spinal Cord Inj Rehabil 2004;9(4):1–10.

12. Dowler R, Richards JS, Putzke JD, et al. Impact of demographic and medical factors on satisfaction with life after spinal cord injury: a normative study. J Spinal Cord Med 2001;24(2):87–91.

13. Krause JS, Saunders LL, Acuna J. Gainful employment and risk of mortality after spinal cord injury: effects beyond that of demographic, injury and socioeconomic factors. Spinal Cord 2012;50(10):784–8.

14. O'Neill J, Ottomanelli L. Vocational rehabilitation for individuals with spinal cord injury. In: Kirshblum S, Lin VW, editors. Spinal cord medicine. 3rd edition. New York: Demos Medical Publishing; 2019. p. 776–88. Available at: https://www.springerpub.com/spinal-cord-medicine-9780826137746.html.

15. Bond GR, Salyers MP, Dincin J, et al. A randomized controlled trial comparing two vocational models for persons with severe mental illness. J Consult Clin Psychol 2007;75(6):968–82.

16. Bond GR, Drake RE, Becker DR. An update on randomized controlled trials of evidence-based supported employment. Psychiatr Rehabil J 2008;31(4):280–90.

17. Drake RE, McHugo GJ, Becker DR, et al. The New Hampshire study of supported employment for people with severe mental illness. J Consult Clin Psychol 1996; 64(2):391–9.

18. Becker DR, Bond GR, McCarthy D, et al. Converting day treatment centers to supported employment programs in Rhode Island. Psychiatr Serv 2001;52(3): 351–7.

19. Becker DR, Smith J, Tanzman B, et al. Fidelity of supported employment programs and employment outcomes. Psychiatr Serv 2001;52(6):834–6.

20. Becker D, Whitley R, Bailey EL, et al. Long-term employment trajectories among participants with severe mental illness in supported employment. Psychiatr Serv 2007;58(7):922–8.

21. Drake R, Becker D, Bond G, et al. A process analysis of integrated and non-integrated approaches to supported employment. J Vocat Rehabil 2003; 18(1):51–8.

22. Trenaman LM, Miller WC, Escorpizo R. Interventions for improving employment outcomes among individuals with spinal cord injury: a systematic review. Spinal Cord 2014;52(11):788–94.

23. Roels EH, Aertgeerts B, Ramaekers D, et al. Hospital- and community-based interventions enhancing (re)employment for people with spinal cord injury: a systematic review. Spinal Cord 2016;54(1):2–7.

24. Ottomanelli L, Goetz LL, Suris A, et al. Effectiveness of supported employment for veterans with spinal cord injuries: results from a randomized multisite study. Arch Phys Med Rehabil 2012;93(5):740–7.

25. Ottomanelli L, Goetz LL, Barnett SD, et al. Individual placement and support in spinal cord injury: a longitudinal observational study of employment outcomes. Arch Phys Med Rehabil 2017;98(8):1567–75.

26. Cotner BA, Ottomanelli L, O'Connor DR, et al. Quality of life outcomes for veterans with spinal cord injury receiving individual placement and support (IPS). Top Spinal Cord Inj Rehabil 2018;24(4):325–35.

27. Ottomanelli L, Barnett SD, Goetz LL. A prospective examination of the impact of a supported employment program and employment on health-related quality of life, handicap, and disability among veterans with SCI. Qual Life Res 2013;22(8):2133–41.

28. Cotner B, Njoh E, Trainor J, et al. Facilitators and barriers to employment among veterans with spinal cord injury receiving 12 months of evidence-based supported employment services. Top Spinal Cord Inj Rehabil 2015;21(1):20–30.

29. Cotner BA, Ottomanelli L, O'Connor DR, et al. Provider-identified barriers and facilitators to implementing a supported employment program in spinal cord injury. Disabil Rehabil 2018;40(11):1273–9.

30. Trexler LE, Trexler LC, Malec JF, et al. Prospective randomized controlled trial of resource facilitation on community participation and vocational outcome following brain injury. J Head Trauma Rehabil 2010;25(6):440–6.

31. Malec JF, Moessner AM. Replicated positive results for the VCC model of vocational intervention after ABI within the social model of disability. Brain Inj 2006;20(3):227–36.

32. Buffington ALH, Malec JF. The vocational rehabilitation continuum: maximizing outcomes through bridging the gap from hospital to community-based services. J Head Trauma Rehabil 1997;12(5):1–13.

33. O'Neill J, Dyson Hudson T, West M, et al. Resource facilitation: early inpatient/assertive outpatient vocational rehabilitation services in SCI [abstract #31]. J Spinal Cord Med 2017;40(5):599–600.

34. Middleton JW, Johnston D, Murphy G, et al. Early access to vocational rehabilitation for spinal cord injury inpatients. J Rehabil Med 2015. https://doi.org/10.2340/16501977-1980.

35. Hilton G, Unsworth CA, Murphy GC, et al. Longitudinal employment outcomes of an early intervention vocational rehabilitation service for people admitted to rehabilitation with a traumatic spinal cord injury. Spinal Cord 2017;55(8):743–52.

36. Krause JS. Years to employment after spinal cord injury. Arch Phys Med Rehabil 2003;84(9):1282–9.

Moving?

Make sure your subscription moves with you!

To notify us of your new address, find your **Clinics Account Number** (located on your mailing label above your name), and contact customer service at:

Email: journalscustomerservice-usa@elsevier.com

800-654-2452 (subscribers in the U.S. & Canada)
314-447-8871 (subscribers outside of the U.S. & Canada)

Fax number: 314-447-8029

Elsevier Health Sciences Division
Subscription Customer Service
3251 Riverport Lane
Maryland Heights, MO 63043

*To ensure uninterrupted delivery of your subscription, please notify us at least 4 weeks in advance of move.

ELSEVIER

Printed and bound by CPI Group (UK) Ltd, Croydon, CR0 4YY

03/10/2024

01040402-0005